Genitourinary Cancer

Cancer Treatment and Research

WILLIAM L MCGUIRE, *series editor*

Livingston RB (ed): Lung Cancer 1. 1981. ISBN 90-247-2394-9.
Bennett Humphrey G, Dehner LP, Grindey GB, Acton RT (eds): Pediatric Oncology 1. 1981. ISBN 90-247-2408-2.
DeCosse JJ, Sherlock P (eds): Gastrointestinal Cancer 1. 1981. ISBN 90-247-2461-9.
Bennett JM (ed): Lymphomas 1, including Hodgkin's Disease. 1981. ISBN 90-247-2479-1.
Bloomfield CD (ed): Adult Leukemias 1. 1982. ISBN 90-247-2478-3.
Paulson DF (ed): Genitourinary Cancer 1. 1982. ISBN 90-247-2480-5.
Muggia FM (ed): Cancer Chemotherapy 1. ISBN 90-247-2713-8.
Bennett Humphrey G, Grindey GB (eds): Pancreatic Tumors in Children. 1982. ISBN 90-247-2702-2.
Costanzi JJ (ed): Malignant Melanoma 1. 1983. ISBN 90-247-2706-5.
Griffiths CT, Fuller AF (eds): Gynecologic Oncology. 1983. ISBN 0-89838-555-5.
Greco AF (ed): Biology and Management of Lung Cancer. 1983. ISBN 0-89838-554-7.
Walker MD (ed): Oncology of the Nervous System. 1983. ISBN 0-89838-567-9.
Higby DJ (ed): Supportive Care in Cancer Therapy. 1983. ISBN 0-89838-569-5.
Herberman RB (ed): Basic and Clinical Tumor Immunology. 1983. ISBN 0-89838-579-2.
Baker LH (ed): Soft Tissue Sarcomas. 1983. ISBN 0-89838-584-9.
Bennett JM (ed): Controversies in the Management of Lymphomas. 1983. ISBN 0-89838-586-5.
Bennett Humphrey G, Grindey GB (eds): Adrenal and Endocrine Tumors in Children. 1983. ISBN 0-89838-590-3.
DeCosse JJ, Sherlock P (eds): Clinical Management of Gastrointestinal Cancer. 1984. ISBN 0-89838-601-2.
Catalona WJ, Ratliff TL (eds): Urologic Oncology. 1984. ISBN 0-89838-628-4.
Santen RJ, Manni A (eds): Diagnosis and Management of Endocrine-related Tumors. 1984. ISBN 0-89838-636-5.
Costanzi JJ (ed): Clinical Management of Malignant Melanoma. 1984. ISBN 0-89838-656-X.
Wolf GT (ed): Head and Neck Oncology. 1984. ISBN 0-89838-657-8.
Alberts DS, Surwit EA (eds): Ovarian Cancer. 1985. ISBN 0-89838-676-4.
Muggia FM (ed): Experimental and Clinical Progress in Cancer Chemotherapy. 1985. ISBN 0-89838-679-9.
Higby DJ (ed): The Cancer Patient and Supportive Care. 1985. ISBN 0-89838-690-X.
Bloomfield CD (ed): Chronic and Acute Leukemias in Adults. 1985. ISBN 0-89838-702-7.
Herberman RB (ed): Cancer Immunology: Innovative Approaches to Therapy. 1986. ISBN 0-89838-757-4.
Hansen HH (ed): Lung Cancer: Basic and Clinical Aspects. 1986. ISBN 0-89838-763-9.
Pinedo HM, Verweij J (eds): Clinical Management of Soft Tissue Sarcomas. 1986. ISBN 0-89838-808-2.
Higby DJ (ed): Issues in Supportive Care of Cancer Patients. 1986. ISBN 0-89838-816-3.
Surwit EA, Alberts DS (eds): Cervix Cancer. 1987. ISBN 0-89838-822-8.
Jacobs C (ed): Cancers of the Head and Neck. 1987. ISBN 0-89838-825-2.
MacDonald JS (ed): Gastrointestinal Oncology. 1987. ISBN 0-89838-829-5.
Ratliff TL, Catalona WJ (eds): Genitourinary Cancer. 1987. ISBN 0-89838-830-9.

Genitourinary Cancer

Basic and Clinical Aspects

edited by

TIMOTHY L. RATLIFF, Ph.D.
Washington University School of Medicine
The Jewish Hospital of St. Louis
216 South Kingshighway Boulevard
P.O. Box 14109, St. Louis, MO 63178
U.S.A.

and

WILLIAM J. CATALONA, M.D.
Washington University School of Medicine
The Jewish Hospital of St. Louis
St. Louis, MO 63178
U.S.A.

1987 **MARTINUS NIJHOFF PUBLISHERS**
a member of the KLUWER ACADEMIC PUBLISHERS GROUP
BOSTON / DORDRECHT / LANCASTER

Distributors

for the United States and Canada: Kluwer Academic Publishers, P.O. Box 358, Accord Station, Hingham, MA 02018-0358, USA
for the UK and Ireland: Kluwer Academic Publishers, MTP Press Limited, Falcon House, Queen Square, Lancaster LA1 1RN, UK
for all other countries: Kluwer Academic Publishers Group, Distribution Center, P.O. Box 322, 3300 AH Dordrecht, The Netherlands

Library of Congress Cataloging in Publication Data

```
Genitourinary cancer.

   (Cancer treatment and research)
   Includes index.
   1. Genito-urinary organs--Cancer. I. Ratliff,
Timothy L.  II. Catalona, William J.  III. Series.
[DNLM: 1. Urogenital Neoplasms.  W1 CA693 /
WJ 160 G33032]
RC280.G4G473  1986        616.99'46        86-18143
```

ISBN 0-89838-830-9 (this volume)
ISBN 90-247-2426-0 (series)

PRINTED IN THE NETHERLANDS

Contents

Cancer Treatment and Research

Foreword

Where do you begin to look for a recent, authoritative article on the diagnosis or management of a particular malignancy? The few general oncology textbooks are generally out of date. Single papers in specialized journals are informative but seldom comprehensive; these are more often preliminary reports on a very limited number of patients. Certain general journals frequently publish good indepth reviews of cancer topics, and published symposium lectures are often the best overviews available. Unfortunately, these reviews and supplements appear sporadically, and the reader can never be sure when a topic of special interest will be covered.

Cancer Treatment and Research is a series of authoritative volumes which aim to meet this need. It is an attempt to establish a critical mass of oncology literature covering virtually all oncology topics, revised frequently to keep the coverage up to date, easily available on a single library shelf or by a single personal subscription.

We have approached the problem in the following fashion. First, by dividing the oncology literature into specific subdivisions such as lung cancer, genitourinary cancer, pediatric oncology, etc. Second, by asking eminent authorities in each of these areas to edit a volume on the specific topic on an annual or biannual basis. Each topic and tumor type is covered in a volume appearing frequently and predictably, discussing current diagnosis, staging, markers, all forms of treatment modalities, basic biology, and more.

In Cancer Treatment and Research, we have an outstanding group of editors, each having made a major commitment to bring to this new series the very best literature in his of her field. Martinus Nijhoff Publishers has made an equally major commitment to the rapid publication of high quality books, and worldwide distribution.

Where can you go find quickly a recent authoritative article on any major oncology problem? We hope that Cancer Treatment and Research provides an answer.

WILLIAM L. MCGUIRE
Series Editor

Preface

The preface to our earlier work in this series (*Urologic Oncology*, Catalona and Ratliff, editors, Martinus Nijhoff Publishing, 1984) began as follows:

The study of genitourinary tumors is an area of recent rapid growth both in the understandign of disease processes and in the development of new diagnostic and therapeutic modalities. During rapid growth phases within any field, it is desirable to reflect on the current 'state of the art'. It is difficult even for experts in reputed areas of advancement to distinguish true advances from false leads, but it is far more difficult yet for those whose expertise lies in other areas to evaluate important advances. Thus, an objective assessment of evolving areas of investigation in the form of a comprehensive review is of considerable value.

In this volume, wa have attempted to provide the reader with an overview of some of the current areas of investigation in urologic oncology by experts in each area. There often is a tendency for invited papers in books of this nature to lack important critical peer review and therefore, suffer from a lack of objectivity. We have attempted to diminish this problem by the selection of two experts to discuss each subject. We believe that this format has improved the overal quality of the book for two reasons: 1) the knowledge of each contributor that his or her work would be reviewed by a peer encourages more rigorous scholarship, and 2) the fact that contributions by two experts, including the individual insights of each, provides a better perspective for the reader.

This volume, entitled *Genitourinary Cancer: Basic and Clinical Aspects*, is an extention of our earlier work. The topics discussed are distinct but naturally complimentary.

The review articles in this book are provided to aid investigators in their attempts to stay abreast of advancements in the field. To provide as critical an evaluation as possible, we have maintained the format of our previous volume in which the insights of two experts are presented for each topic.

X

We gratefully acknowledge the efforts of each contributor. The strength and utility of this volume lies within the individual contributions. Also, we particularly wish to acknowledge the secretarial assistance of Christine Floyd and Kimberly Merritt whose efforts made the completion of this volume possible.

List of contributors

BAHNSON, Robert R., M.D., Assistant Professor, Division of Urology, Washington University School of Medicine, 4960 Audubon Avenue, St. Louis, Missouri 63110 USA.

BANDER, Neil H., M.D., Assistant Professor Surgery/Urology, New York Hospital – Cornell Medical Center, 525 East 68th Street, New York, NY 10021 USA.

BRENDLER, Charles B., M.D., Associate Professor, Johns Hopkins Hospital, Department of Urology, Marburg 145, 600 N. Wolfe St., Baltimore, Maryland 21205.

BULBUL, M., M.D., Urologic Oncology Research, Memorial Sloan-Kettering Cancer Center, 1275 York Avenue, New York NY 100021 USA.

CATALONA, William J., M.D., Professor of Surgery, Division of Urology, Washington University School of Medicine, 4960 Audubon Avenue and The Jewish Hospital of St. Louis, 216 S. Kingshighway, St. Louis, Missouri 63110 USA.

CHUNG, Leland W.K., Ph.D., Associate Professor of Pharmacology Department of Urology, University of Texas System Cancer Center, M.D. Anderson Hospital and Cancer Center, Houston, Texas 77030 USA.

COFFEY, Donald, Ph.D., Professor of Urology, Oncology, Pharmacology and Experimental Therapeutics; Director of Research Laboratories of the Department of Urology, John Hopkins Hospital, Brady Urologic Institute, Baltimore, MD, 21205 USA.

deKERNION, Jean B., M.D., Professor of Surgery/Urology, Director for Clinical Programs, University of California – Los Angeles Jonsson Cancer Center, University of California – Los Angeles Medical Center, 10833 Le Conte Avenue, 66–128CHS, Los Angeles, CA 90024 USA.

DROLLER, Michael J., M.D., Professor and Chairman, Department of Urology, The Mount Sinai Medical Center, One Gustave L. Levy Place, New York, NY 10029 USA.

FAIR, William R., M.D., Chief of Urology, Memorial Sloan-Kettering Cancer Center, Urology Service, 1275 York Avenue, New York, NY 10021 USA.

HAKALA, Thomas R., M.D., Professor and Chief Urologic Surgery, University of Pittsburgh School of Medicine, 4414 Puh, Pittsburgh, PA 15261 USA.

HERR, Harry W., M.D., Associate Attending Surgeon, Urologic Service, Memorial Sloan-Kettering Cancer Center, 1275 York Avenue, New York, NY 10021 USA.

HESTON, Warren D.W., Ph.D., Director, Urologic Oncology Research, Memorial Sloan-Kettering Cancer Center, 1275 York Avenue, New York, NY 10021 USA.

HUFFMAN, Jeffry, M.D., Assistant Professor of Surgery in Resident, University of California – San Diego Medical Center, Division of Urology, H, 897, 225 W. Dickenson Street, San Diego, California 921)3 USA.

JACOBS, Stephen C., M.D., Associate Professor of Urology, The Medical College of Winconsin, 9200 West Wisconsin Avenue, Milwaukee, Wisconsin 53226 USA.

KADMON, Dov, M.D., Assistant Professor-Surgery (Urology), The Jewish Hospital of St. Louis, 216 S. Kingshighway, St. Louis, MO 63110 USA.

KIRSCHENBAUM, Alexander, M.D., Department of Urology, The Mount Sinai Medical Center, One Gustave L. Levy Place, New York, NY 10029 USA.

KLOTZ, Laurence, M.D., F.R.C.S.(C), Consultant, Division of Urology, Sunnybrook Medical Centre, University of Toronto, 2075 Bayview Avenue, Toronto, Ontario, Canada, M4N 3M5.

LABRIE, Fernand, M.D., University of Laval, Department of Molecular Endocrinology and Medicine, 2705, Boulevard Laurier, Quebec GIV 4G2 Canada.

LAMM, Donald L., M.D., Professor and Chairman, Department of Urology, West Virginia University Medical Center, Morgantown, West Virginia 26506 USA.

LYONS, Edward S., M.D., Department of Surgery (Urology), University of Chicago School of Medicine, Box 403, 950 E. 59th Street, Chicago, ILL 60637 USA.

MORALES, Alvaro, M.D., Professor and Chairman, Department of Urology, Queen's University, Kingston General Hospital, Kingston, Ontario, Canada K7L 2V7.

RATLIFF, Timothy L., Ph.D., Associate Professor of Surgery (Urology), Washington University School of Medicine and Director of Urologic Research at The Jewish Hospital of St. Louis, 216 S. Kingshighway, St. Louis, MO 63110 USA.

RESNICK, Martin I., M.D., Professor and Chairman, Division of Urology, Case Western Reserve University, 2065 Adelbert Road, Cleveland, Ohio 44106 USA.

SAGALOWSKY, Arthur I., M.D., Associate Professor, Division of Urology, The University of Texas Health Science Center, Southwestern Medical School, 5323 Harry Hines Blvd., Dallas, TX 75235 USA.

SMITH, Joseph A., Jr., M.D., Associate Professor, Division of Urology, The University of Utah, 50 N. Medical Drive, Salt Lake City, Utah 84132 USA.

STONE, Kenneth R., Ph.D., Reserach Assistant Professor in the Department of Pathology, The Jewish Hospital of St. Louis, 216 S. Kingshighway, St. Louis, MO 63110 USA.

STORY, Michael T., Ph.D., Assistant Professor, Department of Urology, Medical College of Wisconsin, 9200 West Wisconsin Avenue, Milwaukee, Wisconsin 53226 USA.

WILLIAMS, Richard D., M.D., Professor and Chairman, The University of Iowa Hospital and Clinics, Department of Urology, Iowa City, Iowa 52242 USA.

WINFIELD, Howard N., M.D., Assistant Professor, Department of Urology, McGill University, 687 Pine Avenue West, Montreal, Quebec, Canada.

1. Isoenzymes in prostate cancer

CHARLES B. BRENDLER

Introduction

The human prostate is a rich source of both hydrolytic enzymes that are secreted in seminal plasma and of intracellular enzymes that regulate the metabolism of the glandular epithelium. Prostatic enzymatic activities may be altered both within the prostate and also in other tissues by neoplastic transformation and subsequent metastatic spread. Thus determination of enzymatic activities can be useful in the diagnosis and subsequent clinical evaluation of prostatic carcinoma. In the past, clinical enzymology of the prostate focused primarily on measurement of serum acid and alkaline phosphatase. More recently, however, other enzymes have attracted attention as potential biologic markers of prostatic carcinoma.

Since most enzymes within the prostate are found in other tissues as well, it may be difficult to assess the significance of an altered serum enzymatic level. The characterization and measurement of isoenzymes that are specific for the prostate enhances the accuracy of enzymatic measurements as biologic markers of prostatic disease. Isoenzymes are enzymatically active proteins that catalyze the same biologic reaction but differ in certain physicochemical properties. In the strict sence of the definition, isoenzymes should catalyze the same physiologic reaction in vivo. However, since the physiologic function and natural substrates of many prostatic enzymes are unknown, prostatic isoenzymes usually are distinguished and measured using artifical substrates reacting under somewhat empiric conditions [1].

Isoenzymes are usually separated by electrophoresis. Electrophoretic mobility may be altered by amino acid substitutions or other variations in charged side groups of the enzyme molecule that are not part of the integral polypeptide chain. Such alterations can occur without effecting either the catalytic function or the antigenicity of the enzyme molecule. Isoenzymes can also be separated by immunologic techniques.

The remainder of this chapter will discuss the current state of isoenzyme measurements in prostatic carcinoma.

Ratliff, T.L. and Catalona, W.J. (eds), Genitourinary Cancer. ISBN 0–89838–830–9
© *1987, Martinus Nijhoff Publishers, Boston. Printed in the Netherlands.*

Isoenzymes of acid phosphatase

The phosphatases are a group of enzymes capable of hydrolyzing phosphate esters. If active mainly at pH less than 7.0, they are called acid phosphatases; if active mainly at pH greater than 7.0 they are called alkaline phosphatases. The group of enzymes known as acid phosphatase was first identified in erythrocytes in 1924 [2]. During the next decade acid phosphatase activity was recognized in liver, spleen, and prostate. In 1941 Huggins and Hodges observed that serum acid phosphatase activity decreased in patients with advanced prostate cancer following hormonal therapy [3]. Since that time considerable effort has been expended attempting to develop assays that would differentiate between the various fractions of acid phosphatase and that would measure prostatic acid phosphatase specifically. Earlier efforts to distinguish prostatic acid phosphatase involved the use of different enzymatic inhibitors and substrates. More recently, prostatic acid phosphatase has been characterized and quantitated by electrophoresis and immunologic techniques. Each of these methods will be discussed.

Separation of acid phosphatase by inhibitors

Since acid phosphatase was first identified in red blood cells, inhibitors initially were used to differentiate between the erythrocytic and prostatic fractions of the

Table 1. % Inhibition or activation (phenyl phosphate in pH-5.0 acetate buffer)[a]

Substance	Prostate in saline	Red cells in water
Arsenate, 0.001 M	− 66	− 80
Citrate, 0.001 M	+ 8	+ 5
Cyanide, 0.001 M	+ 12	+ 8
Fluoride, 0.001 M	− 96	− 8
Formate, 0.001 M	8	0
Oralate, 0.001 M	− 22	− 27
Salicylate, 0.001 M	0	0
Tartrate (L), 0.001 M	− 94	0
Tartrate (D), 0.001 M	0	0
Tauroglycocholate, 0.01 M	− 76	− 77
Ethanol preincubation, 40%	− 80	− 75
Formaldehyde, 0.5%	0	− 100
Stilbestrol	0	0
Acetone preincubation, 40%	− 100	− 70
Copper[b], 0.0002 M	− 8	− 96
Iron[b], 0.0005 M	− 80	− 9

[a] Selectively compiled from Abul-Fadl and King [6].
[b] No effect in citrate buffer.

enzyme. In 1941 Gutman and Gutman reported that fluoride inhibited prostatic acid phosphatase but did not inhibit the erythrocytic fraction [4]. In 1945 Herbert reported selective inhibition of prostatic acid phosphatase with ethanol [5]. In 1949 Abul-Fadul and King confirmed these observations and reported the effects of various ions and organic compounds on prostatic and erythrocytic acid phosphatase [6]. These observations were summarized by Moncure [1], and are shown in Table 1.

Of the inhibitors of acid phosphatase, L(+) tartrate has received the most clinical attention. Because L(+) tartrate produces almost complete inhibition of prostatic acid phosphatase and only negligible inhibition of erythrocytic acid phosphatase, the tartrate inhibited fraction of the enzyme has often been regarded as prostate specific. In fact, other tissues including liver, spleen, kidney, and platelets all contain tartrate inhibitable acid phosphatase [7]. Nevertheless, because the prostate has such a high content of the enzyme, elevated serum levels of tartrate inhibitable acid phosphatase almost always result from prostatic acid phosphatase activity.

Separation of acid phosphatase by substrate selectivity

Because the natural substrates of acid phosphatase are unknown, all in vitro assays and histochemical stains use synthetic phosphate esters to measure enzymatic activity. The rates of hydrolysis of these esters vary with the different acid phosphatases from various tissues. Once again, because of potential false elevations of serum acid phosphatase by red blood cell hemolysis, substrates generally have been chosen because of their ability to distinguish between the prostatic and erythrocytic fractions of the enzymes [1].

Substrates that have been used to measure prostatic acid phosphatase activity include phenylphosphate [8], para-nitrol phenylphosphate [9], beta-glycerophosphate [10], phenolphthalein phosphate [11], alpha-naphthyl phosphate [12], beta-naphthyl phosphate [13], and thymolphthalein monophosphate [14]. Of all these substrates, thymolphthalein monophosphate appears to have the greatest specificity for prostatic acid phosphatase, and there is a close correlation between prostatic acid phosphatase activity measured with thymolphthalein monophosphate and radioimmunoassay techniques. Nevertheless, electrophoretic analysis has demonstrated that none of the currently employed substrates is truly prostate specific [15].

Separation of acid phosphatase by electrophoresis

Electrophorectic separation of acid phosphatase isoenzymes has been accomplished in serum and numerous tissue extracts. Initially there was considerable variation in the methodology, and no standard diagnostic technique or isoenzyme pattern geined widespread acceptance. However, these early studies did suggest that there were four major subgroups of acid phosphatase. These subgroups included: 1) intracellular red blood cell acid phosphatases, 2) intracellular lysosome-associated acid phosphatases, 3) intracellular non-lysosome associated but membrane-bound acid phosphatases, and 4) secretory acid phosphatases with extracellular functions [1].

In 1968 Smith and Whitby performed electrophoretic separation of human prostate extract on starch gel and identified 20 consecutive bands. They postulated that the heterogeneous appearance of acid phosphatase was due to variable carbohydrate moieties that were present within the same protein molecule. This hypothesis was supported by the observation that removal of carbohydrate residues from the acid phosphatase molecule with sialidase reduced the electrophoretic mobility of the enzyme [16].

In 1973 Lam and associates, using acrylamide gel electrophoresis, identified 5 acid phosphatase isoenzyme bands. They analyzed 20 different tissues and found that prostate is the only tissue with a high activity of isoenzyme 2, while pancreas, spleen, and leukocytes contain low amounts of isoenzyme 2 [17]. In 1980 these investigators reported that prostatic acid phosphatase contains only isoenzymes 2 and 4. Isoenzyme 2 is a glycoprotein with slow electrophoretic mobility. Treatment with sialidase removes most of the carbohydrate moieties on isoenzyme 2 and increases its electrophoretic mobility to approach that of isoenzyme 4 which contains no carbohydrate. Furthermore, antigenic studies revealed that isoenzymes 2 and 4 have an identical protein structure. These observations suggest that isoenzyme 4 may be a precursor of the final secretory product isoenzyme 2 that is formed by the addition of a carbohydrate moeity. This observation is further supported by the fact that seminal acid phosphatase contains only isoenzyme 2 [18].

Lam and coworkers also reported that the isoenzyme 2 and 4 pattern is not unique to the prostate. Leukocytes also contain acid phosphatase isoenzymes 2 and 4 exclusively. However, these isoenzymes are found in much higher concentration in the prostate than in any other tissue, thus emphasizing their value as markers for prostatic carcinoma. These same investigators also determined that acid phosphatase isoenzyme 5, which is frequently found in high concentrations in the bone marrow of patients with metastatic prostate cancer, is a different protein species with no antigenic relationship to isoenzymes 2 and 4. Isoenzyme 5 is produced by bone osteoclasts and is not of prostatic origin [18].

Lin and associates, using polyacrilamide gel electrophoresis, determined that human prostatic acid phosphatase has a molecular weight of 100,000 and is composed of two subunits each of molecular weight 50,000. Prostatic acid phosphatase has multiple isoelectric points due in part to variable sialic acid content within the molecule [19].

McTigue and Van Etten have further characterized human prostatic acid phosphatase. Starting with purified human prostatic acid phosphatase, they identified two forms of the enzyme by gradient elution DEAE-cellulose chromatography. The two isoenzymes have an identical amino acid composition and V-max values but differ in certain properties such as circular dichroism spectra, relative fluorescence intensities, K_m values, and carbohydrate compositions. The major difference between the two isoenzymes appears to be in their carbohydrate side chain composition, and this is due in part to variation in sialic acid composition. They observed spontaneous interconversion between the two isoenzymes under certain storage conditions [20].

Tage and coworkers have recently reported that the electrophoretic heterogeneity of human prostatic acid phosphatase is not due totally to variability in sialic acid content. Treatment with neuraminidase which completely removes the sialic acid reduces but does not abolish the observed heterogeneity. These investigators agree that the two enzyme forms identified by polyacrilamide gel electrophoresis probably correspond to isoenzymes 2 and 4 previously described by Lam. However, the complete explanation for the electrophoretic heterogeneity between the two isoenzymes remains to be established [21].

Lin and associates have recently reported a new prostatic acid phosphatase molecule which they have designated prostatic acid phosphatase II (PAP-II). PAP-II has a molecular weight of 120,000, and is composed of two subunits of molecular weight 55,000 each. Although immunologically similar, PAP-II appears to have a different amino acid and carbohydrate composition as well as different isoelectric points, suggesting that it is different from the originally identified prostatic acid phosphatase. Further studies are underway to characterize this newly identified ensyme [22].

Separation of acid phosphatase by immunologic methods

The development of a reliable antibody to human prostatic acid phosphatase has permitted the development of several immunochemical techniques to characterize and measure prostatic acid phosphatase. In 1974 Cooper and Foti used a double antibody technique to measure prostatic acid phosphatase activity in serum. This technique involves immunizing rabbits with purified human prostatic acid phosphatase obtained from prostatic fluid and producing a prostatic acid phosphatase anti-serum. Acid phosphatase activity is determined by a competitive assay of unlabelled antigen and radioactive iodine-labelled antigen that compete for antibody binding sites. Acid phosphatase activity is determined from a standard curve [23].

In 1975 Foti, Herschman, and Cooper described a solid phase radioimmunoassay technique in which the antibody is absorbed to a fixed surface allowing more rapid and accurate separation of the antigen-antibody complex from excess antigen [24].

In 1978 Chu and coworkers adapted the technique of counter-immunoelectrophoresis to measure prostatic acid phosphatase. When an appropriate electrical current is applied, the prostatic acid phosphatase antigen and antibody (raised in rabbit serum) move in opposition directions. The enzymatic activity of the preciptin line that is formed is evaluated using alpha-naphthylphosphate as the substrate [25].

Clinical application

Serum acid phosphatase has been used as a marker for metastatic carcinoma of the prostate for 50 years. In 1936 Gutman and associates reported increased acid phosphatase activity at the site of a skeletal metastasis from carcinoma of the prostate [26]. In 1938 Gutman and Gutman reported that 11 of 15 (73%) of patients with metastatic prostate cancer had elevated serum levels of acid phosphatase [27]. In 1941 Huggins and Hodges reported that acid phosphatase activity decreased in patients with metastatic prostate cancer following castration or estrogen therapy [3].

Since these early observations, measurement of serum acid phosphatase has been used as a marker for metastatic disease and to assess response to hormonal therapy. Unfortunately, serum acid phosphatase is elevated in only about 75% of patients with radiographically proven skeletal metastases [28]. Furthermore, prostatic acid phosphatase can be falsely elevated by other conditions such as osteosarcoma, carcinoma of the pancreas, Gaucher's disease, thromboembolism, and thrombocytopenia [29].

The mechanism by which serum acid phosphatase becomes elevated in metastatic prostate cancer remains unclear. It is not on the basis of an increased cellular content of acid phosphatase, because individual prostate cancer cells contain less acid phosphatase than normal or hyperplastic prostate cells [30]. Alternative explanations include: 1) prostatic cancer cells become disorganized, form irregular acini, and lose their connection with the prostatic ductal system, thus preventing secretion of acid phosphatase into the seminal fluid; 2) the tumor may compress the prostatic ductal system blocking secretion of acid phosphatase; 3) the tumor load is so large that even though individual cells secrete less acid phosphatase, the overall serum activity becomes elevated [31].

Over the years determination of serum acid phosphatase by colorimetric techniques has become increasingly specific for the prostatic fraction because of both tartrate inhibition and more accurate substrates. The substrate that appears most specific for prostatic acid phosphatase is thymolphthalein monophosphate [14]. Many clinicians regard an elevated serum acid phosphatase determined with this substrate as diagnostic of advanced disease. However, although virtually 100% specific, the assay will detect only about 75–80% of patients with radiograhically proven metastatic disease.

In the 1970s, enthusiasm arose over the use of immunologic techniques to measure serum acid phosphatase because of initial reports that these methods were both more sensitive and specific than standard colorimetric assays. It was hoped that these new assays could be used not only as markers of metastatic prostate cancer, but also to detect early disease. In 1974 Cooper and associates reported that, using a double antibody radioimmunoassay (RIA) technique, serum prostatic acid phosphatase (SPAP) was elevated in 43% of men with localized prostate cancer and in 94% of men with metastatic prostate cancer. They reported a false positive rate of less than 6% [23]. Subsequently, Lee and coworkers, using a solid-phase fluorescent immunoassay, reported elevated SPAP levels in 73% of patients with stage A prostate cancer, 56% in stage B, 82% in stage C, and 86% in stage D [32]. Murphy and associates, using a counter-immunoelectrophoresis technique, reported elevated SPAP activity in 39% of patients with stage A disease and in 35% of patients with stage B disease [33].

Despite these early reports, subsequent studies have shown that these immuno-chemical methods are less accurate in detecting early prostate cancer than original-ly reported. Bruce and coworkers reported that RIA SPAP was elevated in only 14% of patients with clinical stage A disease and in 29% of patients with clinical stage B disease. Furthermore, when they compared 3 RIA techniques to measure SPAP, they found that, with all three techniques, SPAP levels were elevated in only a slightly greater percentage of men with prostate cancer than in men with benign prostatic hyperplasia [34]. Wajsman and associates reported that SPAP measured by counterimmunoelectrophoresis was elevated in 35% of patients with clinically localized prostate cancer, but there was a false positive rate of 14% [35]. Lindholm and associates found that SPAP levels were elevated in only 22% of clinical stage A patients, and in 29% of clinical stage B patients. Furthermore, SPAP levels were normal in 7 of 7 patients with pathologically confirmed stage A and B tumors, suggesting that elevation of SPAP measured by RIA may reflect early metastatic disease rather than increased assay sensitivity [36]. Similarly, Pontes and coworkers reprted that 20 of 20 patients with clinically localized prostate cancer and elevated RIA SPAP levels preoperatively all had lymph node metastases at the time of surgery [37].

Thus, while immunochemical methods may be more sensitive than standard colorimetric techniques in detecting localized disease, they do not appear to be specific enough to be used as a screening test for early prostate cancer. The use of immunochemical methods to measure SPAP to detect metastatic prostate cancer suffers from the same limitation. Although these methods appear more sensitive than colorimetric techniques, they are unreliable because of the high false positive rate.

Acid phosphatase activity in bone marrow aspirates obtained from the posterior iliac crest also has been evaluated as a marker for metastatic prostate cancer using both colorimetric and immunochemical techniques. In 1970 Chua and associates reported that colorimetric bone marrow acid phosphatase (BMAP) was normal in 12 of 12 patients with BPH and elevated as the only evidence of metastatic disease in 4 of 12 patients with prostate cancer [38]. Similar observations were reported by Reynolds and associates in 1973 [39] and Gursel and associates in 1974 [40], suggesting that determination of BMAP might be useful to detect early metastatic disease. In 1975 Pontes and coworkers reported that BMAP was elevated in 4 of 20 patients with prostate cancer, all of whom had a normal serum prostatic acid phosphatase and radionuclide bone scan [41].

Subsequent studies, however, by Khan and associates in 1977 [42] and Dias and Barnett in 1977 [43] have revealed that colorimetric measurement of BMAP is falsely elevated in a percentage of patients without prostate cancer. These false positives are thought to be due to the fact that the acid phosphatase in bone marrow may be derived from a variety of sources other than prostate cancer cells. Indeed, Lam and coworkers have reported that the major acid phosphatase isoenzyme in bone marrow is isoenzyme 5 which is derived from osteoclasts and not prostate cells [18]. In 1978 Pontes and coworkers reported that BMAP was elevated in 61% of patients without prostate cancer [44], and substantiated this observation in a subsequent paper in 1979 that compared BMAP levels in 20 patients with prostate cancer and 20 patients with BPH [45].

Immunochemical measurement of BMAP appears no more specific than SAP determinations. In 1981 Belville and associates, using an RIA technique to measure BMAP, reported that 4 of 11 (36%) of patients with elevated BMAP levels developed metastatic disease within 2 years compared to only 3 of 86 (3%) of patients with normal BMAP levels. However, serum PAP levels were not reported in these patients [46]. In 1982 Shellhammer and coworkers found that SPAP was normal in only 3 of 55 patients who had an elevated BMAP, and concluded that determination of BMAP was of limited clinical value [47]. In 1982 Vihko and associates reported that BMAP measurements were no more useful than SPAP determinations [48]. Thus, routine determination of BMAP whether done colorimetrically or by immunochemical techniques, appears no more helpful than SPAP in staging prostatic cancer.

In summary, the measurement of serum prostatic acid phosphatase by routine colorimetric assay employing thymolphthalein monophosphate as the substrate remains a very useful marker for metastatic carcinoma of the prostate. Measurement of SPAP by immunological techniques has not proved useful either in detecting early disease or as a marker for advanced disease because of the high incidence of false positive elevations. Measurement of bone marrow acid phosphatase activity whether done colorimetrically or by immunochemical methods has proved similarly unreliable, and has been for the most part abandoned.

Isoenzymes of alkaline phosphatase

The measurement of alkaline phosphatase as a tumor marker for carcinoma of the prostate preceded the measurement of acid phosphatase. In 1933 Bodansky reported a method for measuring serum alkaline phosphatase in patients with prostate cancer [49]. In 1936 Gutman and coworkers, while studying alkaline phosphatase activity in prostate cancer, incidentally discovered increased acid phosphatase activity at the site of an osteoblastic metastasis [26]. In 1941 Huggins and Hodges observed that, in patients undergoing going hormonal therapy for carcinoma of the prostate, there was a transient rise in serum alkaline phosphatase levels followed by a gradual decline in response to therapy. They termed this the 'flare phenomenon' [3].

Alkaline phosphatase has been recognized as a tumor marker for bone tumors such as osteogenic sarcomas for many years. However, it is a non-specific tumor marker and is neither organ nor tumor specific. Its elevation in patients with metastatic prostate cancer reflects either or both skeletal or hepatic metastases. It does not result directly from tumor activity [50]. There are four known isoenzymes of alkaline phosphatase that are secreted by bone, liver, intestine, and placenta. The immunologic specificity of these enzymes has not been fully evaluated, but there appear to be at least three major antigenic forms of the enzyme in man. As with acid phosphatase, part of the electrophoretic heterogeneity of alkaline phosphatase is due to variation in the sialic acid content of the isoenzymes [51].

It is important to distinguish the bone isoenzyme of alkaline phosphatase (BAP) from other forms of the enzyme in evaluating patients with prostate cancer, since BAP is the isoenzyme most often elevated in metastatic disease. Although immunological methods have been developed for this purpose, the isoenzymes are easily separable by ordinary physicochemical methods. The placental and intestinal isoenzymes are inhibited by 0.005 M L-phenylalanine while the bone and liver fractions are not. The bone isoenzyme is inhibited both by heating at 56° for five minutes and by denaturation with urea. The liver isoenzyme is more resistant both to heat and urea [52].

Although alkaline phosphatase is a non-specific tumor marker, it is elevated in 60% of patients with untreated prostate cancer and in over 90% of prostate cancer patients with radiographically proven skeletal metastases [53]. It is therefore a more sensitive but less specific marker for metastastic disease than acid phosphatase. Although routine measurement of alkaline phosphatase has little value in the diagnosis of prostate cancer, serial measurements of the enzyme are important both in staging the disease and in assessing response to therapy.

In 1978 Wajsman and associates reported a study of serum alkaline phosphatase in 357 patients stage D carcinoma of the prostate who entered the National Prostatic Cancer Project (NPCP) for chemotherapy. All had developed tumor relapse following previous orchiectomy, and all had radiographically proven skeletal mctastases. 305 patients (85%) had an elevated total serum alkaline phosphatase (TAP). Fifty-two (15%) had a normal TAP, but 22 of these 52 (44%) had elevated levels of BAP, indicating that BAP is a more sensitive marker of metastatic prostate cancer than TAP [54].

In the same study, 105 of these 357 patients underwent serial TAP and BAP determinations which were then correlated to response chemotherapy. There was a close correlation between initial TAP and BAP levels and response to treatment. All patients with TAP levels less than 200 mU/ml and BAP levels less than 100 mU/ml responded to therapy. All patients with TAP levels greater than 500 mU/ml and BAP levels greater than 400 mU/ml failed to respond to therapy. In a subgroup of 46 patients, there was a similar correlation between changes in alkaline phosphatase levels after starting treatment and response to chemotherapy. Of 24 patients who demonstrated a partial regression or stabilization of disease, 12 (56%) had at least a 25% decrease in serum TAP and 17 (71%) had a similar decrease in serum BAP. Conversely, of 22 patients who did not respond to therapy, 20 (90%) had less than a 25% decrease in TAP and 16 (72%) had less than a 25% decrease in BAP [54].

In another NPCP study reported by Killian and coworkers in 1981, the tumor burden of 98 patients with metastatic prostatic cancer was compared longitudinally with the activities of TAP, BAP and liver alkaline phosphatase (LAP) as well as total acid phosphatase and prostate-specific acid phosphatase. High pretreatment levels of BAP and TAP correlated with a greater tumor burden and a poorer prognosis. LAP levels that were increased more than three times above normal were suggestive of liver metastases and a poor prognosis. The bone and liver tumor burden of patients could be predicted from BAP and LAP levels provided these levels correlated with prostatic acid phosphatase activity. Finally, erratic fluctuations of BAP and LAP levels did not necessarily indicate a poor prognosis and sometimes resulted from unrelated diseases [55].

Taken together, these two studies suggest that measurement of serum alkaline phosphatase, particularly the bone fraction, is valuable in assessing tumor burden and in assessing response to chemotherapy in patients with metastatic carcinoma of the prostate. Patients with low pretreatment levels of TAP and BAP are likely to respond to therapy, whereas patients with high levels of TAP and BAP are unlikely to respond. There is also a close correlation following treatment between changes in serum levels of TAP and BAP and clinical response to therapy.

There is a third isoenzyme of alkaline phosphatase besides BAP and LAP that deserves further mention in regard to carcinoma of the prostate. In 1968 Fishman and associates reported the presence of a placental-type alkaline phosphatase in the tumor cells of a patient (Regan P) with bronchogenic carcinoma of the lung [56]. This has subsequently been termed the Regan isoenzyme. This isoenzyme is an oncofetal protein that is expressed in about 20% of patients with a wide variety of tumors. It is most commonly elevated with gonadal tumors, particularly seminomas [57].

The Regan isoenzyme has been evaluated as a potential biochemical marker for prostatic carcinoma. In 1981 Slack and coworkers reported that this isoenzyme was elevated in 14/98 (18%) of stage D NPCP patients receiving chemotherapy. Isoenzyme activity did not correlate with patient age, tumor grade, previous surgical history, or associated diseases [58]. In 1982 Schmidt and associates reported elevated Regan isoenzyme levels in 19/96 (20%) of prostate cancer patients of varying stages. Fifteen patients had clinical stage D2 disease, 1 had stage B1 disease, 2 had stage B2 disease, and 1 had stage D1 disease. Once again there was no correlation between elevated isoenzyme levels with either the stage of disease or subsequent response to therapy [59]. Therefore, the Regan isoenzyme appears to be a nonspecific tumor marker with no apparent value at present in assessing patients with prostate cancer.

Isoenzymes of lactate dehydrogenase

Lactate dehydrogenase (LDH) is an enzyme that reversibly catalyzes the conversion of pyruvate to lactate in anaerobic glycolysis. The enzyme is comprised of two major subunits designated M and H. Five isoenzymes have been identified, all of which are tetrameric combinations of these two major subunits. LDH 1 is comprised of 4 H subunits and LDH 5 of 4 M subunits. The intermediate LDH isoenzymes are hybrids of M and H [60].

The value of LDH measurements in a variety of cardiac, hepatic, and muscle disorders is well recognized. Malignant diseases may produce an elevation in total serum LDH and/or an alteration in isoenzyme activity. In general, neoplastic transformation results in a shift from H to M subunits resulting in an increase in LDH 5 content within malignant tissues. This alteration probably results from increased glycolytic activity [61].

In 1963 Denis and Prout reported that serum levels of LDH 5 were elevated in patients with prostatic cancer compared to those with benign prostatic hyperplasia [62]. In 1965 Prout and associates reported consistent alterations in serum LDH isoenzymes 4 and 5 in patients with metastatic prostate cancer, and found that these levels returned to normal after successful treatment [63].

Because of the ubiquitous nature of LDH and the fact that none of its isoenzymes is prostate specific, most studies have focused on LDH isoenzyme content either within prostatic tissue or within prostatic fluid rather than in serum. In 1970 Oliver and coworkers analyzed over 600 surgical prostate specimens by LDH electrophoresis. They reported that the ratio of LDH 5/LDH 1 was greater than 1 in 78% of patients with prostate cancer and was less than 1 in 86% with benign prostatic disease [64]. In 1972 Flocks and Schmidt reported a similar elevation in the LDH 5/LDH 1 ratio in the prostatic tissue of patients with carcinoma. They also described two patients whose initial prostatic biopsy was benign who, because of an elevated LDH 5/LDH 1 ratio, were rebiopsied and found to have carcinoma [65]. Conversely, in 1973 Clark and Srinivasan reported that LDH 5/LDH 1 determinations in prostatic tissue were of little value in the initial clinical diagnosis of prostate cancer when compared to digital rectal examination and serum acid phosphatase [66].

In 1967 Elhilali and associates analyzed LDH isoenzymes in prostatic fluid and urine and reported a marked elevation in the LDH 5/LDH 1 ratio in patients with prostate cancer [67]. In 1970 Belitsky and coworkers reported that the serum LDH 5/LDH 1 ratio increased following prostatic massage in 36 patients with prostatic cancer [68].

These earlier studies stimulated Grayhack and associates to analyze prostatic fluid for LDH isoenzyme content as well as other biochemical factors in an attempt to identify markers for the early diagnosis of prostate cancer. In 1977 these investigators reported LDH 5/LDH 1 ratios in prostatic fluid from over 1,000 patients. The LDH 5/LDH 1 ratios were as follows: normal- 0.48 ± 0.09, BPH- 1.36 ± 0.17, and carcinoma- 5.21 ± 0.79. The mean values for the three histologic groups were all statistically different ($p < 0.001$). 25 of 30 (85%) patients with histologically proven carcinoma of the prostate had an LDH 5/LDH 1 ratio greater than 2. 50 of 57 (88%) patients with BPH had a ratio of less than 2. Patients with significant prostatic inflammation (greater then 10 leukocytes per high powered field in the prostatic fluid) were excluded from analysis because of the high content of LDH 5 within granulocytes. These authors concluded that prostatic fluid with an LDH 5/LDH 1 ratio greater than 2 in the absence of prostatic inflammation was suggestive of prostatic carcinoma [69].

Subsequent reports have confirmed that there is a shift in the LDH 5/LDH 1 ratio in the prostatic fluid of patients with carcinoma of the prostate. Nevertheless, there is considerable overlap among individual patients with prostate carcinoma and BPH. In a recent update Schacht and coworkers reported that the LDH 5/LDH 1 ratio in prostatic fluid was greater than 2 in 76 of 92 (83%) patients with prostatic cancer, but the ratio also was greater than 2 in 39 of 117 (33%) men with BPH, and in 70% of men with BPH and associated prostatic inflammation [70]. Therefore, this test does not appear sufficiently specific to be used as a screening test for early prostate carcinoma.

Isoenzymes of creatine kinase

Creatine kinase is an enzyme that catalyzes the reversible transfer of a phosphate group from phosphocreatine to ADP producing creatine and ATP. The enzyme is dimeric and consists of two 40,000-Dalton subunits which can combine to form three active hybrid isoenzymes designated MM, MB, and BB. The major isoenzyme in cardiac and skeletal muscle is MM. Cardiac muscle also has a significant amount of MB, while skeletal muscle contains only trace amounts of MB. The BB isoenzyme is found in high concentrations in brain, genitourinary tissues, gastrointestinal organs, and most other visceral organs. Within the prostate, creatine kinase BB (CK-BB) is localized in the cytoplasm of both benign and malignant prostatic epithelium [71] .

Elevated levels of CK-BB were first reported in 1977 by Feld and Witte. They found that 9 of 19 (47%) patients with stage D prostate cancer had elevated levels of CK-BB, and only 3 of the 9 had elevated levels of total creatine kinase. All 9 patients with elevated CK-BB levels had normal serum acid phosphatase and alkaline phosphatase levels [72]. Interest in CK-BB as a potential tumor marker for metastatic prostate cancer was further aroused by Forman in 1979 who reported elevated CK-BB levels in 2 of 3 patients with metastatic carcinoma of the prostate [73].

The source of elevated CK-BB levels in patients with prostatic cancer is not known. It is unclear whether such elevations result from an increased release of the isoenzyme from prostatic tissue or whether they are due to release of a fetal form of the enzyme from dedifferentiated tumor tissue. It seems unlikely that the isoenzyme is released directly from the prostate itself, since CK-BB levels are seldom elevated in patients with early stage disease. Additionally, Pretlow and associates have reported that CK-BB activity is lower in malignant prostatic tissue than in benign hyperplastic tissue [74].

In 1979 Silverman and coworkers reported that serum CK-BB levels were elevated in 15 of 17 (88%) patients with untreated carcinoma of the prostate and in 0 of 18 (0%) patients with previously treated carcinoma of the prostate who were in remission [75]. In 1981, Silverman and associates reported that serum CK-BB levels were elevated in 70% of patients with carcinoma of the prostate and in only 10% with benign prostatic hyperplasia [71]. Subsequent studies, however, have yielded less impressive results. In 1981 Zweig and associates found that, in a group of untreated prostatic cancer patients, CK-BB was elevated in only 29% compared to 65% who had an elevated serum prostatic acid phosphatase [76]. In 1982 Huber and coworkers reported that CK-BB either alone or in combination with serum prostatic acid phosphatase was not a reliable marker to detect prostatic cancer [77]. In the same year Fair and associates reported that CK-BB was elevated only in patients with advanced prostate cancer [78].

It appears that CK-BB is not useful to detect prostate cancer, and that its only potential clinical application is as a marker for metastatic disease. Even in this regard, it does not appear either sufficiently sensitive or specific. In 1980 Aleyassine and MacIsaac reported that CK-BB was elevated in only 8/30 (27%) of patients with histologically proven carcinoma of the prostate. All 8 patients had poorly differentiated tumors; 7 had clinical stage C disease, and 1 had clinical stage D disease. Of 19 patients with clinical stage D disease, only 7 (37%) had elevated CK-BB levels [79]. In the same year Feld and associates reported that CK-BB levels were elevated in only 1 of 26 (4%) patients with clinical stage B disease, 0 of 35 (0%) patients with clinical stage C disease, and 11 of 46 (24%) patients with clinical stage D disease [80]. In 1982 Fair and associates reported that serum CK-BB levels were elevated in 4 of 26 (15%) patients with clinical stage C disease, and 4 of 19 (21%) patients with clinical stage D disease. Again, almost all patients with elevated CK-BB levels not only had advanced disease, but had also poorly differentiated tumors [78].

Silverman and associates have suggested that the specificity and sensitivity of CK-BB as a tumor marker may increase when a specific antiserum raised against prostatic CK-BB is developed. At present, brain antiserum is used to measure the prostatic fraction. These investigators have reported that the CK-BB in prostatic fluid and tissue is antigentically different from the CK-BB found in brain. Antisera raised against brain CK-BB reacts less strongly toward CK-BB of prostatic origin [71]. If a specific antiserum could be developed against CK-BB of prostatic origin for use in immunoassays, such a modification might increase both the sensitivity and specificity of serum CK-BB measurements.

Isoenzymes of leucine aminopeptidase

Leucine aminopeptidase (LAP) is an acrylamidase that hydrolyzes L-leucylbeta-naphthylamide. In 1960 Lawrence and associates demonstrated electrophoretic heterogeneity of LAP [81]. However, no standard isoenzyme nomenclature has yet been established for this enzyme. Normal serum contains a single zone of activity that varies somewhat in its location with the electrophoretic technique employed. On starch gel most investigators report LAP in the fast alpha 2 region. On paper or cellulose acetate electrophoresis, LAP shows activity in the alpha 1 region [82].

Beckman and associates demonstrated multiple forms of LAP in numerous human tissues including 4 bands in placenta, 3 in kidney, 2 each in liver, lung, spleen, and heart, a single slow band in intestine, and a single fast band in erythrocytes and brain [83].

The prostate is known to be rich in LAP, but little is known about the serum levels or isoenzyme patterns of LAP in patients with carcinoma of the prostate. Two apparently antigenically distinct forms have been identified within prostatic tissue, but tissue specificity of prostatic LAP has not been thoroughly investigated. Immunologic studies suggest that prostatic LAP may be present in very low concentrations in other tissues, but may, nonetheless, be of diagnostic value owing to its high concentration in the prostate [84]. To date, however, there has been little clinical application of LAP measurement in human prostatic carcinoma.

Conclusions

Despite recent investigations, acid and alkaline phosphatase are the only enzymes routinely measured at present in the evaluation of patients with prostatic carcinoma. Other isoenzymes have not proved clinically useful, mainly because of a lack of specificity. In the future, we must continue to search for isoenzymes and other biochemical markers that are specific for prostatic carcinoma. A particular challenge is to identify a marker that could be used to detect early carcinoma of the prostate and be applied as a screening test in the general population. Since most men with carcinoma of the prostate present with advanced disease, identification of such a marker that would allow earlier diagnosis would represent a major advance in this disease.

Reference

1. Moncure CW: Isoenzymes in prostatic carcinoma. In: Urologic Pathology: The Prostate, M Tannenbaum (ed). Lea and Febiger, Philadelphia, 141–155, 1977
2. Martland M, Hansman FS, Robinson R: The phosphoric-esterase of blood. Bioche J 18: 1152, 1924
3. Huggins C, Hodges CV: Studies on prostatic cancer. I. The effect of castration, of estrogen and of androgen injection on serum phosphatases in metastatic carcinoma of the prostate. Cancer Res 1: 293, 1941
4. Gutman EB, Gutman AB: Erythrocyte phosphatase activity in hemolyzed sera and estimation of serum acid phosphatases. Proc Soc Exp Biol Med 47: 513, 1941
5. Herbert FK: The differentiation between prostatic phosphatase and other acid phosphatases in pathological human sera. Biochem J 39: iv, 1945
6. Abul-Fadl MAM, King EJ: properties of the acid phosphatases of erythrocytes and of the human prostate gland. Biochem J 45: 51, 1949
7. Yam LT: Clinical significance of the human acid phosphatases: A review. Am J Med 56: 604, 1974
8. Gutman EB, Gutman AB: Estimation of 'acid' phosphatase activity of blood serum. J Biol Chem 136: 201, 1940
9. Modder CP: Investigations on acid phosphatase activity in human plasma and serum. Clin Chim Acta 43: 205, 1973
10. Woodard HQ: The clinical significance of serum acid phosphatase. AM J Med 27: 902, 1959
11. Huggins C, Talalay P: Sodium phenolphthalein phosphatase as a substrate for phosphatase tests. J Biol Chem 159: 399, 1945
12. Babson AL, Read PA: A new assay for prostatic acid phosphatase in serum. Am J Clin Pathol 32: 88, 1959
13. Seligman AM, et al 1951: The colorimetric determination of phosphatases in human serum. J Biol Chem 190: 7, 1951
14. Roy AV, et al: Sodium thymolphtalein monophosphate: A new acid phosphatase substrate with greater specificity for the prostatic enzyme in serum. Clin Chem 17: 1093, 1971
15. Li CY, et al: Acid phosphatases in human plasma. J Lab Clin Med 82: 446, 1973
16. Smith JK, Whitby LG: The heterogeneity of prostatic acid phosphatase. Biochem Biophys Acta 151: 607, 1968
17. Lam KW, Li O, Li CY, et al: Biochemical properties of human prostatic acid phosphatase. Clin Chem 19: 483, 1973
18. Lam KW, Lee P, Eastlund T, Yam LT: Antigenic ans molecular relationship of human prostatic acid phosphatase isoenzymes. Invest Urol 18: 209, 1980
19. Lin MF, Lee CL, Wojcieszyn JW, Wang MC, Valenzuela LA, Murphy GP, Chu TM: Fundamen-

tal biochemical and immunological aspects of prostatic acid phosphatase. The Prostate 1: 415, 1980

20. McTigue JJ, Van Etten RL: Isolation, characterization, and spontaneous interconversion of two forms of human prostatic acid phosphatase. The Prostate 3: 165, 1982
21. Taga EM, Moore DL, Van Etten RL: Studies on the structural basis of the heterogeneity of human prostatic and seminal acid phosphatases. The Prostate 4: 141, 1983
22. Lin MF, Lee CL, Li SSL, Chu TM: Purification and characterization of a new human prostatic acid phosphatase isoenzyme. Biochemistry 22: 1055, 1983
23. Cooper JF, Foti A: A radioimmunoassay for prostatic acid phosphatase. I. Methodology and range of normal male serum values. Invest Urol 12: 98, 1974
24. Foti AG, Herschman H, Cooper JF: A solid-phase radio-immunoassay for human prostatic acid phosphatase. Cancer Res 35: 2446, 1975
25. Chu TM, Wang MC, Scott WW, et al: Immunochemical detection of serum prostatic acid phosphatase. Methodology and clinical evaluation. Invest Urol 15: 319, 1978
26. Gutman EB, Sproul EE, Gutman AB: Significance of increased phosphatase activity of bone at the site of osteoplactic metastases secondary to carcinoma of the prostate gland. Am J Cancer 28: 485, 1936
27. Gutman AB, Gutman EB: An 'acid' phosphatase occuring in the serum of patients with metastasizing carcinoma of the prostate gland. J Clin Invest 17: 473, 1938
28. Woodard HQ: Factors leading to elevations in serum acid glycerophosphate. Cancer 5: 236, 1952
29. Henneberry MO, Engel G, Grayhack JT: Acid phosphatase. Urol Clin of North America 6: 3, 629, 1979
30. Brendler CB, Follansbee AL, Isaacs JT: Discrimination between normal, hyperplastic, and malignant human prostatic tissues by enzymatic profiles. J Urol 133: 495, 1985
31. Catalona WJ: Prostate Cancer. Grune and Stratton INc, Orlando, 61–62, 1984
32. Lee CL, Chu TM, Wajsman LZ, Slack NH, Murphy GP: Value of a new fluorescent immunoassay for human prostatic acid phosphatase in prostate cancer. Urology 15: 338, 1980
33. Murphy GP, Chu TM, Karr JP: Prostatic acid phosphatase the developing experience. Clin Biochem 12: 226, 1979
34. Bruce AW, Mahan DE, Sullivan LD, Goldenberg L: The significance of prostatic acid phosphatase in adenocarcinoma of the prostate. J Urol 125: 357, 1981
35. Wajsman Z, Chu TM, Saroff J, Slack N, Murphy GP: Two new direct and specific methods of acid phosphatase determination; national field trial. Urology 13: 8, 1979
36. Lindholm GR, Stirton MS, Liedtke RJ, Batjer JD: Prostatic acid phosphatase by radioimmunoassay. Sensitivity compared with enzymatic assay. JAMA 244: 2071, 1980
37. Pontes JE, Choe BK, Rose NR, Ercole C, Pierce Jr JM : Clinical evaluation in immunological methods for detection of serum prostatic acid phosphatase. J Urol 126: 363, 1981
38. Chua DT, Veenema RJ, Muggia F, Graff A: Acid phosphatase levels in bone marrow: value in detecting early bone metastases from carcinoma of the prostate. J Urol 103: 462, 1970
39. Reynolds RD, Greenberg BR, Martin ND, Lucas RN, Gaffney CN, Hawn L: Usefulness of bone marrow serum acid phosphatase in staging carcinoma of the prostate. Cancer 32: 181, 1973
40. Gursel EO, Rezvan M, Sy FA, Veenema RJ: Comparative evaluation of bone marrow acid phosphatase and bone scanning in staging of prostatic cancer. J Urol 111: 53, 1974
41. Pontes JE, Alcorn SW, Thimas Jr AJ, Pierse Jr JM: Bone marrow acid phosphatase in staging prostatic carcinoma. J Urol 114: 422, 1975
42. Khan R, Turner B, Edson M, Dolan M: Bone marrow acid phosphatase: another look. J Urol 117: 79, 1977
43. Dias SM, Barnett RN: Elevated bone marrow acid phosphatase: the problem of false positives. J Urol 117: 749, 1977
44. Pontes JE, Choe BK, Rose NR, Pierce Jr JM: Bone marrow acid phosphatase in staging prostatic cancer: how reliable is it? J Urol 119: 772, 1978

45. Pontes JE, Choe B, Rose N, Pierce Jr JM: Reliability of bone marrow acid phosphatase as a parameter of metastatic prostatic cancer. J Urol 122: 178, 1979
46. Belville WD, Mahan DE, Sepulveda RA, Bruce AW, MIller CF: Bone marrow acid phosphatase by radioimmunoassay: 3 years of experience. J Urol 125: 809, 1981
47. Schellhammer PF, Warden SS, Wright GL, Sieg S: Bone marrow acid phosphatase by counterimmune electrophoresis: Pre-treatment and post-treatment correlations. J Urol 127: 66, 1982
48. Vihko P, Kontturi M, Lukkarinen O, Vihko R: Radioimmunoassayable prostatic-specific acid phosphatase in peripheral and bone marrow sera compared in diagnosis of prostatic cancer patients. J Urol 128: 739, 1982
49. Bodansky A: Phosphate studies. II. Determination of serum phosphatase. Factors influencing the accuracy of the determination. J Biol Chem 101: 93, 1933
50. Killian C, Chu TM, Drzewiecki G, et al: A simple and reliable method for alkaline phosphatase isoenzymes in prostatic cancer. Clin Chem 22: 1174, 1976
51. Robinson JC, Pierce JE: Differential action of neuraminidase on human serum alkaline phosphatases. Nature 204: 472, 1964
52. Ewen LM: Separation of alkaline phosphatase isoenzymes and evaluation of the clinical usefulness of this determination. Amer J Clin Path 61: 142, 1974
53. Goldberg DM, Ellis G: An assessment of serum acid and alkaline phosphatase determination in prostate carcinoma with clinical validation of acid phosphatase assay utilizing adenosine 3-monophosphate as substrate. J Clin Pathol 27: 140, 1974
54. Wajsman Z, Chu JM, Bross D, et al: Clinical significance of serum alkaline phosphatase isoenzymes in advanced prostate carcinoma. J Urol 119: 244, 1978
55. Killian CS, Vargas FP, Pontes EJ, Beckley S, Slack NH, Murphy GP, Chu TM: The use of serum isoenzymes of alkaline and acid phosphatase as possible quantitative markers of tumor load in prostate cancer. Prostate 2: 187, 1981
56. Fishman WH, INglis NR, Stolbach LL, et al: A serum alkaline phosphatase isoenzyme of human neoplastic cell origin. Cancer Res 28: 150, 1968
57. Fishman WH, Inglis NR, Vaitukaitis J, et al: Regan isoenzyme and human chorionic gonadtropin in ovarian cancer. Natl Cancer Inst Monogr 42: 63, 1975
58. Slack NH, Chu TM, Wajsman LZ, Murphy GP: Carcinoplacental isoenzyme (Regan) in carcinoma of the prostate. Cancer 47: 146, 1981
59. Schmidt JD, Slack NH, Chu TM, Murphy GP: Placentalike isoenzyme of alkaline phosphatase in prostatic cancer. J Urol 127: 457, 1982
60. Dietz AA, Lubrano T: LDH isoenzymes. Standard Meth Clin Chem 1: 49, 1972
61. Goldman RD, Kaplan NO, Hall TC: Lactic dehydrogenase in human neoplastic tissues. Cancer Res 24: 389, 1964
62. Denis LJ, Prout Jr GR: Lactic dehydrogenase in prostatic cancer. Invest Urol 1: 101, 1963
63. Prout Jr GR, Macalalag Jr EV, Denis LJ, Preston Jr LW; Alterations in serum lactate dehydrogenase and its fourth and fifth isoenzymes in patients with prostatic cancer. J Urol 94: 451, 1965
64. Oliver JA, et al: LDH isoenzymes in benign and malignant prostate tissue. The LDH V/I ratio as an index of malignancy. Cancer 25: 863, 1970
65. Flocks RH, Schmidt JD: Lactate dehydrogenase isoenzyme patterns of prostatic cancer and hyperplasia. J Surg Oncol 4: 161, 1972
66. Clark SS, Srinivasan C: Correlation of lactic dehydrogenase isoenzymes in prostatic tissue with serum acid phosphatase, digital examination and histological diagnosis. J Urol 109: 444, 1973
67. Elhilali MM, Oliver JH, Sherwin AL, MacKinnon KJ: Lactate dehydrogenase isoenzymes in hyperplasia and carcinoma of the prostate: a clinical study. J Urol 98: 686, 1967
68. Belitsky P, et al: The effect of stilbesterol on the isoenzymes of lactic dehydrogenase in benign and malignant prostatic tissue. J Urol 104: 453, 1970
69. Grayhack JT, Wendel EF, Lee C, OLiver L, Cohen E: Lactate dehydrogenase isoenzymes in human prostatic fluid: an aid in recognition of malignancy? J Urol 118: 204, 1977

70. Schacht MJ, Garnett JE, Grayhack JT: Biochemical markers in prostatic cancer. Urologic Clinics of North America 11: 2, 253, 1984

71. Silverman L, Chapman J, Jones M, et al: Creatine kinase BB and other markers of prostatic carcinoma. Prostate 2: 109, 1981

72. Feld RD, Witte DL: Presence of creatine kinase BB isoenzyme in some patients with prostatic carcinoma. Clin Chem 23: 1930, 1977

73. Forman DT: The significance of creatine kinase (CKBB) in metastatic cancer of the prostate. Ann Clin Lab Sci 9: 333, 1979

74. Pretlow II TG, Whitehurst GB, Pretlow TP, Hunt RS, Jacobs JM, McKenzie DR, McDaniel HG, Hall LM, Bradley Jr EL: Decrease in creatine kinase in human prostatic carcinoma compared to benign prostatic hyperplasia. Cancer Res 42: 4842, 1982

75. Silverman L, Dermer G, Zweig M, et al: Creatine kinase BB: A new tumor-associated marker. Clin Chem 25: 1432, 1979

76. Zweig MH, Van Steirteghem AC: Assessment of radioimmunoassay of serum creatine kinase BB (CK-BB) as a tumor marker: studies in patients with various cancers and a comparison of CK-BB concentrations to prostate acid phosphatase concentrations. J Natl Cancer Inst 66: 659, 1981

77. Huber PR, Zaugg Th, Linder E, Hagmaier V, Rutishauser G: Creatine kinase isoenzyme (CK-BB) in combination to prostatic acid phosphatase measured by RIA in the diagnosis of prostatic cancer. Urol Res 10: 75, 1982

78. Fair WR, Heston WDW, Kadmon D, Crane DB, et al: Prostatic cancer, acid phosphatase, creatine kinase-BB and race: a prospective study. J Urol 128: 735, 1982

79. Aleyassine H, MacIsaac SG: The diagnostic significance of serum creatine kinase-BB isoenzyme in adenocarcinoma of prostate. Clin Biochem 13: 109, 1980

80. Feld RD, Van Steirteghem AC, et al: The presence of creatine kinase BB isoenzyme in patients with prostatic cancer. Clinia Chimica Acta 100: 267, 1980

81. Lawrence SH, et al: A species comparison of serum proteins and enzymes by starch gel electrophoresis. Proc Soc Exp Biol Med 105: 572, 1960

82. Kowlessar OD, et al: Localization of serum leucine aminopeptidase, 5-nucleotidase and nonspecific alkaline phosphatase by starch-gel electrophoresis: clinical and biochemical significance in disease states. Ann NY Acad Sci 94: 836, 1961

83. Beckman L, et al: Multiple molecular forms of leucine aminopeptidase in man. Acta Genet Stat Med 16: 223, 1966

84. Mattila S: Further studies on the prostatic tissue antigens. Separation of two molecular forms of aminopeptidase. Invest Urol 7: 1, 1969

Editorial Comment

Leland W.K. Chung

Isoenzymes in the human prostate gland are reviewed in depth by Dr. C.B. Brendler in the preceding chapter. The author focused his attention on the marker enzymes of clinical importance, i.e., acid and alkaline phosphatases, lactate dehydrogenase, creatine kinase and leucine aminopeptidase. Valuable information on the comparative aspect of prostatic and erythrocytic prostatic acid phosphatases was presented in Table I, in which the biochemical characteristics of the various forms of acid phosphatases were cited. It would, however, have perhaps been more beneficial to the readers if the author had provided similar tables for each of the other isoenzymes discussed. Nonetheless, this chapter successfully conveys the current status of isoenzymes in the human prostate gland, the general biochemical methodologies that have been used to characterize them, and the application of quantitative procedures for these isoenzymes pertinent to prostatic cancer. The author points out the potential and future challenge for urological researchers to discover markers that would have clinical value in diagnosing and staging of prostatic cancer in man, particularly in the early phases.

The study of various forms of isoenzymes in tissues has no doubt contributed to their direct application in clinical medicine. These isoenzymatic markers may also have helped the cancer biologists probe the significance of these marker enzymes in biological processes. For example, the human prostatic acid phosphatase was characterized by Li et al. [1] as a form of phosphoprotein phosphatase that catalyzed specifically the dephosphorylation of protein that contained tryosine phosphate. A number of the oncogenes that produce transforming proteins have been shown to possess phosphotyrosyl-protein kinase activity [2–4]. The balance between protein kinase and phosphoprotein phosphatase activities has long been recognized as a primary factor in controlling the rates of many critical biological processes. Although the role of prostatic acid phosphatase remains obscure, the potential significance of this isoenzyme in prostatic cancer development at the level of protein dephosphorylation requires additional investigation.

The literature on the usefulness of isoenzymes and other biochemical markers for the investigation of prostatic carcinoma is steadily expanding. Specific cellular protein and enzyme markers have been prepared from normal, hyperplastic, and carcinomatous human prostatic tissues [5–7]. It is anticipated that modern molecular biology techniques will lead to rapid development of unique DNA and RNA probes which recognize specific nucleic acid sequences in normal and cancerous prostatic cells [8–11], These molecular probes will undoubtedly contribute to our further understanding of the biology of prostatic cancer and assist oncologists in diagnosing, staging and predicting therapeutic responses of prostatic cancer in man.

20

References

1. Li HC, Chernoff J, Chen LB, Kirschenbauw A: A phosphotyrosylprotein phosphatase activity associated with acid phosphatase from human prostate gland. European Journal of Biochem 138, 45–51, 1984
2. Hunter T, Sefton BM: Transforming gene product of rous sarcoma virus phosphorylates tyrosine. Proc Natl Acad Sci USA 77, 1311–1315, 1980
3. Collett MS, Purchio AF, Erikson RL: Avian sarcoma virus-transforming protein, p 60,shows protein kinase activity specific for tyrosine. Nature 285: 167–169, 1980
4. Levinson AD, Oppermann H, Varmus HE, Bishop JM: The purified product of the transforming gene of avian sarcoma virus phosphorylates tyrosine. J of Biol Chem 255: 11973–11979, 1980
5. Wang MC, Pepsidero LD, Kuriyama M, Valenzuela LA, Murphy GP: Prostate antigen: a new potential marker for prostatic cancer. The Prostate 2: 89–96, 1981
6. Silverman LM, Chapman JF, Jones ME, Dermer GB, Pullano T, Tokes ZA: Creatine kinase BB and other markers of prostatic carcinoma. The Prostate 2: 109–119, 1981
7. Fishman WH: Immunology and biochemistry of the Regan isoenzyme. The Prostate 1: 399–410, 1980
8. Parker MG, Mainwaring WIP: Effects of androgens on the complexity of poly (A) RNA from rat prostate. Cell. 12: 401–407, 1977
9. Montpetit ML, Lawless KR, Tenniswood M: Androgen repressed messages in the rat ventral prostate. The Prostate 8: 25–36, 1986
10. Smith RG, Nag A: Regulation of c-sis expression in tumors of the male reproductive tract: In Assessment of Current Concepts and Approaches to the Study of Prostatic Cancer, Coffey DS, Chiarodo A, Karr J (eds). Prouts Neck Maine October 18–20, 1985
11. Fleming WH, Hamel A, MacDonald R, Ramsey E, Pettigraw NM, Johnston B, Dodd JG, Matusik RJ: Expression of the c-myc protooncogene in human prostatic carcinoma and benign prostatic hyperplasia. Cancer Research 46: 1535–1538, 1986

2. Potency-sparing modification of radical retropubic prostatectomy

WILLIAM J. CATALONA

In recent years efforts have been made in surgical oncology to achieve cancer control while minimizing morbidity and functional sacrifices for patients. To this end the potency-sparing modification of radical retropubic prostatectomy was developed by Walsh (1983). This operation preserves erectile function in the great majority of patients.

Erectile impotency following standard radical retropubic prostatectomy occurs because of injury to the sacral parasympathetic neurovascular bundles that innervate the arteries of the corpora cavernosa (Walsh, 1982). These nerves arise from the second, third and fourth sacral segments and join the pelvic nerve plexus. The pelvic nerves are situated immediately adjacent tot the prostate and are susceptible to injury during the separation of the prostate and urethra from the rectum, and during the securing of the lateral prostatic vascular pedicles (Fig. 1).

The staging pelvic lymphadenectomy performed in association with radical retropubic prostatectomy is a modified node dissection including only the lymph nodes medial to the external iliac veins. This has been shown to be a reasonably accurate staging procedure and is associated with minimal morbidity.

The radical prostatectomy is begun by sweeping the fatty arealor tissue off the anterior surface of the porstate and exposing the endopelvic fascia and the puboprostatic ligaments (Fig. 2). Usually the puboprostatic ligaments can be palpated in the fatty tissue. Care should be taken not to injure the superficial branch of Santorini's plexus which perforates the endopelvic fascia between the puboprostatic ligaments and courses cephalad on the anterior surface of the prostate (Fig. 2).

The endopelvic fascia is incised by inserting the tips of dissecting scissors through the fascia in the groove between the prostate and the urogenital diaphragm (Fig. 2). If the proper plane is entered, the prostate is found to be covered with a smooth glossy membrane overlying the venous plexus. Laterally the urogenital diaphragm muscle fibers should are seen. The diaphragmatic fibers should be swept off the prostate on to the pelvic diaphragm. Near the puboprostatic ligaments there may be muscular attachments from the urogenital diaphragm

Ratliff, T.L. and Catalona, W.J. (eds), Genitourinary Cancer. ISBN 0–89838–830–9
© *1987, Martinus Nijhoff Publishers, Boston. Printed in the Netherlands.*

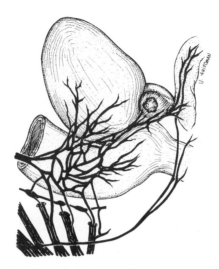

Figure 1. The anatomic relationship between the sacral 2, 3, 4 parasympathetic neurovascular bundle that is situated lateral to the bladder and prostate and innervates the corpora cavernosa. This neurovascular bundle is susceptible to injury during radical retropubic prostatectomy at the time of transection of the membranous urethra and in securing the vascular pedicles of the prostate.

to the apex of the prostate. These fibers may be incised so that they will not tether the apex of the prostate to the urogenital diaphragm and risk injury to the diaphragm during mobilization of the prostatic apex. Occasionally there are small blood vessels that accompany these muscle fibers. These vessels can be spot cauterized or ligated and divided.

After the endopelvic fascia has been opened on both sides, the superficial branch of the dorsal venous complex is retracted medially and the puboprostatic ligaments are incised near their insertion on the pubic symphysis (Fig. 3), taking care not to cut too medially nor too far under the pubic symphysis as this may result in injury to the dorsal venous complex or the urogenital diaphragm.

The plane anterior to the urethra can be identified by palpating a # 22 Fr catheder in the urethra. A pinching motion with the thumb and index finger demonstrates a plane between the urethra and the dorsal venous complex. A right angle clamp is then passed anterior the urethra and a heavy ligature is grasped, pulled through and tied (Fig. 4). A suture ligature is then placed more cephalad around the superficial branch of the dorsal venous complex on the anterior surface of the prostate. The right angle clamp is then passed posterior to the dorsal venous complex and the jaws of the clamp are spread while the venous complex is transected with a knife (Fig. 4).

In patients who have had a prior transurethral resection of the prostate, particularly those in whom the anterior portion of the prostate has been well resected, the venous complex may be adherant to the anterior surface of the prostate. In this case, it is possible to tent up the attenuated anterior portion of

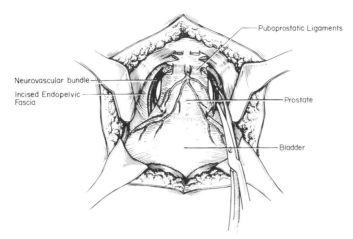

Figure 2. The endopelvic fascia is opened lateral to the prostate and neurovascular bundles. The puboprostatic ligaments and superficial branch of Santorini's plexus are depicted. (Catalona WJ: Radical prostatectomy: In *Prostate Cancer.* Grune & Stratton Inc. New York, 1984, with permission).

the prostatic capsule which may be incised inadvertantly while transecting the dorsal venous complex. Therefore, the venous complex should be transected as caudally as possible without jeapordizing the distal ligature.

After the dorsal venous complex has been transected, there is usually back bleeding from veins that drain along the lateral surface of the prostate. These veins are suture ligated with a 2–0 chromic catgut suture.

Because the ligature may slip off the dorsal venous complex at an inopportune time, it is prudent to suture ligate the venous complex routinely. The stump of the venous complex can best be secured with a suture ligature (placed while holding the needle holder in a vertical position) passing the needle first through the anterior portion of the venous complex, then passing it through the middle portion of the complex and finally passing it through the posterior portion of the venous complex before tieing the ligature. This assures good hemostasis for the remainder of the operation.

The apex of the prostate and the urethra with its adjacent neurovascular bundles can be identified after the venous complex has been ligated. The catheter can be palpated in the urethra at the apex of the prostate. On either side of the urethra is a groove and lateral to the grooves are the neurovascular bundles which are palpable as firm tissue bands. A plane between the urethra and the neurovascular bundles is developed on each side by spreading with the dissecting scissors parallel to the urethra. These planes can be further developed by blunt dissection with the tip of the index finger. The urethra is then isolated between both neurovascular bundles with a right angle clamp and a vessel loop is pulled through to elevate the urethra. The anterior wall of the urethra is then icised just distal to the apex of the prostate (Fig. 5). The catheter is then hooked with a right

24

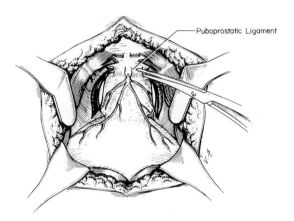

Figure 3. The puboprostatic ligaments are incised just lateral to the superficial branch of Santorini's venous plexus. The superficial branch may be retracted medially to avoid injury. (Catalona WJ: Radical prostatectomy: In *Prostate Cancer*. Grune & Stratton Inc, New York, 1984, with permission).

angle clamp and pulled through the opening in the urethra. The catheter is then clamped with a Kelly clamp and is then transected distal to the clamp pulling the transected end of the catheter cephalad to use as a tractor on the prostate. Finally, the posterior wall of the urethra is transected.

After transection of the urethra, the rectourethralis muscle fibers must be separated and incised to the develop the plane between the prostate and the rectum (Fig. 6). The rectourethralis fibers form a broad, thin, dense band that passes from the apex of the prostate to the rectum. With the apex of the prostate retracted cephalad, the rectourethralis fibers have a whitish appearance similar to a muscle facia. The tips of long pointed dissecting scissors are placed in the midline and spread until the plane between the prostate and rectum is entered. This plane is further developed bluntly with the tip of the index finger until the posterior lip of the prostatic apex is palpable. After the rectourethralis fibers have been incised, the plane between the prostate and the rectum is developed in the midline (Fig. 7). The lateral pelvic fascia is incised on the anterior surface of the prostate to develop a plane between the prostate and the neurovascular bundle. This vascia is incised sharply from the apex to the base of the prostate (Fig. 7). This maneuver frees the neurovascular bundles from the posterolateral surface of the prostate.

If there is tumor invasion into a neurovascular bundle, the bundle may be sacrified on one side without jeopardizing preservation of erectile function. After the apex of the prostate has been mobilized back to the prostatic pedicles, the vascular pedicles are secured by passing a right angle clamp around the pedicle and spreading. A 2–0 silk ligature is passed and tied around the pedicle and the pedicle is transected close to the prostate (Fig. 8). Bleeding from the prostatic side of the pedicles can be controlled with a suture ligature. The neurovascular bundles

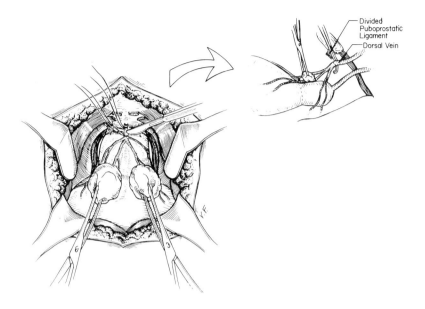

Figure 4. The deep dorsal complex has been ligated distally with a free ligature and proximally with a suture ligature. The free ligature was passed with a right-angle clamp as shown in the inset. The dorsal venous complex is then sharply divided between the ligatures. (Catalona WJ: Radical prostatectomy: In *Prostate Cancer.* Grune & Stratton Inc, New York, 1984, with permission).

pass immediately adjacent to the seminal vesicles and care must be taken to avoid injuring the bundles during the dissection of the prostatic pedicles and seminal vesicles. The prostate is mobilized on the posterior surface until the ampullary portions of the vasa deferentia and the seminal vesicles have been visualized.

Attention is then directed to the anterior surface of the prostate. Indigo carmen is injected intravenously and the bladder neck is transected in the groove just superior to the prostate (Fig. 9). The bladder neck is opened, the catheter balloon is deflated and the catheter is looped through the opening in the bladder neck to serve as a tractor on the prostate. The posterior bladder neck is incised and dissection is carried down to the plane anterior to the seminal vesicles. Then the seminal vesicles and ampullary portions of the vasa deferentia can be dissected on the anterior and lateral surfaces of the prostate. The seminal vesicles are dissected out by sharp and blunt dissection. There is usually a small artery entering the tip of the seminal vesicles which can be secured with a hemostatic clip. It is often necessary also to incise Denonvillier's fascia between the ampullary portions of the vasa. The specimen is then removed (Fig. 10).

The pelvis is inspected for adequacy of hemostasis. It is important to avoid using electrocautery on vessles or the neurovascular bundles because of the possibility of thermal damage to the parasympathetic nerves. Most of the bleeding in the neurovascular bundles will stop spontaneously; however, any bleeding that

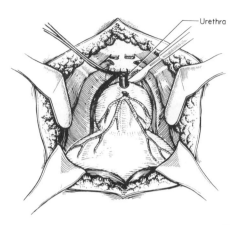

Figure 5. The anterior surface of the membranous urethra is transected. (Catalona WJ: Radical prostatectomy: In *Prostate Cancer*. Grune & Stratton Inc, New York, 1984, with permission).

does not stop may be scured by placing a suture ligature of fine absorbable suture material and tieing it only tightly enough to stop the bleeding. If a nerve is entrapped in the ligature, it may regenerate through the nerve sheath when the suture is absorbed.

After hemostasis has been obtained, a pack is placed in the pelvis, and the bladder neck is reconstructed. A tennis-recket shaped bladder neck closure with the handle of the racket directed posteriorly offers several theoretical advantages (Fig. 11). It recesses the ureteral orifices away from the vesicourethral anastomosis, allows the bladder neck to come down to the urethra more easily and provides for nearly circular muscle fibers at the anastomotic site. The bladder neck is closed in two layers, the first layer utilizing a running 3–0 chromic catgut suture and the second layer using interrupted 2–0 chromic catgut sutures. In placing the second layer of sutures, care must be taken to avoid inverting the bladder mucosa. The mucosa should be included in the anastomosis to avoid incontinence and stricture formation of the vesicourethral anastomosis. The bladder neck should be closed to the size of a # 20 Fr catheter.

The vesicourethal anastomosis is performed by placing 4 sutures of 2–0 chromic catgut on a 5/8th's circle (horseshoe) needle (Fig. 11). The sutures are first placed from inside out on the anterior lip of the urethra tagging these sutures with a curved mosquito clamp. Gentle traction is used on the anterior sutures while the posterolateral sutures are placed. The posterior sutures are tagged with straight mosquito clamps. The tails of the sutures are then rethreaded on a needle and passed through the bladder neck from inside to outside. A # 18 Fr Foley catheter is passed through the urethra into the bladder neck and the sutures are tied (Fig. 12). The bladder is irrigated free of clots and the pelvis is drained with a suction drain that remains in place for 7 days. The Foley catheter is removed on the 14th postoperative day.

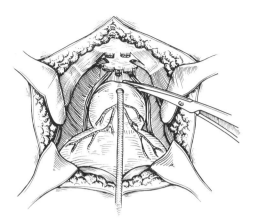

Figure 6. The rectourethralis fibers are separated from the posterior surface of the prostatic apex by spreading with a dissecting scissors in the midline and incising the fibers at their junction with the prostate. (Catalona WJ: Radical Prostatectomy: In *Prostate Cancer*. Grune & Stratton Inc, New York, 1984, with permission).

The potency-sparing technique of radical retropubic prostatectomy requires that the surgeon become throroughly familiar with the precise details of the anatomy of this region. If the operation is performed anatomically, operative blood loss and postoperative morbidity are minimal. The operation can be performed under epidural anesthesia in approximately 3 hours after familiarity with the technique has been gained.

Concern has been expressed about whether the nerve-sparing modification is an adequate cancer operation in terms possible compromise of the posterolateral margins of the prostate that lie close to the neurovascular bundles. Histopathologic studies by Walsh (1983) and Eggleston and associates (1985) suggest that the nerve-sparing modification for surgical margins that are more generous than those obtained with standard radical perineal prostatectomy but somewhat less generous than those obtained with standard radical retropubic prostatectomy. These investigators reported that 41 of 100 patients undergoing the nerve-sparing radical retropubic prostatectomy had established tumor in the periprostatic tissue and an additional 21 had focal microscopic soft tissue involvement. However, only 7 of 41 patients with established soft tissue involvement had positive surgical margins and all 7 had positive margins at sites other than the nerve-sparing modification.

We (Catalona, in press) also have reported on histopathologic findings in 52 patients who underwent the potency-sparing modification of radical retropubic prostatectomy. The incidence of positive surgical margins was not significantly different from the incidence of positive margins in a series of patients previously treated with standard radical retropubic prostatectomy. In both Walsh's and our series, erectile function has been preserved in the majority of patients. Walsh (1985) reported that among 64 preoperatively potent patients with sexual partners, potency returned in three months in 30%, six months in 40%, nine months in 60%

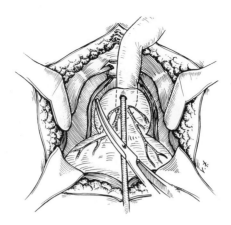

Figure 7. After the posterior portion of the prostatic apex has been exposed, the prostate is mobilized off the rectum in the midline by blunt dissection. The lateral pelvic fascia is then incised between the neurovascular bundles and the prostate. (Catalona WJ: Radical prostatectomy: In *Prostate Cancer.* Grune & Stratton Inc, New York, 1984, with permission).

and one year in 85%. In our series among 42 sexually potent patients followed for four months or more, 98% had partial erections and 52% had erections sufficient for vaginal penetration.

In conclusion, the available data suggest that with the potency-sparing modification of radical retropubic prostatectomy, postoperative sexual function can be preserved in the great majority of patients having clinical stages A or B prostate cancer without compromising the adequacy of tumor excision.

References

1. Catalona WJ, Dresner SM: Nerve-sparing radical prostatectomy: Extraprostatic tumor extension and preservation of erectile function. J Urol (in press)
2. Eggleston JC, Walsh PC: Nerve-sparing radical retropubic prostatectomy: pathologic findings in the first 100 cases. American Urological Association Eightieth Annual Meeting abstract 511, 1985
3. Walsh PC, Donker PJ: Impotence following radical prostatectomy: insight into etiology and prevention. J Urol 128: 492, 1982
4. Walsh PC, Lepor H, Eggleston JC: Radical prostatectomy with preservation of sexual function: anatomical and pathological considerations. Prostate 4: 1983

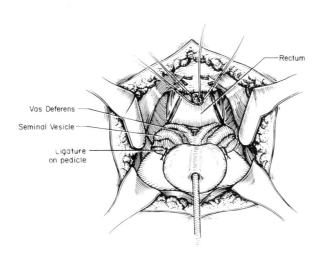

Figure 8. The prostatic pedicles are divided close to the seminal vesicles to preserve the neurovascular bundles. The ampullary portions of the vasa deferentia and seminal vesicles are exposed, and the prostate is retracted cephalad. (Catalona WJ: Radical prostatectomy: In *Prostate Cancer*, Grune & Stratton Inc, New York, 1984, with permission).

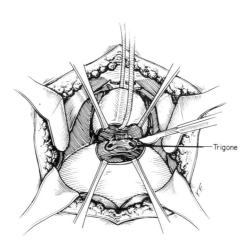

Figure 9. The bladder neck is incised cephalad to the prostate. The posterior bladder neck is transected caudal to the ureteral orifices. (Catalona WJ: Radical prostatectomy: In *Prostate Cancer*. Grune & Stratton Inc, New York, 1984, with permission).

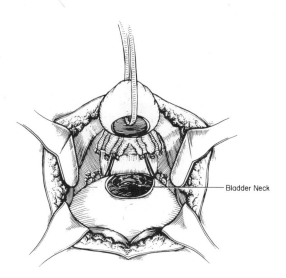

Figure 10. The seminal vesicles and vasa deferentia are divided, and the surgical specimen is removed. (Catalona WJ: Radical prostatectomy: In *Prostate Cancer*. Grune & Stratton Inc, New York, 1984, with permission).

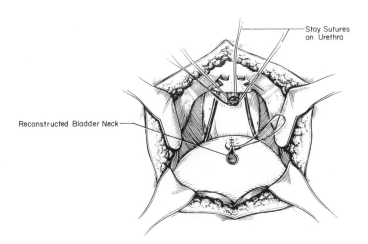

Figure 11. The bladder neck is closed in the shape of a tennis racket with a handle of the racket directed posteriorly. Sutures have been placed in the stump of the membranous urethra. (Catalona WJ: Radical prostatectomy: In *Prostate Cancer*. Grune & Stratton Inc, New York. 1984, with permission).

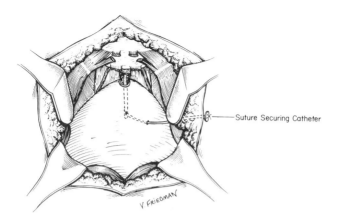

Figure 12. Completion of the vesicourethral anastomosis. (Catalona WJ: Radical prostatectomy: In *Prostate Cancer*. Grune & Stratton Inc, New York, 1984, with permission).

Editorial Comment

RICHARD D. WILLIAMS

Description of the cavernous nerves responsible for erectile potency and the subsequent development of a potency-sparing modification of radical retropubic prostatectomy by Walsh and co-workers is one of the true urologic surgical advances in the last decade. Corroboration of Walsh's results has been described by several urologic surgeons including the fine depiction presented here by Dr. Catalona. I will discuss only those areas in which I approach the operation in a different manner.

First, I think it is helpful to visualize the neurovascular bundles as very friable structures that course lateral to the urethra just distal to the prostatic apex at 3 and 9 o'clock and then dive posteriolateral on the prostate at 5 and 7 o'clock. The bundles are in close approximation to the prostatic capsule at the apex and posteriorly. Surgical damage to the bundles will most likely occur at 3 places: the apex of the prostate; the junction of the prostatic vessels with the prostate; and lateral to the seminal vesicles where they meet the prostate and thus special care must be excercised particularly during dissection at these areas.

I approach the puboprostatic ligaments as does Dr. Catalona, however, I would make a stronger point of caution about the vessels accompanying the muscles lateral to the puboprostatic ligaments from the urogenital diaphragm. I find that these vessels are present quite often and that they can be the source of troublesome bleeding if not carefully ligated prior to incising the puboprostatic ligaments. Indeed, once these vessels begin bleeding they may retract deep into the pelvis and cause considerable difficulty in maintaining the vision necessary for preservation of the cavernous nerves. I also use a large catheter, 22 or 24 French, to aid in palpation of the urethra but do not attempt to make a plane between the dorsal vein complex and the urethra with fingers but merely place a right angle clamp just above the urethra underneath the dorsal vein complex and then pull through a 1–0 silk suture. It should be noted that this tissue is quite thick and fibrous and considerable effort may be required to pass the right angle tip through it. I often place 2 sutures using the first as a traction suture to allow more proximal (on the vein) placement of the second. Directly following placement of this suture I place a suture around each branch of the dorsal vein on the surface of the prostate. A 2–0 chromic on a 5/8 curved needle is perfect for this and should be placed around the venous branches directing the needle right into the prostatic substance. This maneuver eliminates back bleeding before it occurs in most instances. Transection of the dorsal vein complex in my hands is done with heavy scissors, cutting directly toward the apex of the prostate between the 3 (or 4) sutures previously placed. The index finger is used liberally after small cuts to push the vein complex tissue distally and thus exposing the prostatic apex. I rarely see the dorsal vein itself until it has been transected due to the broad band of fibrofatty tissue surrounding it. At this point quite often, as Dr. Catalona has described, the dorsal vein ligature falls off (particularly if only one was placed), however, use of the 5/8 curve needle and 2–0 chromic with a figure-of-8 suture ligature through and through the vein complex deep up against the pubis will reliably accomplish hemostasis.

Once the apex of the prostate is identified, the neurovascular bundles can be separated from the urethra using metzenbaum scissors as described. It is important to begin the dissection of the lateral pelvic fascia on the prostate at the apex first and then along the lateral edge of the prostate initially as it allows blunt finger dissection of the neurovascular bundles to proceed smoothly as described in Figure 7. Note that the nerves are not well seen but the veins on the surface of the bundles are. I use finger dissection to complete the plane around the urethra. Care must be taken during this dissection to tease off the neurovascular bundle, from the prostate and urethra without undue tension which may rip the relatively friable structures. At the time of transection of the urethra, I place four to six 2–0 chromic sutures inside-out using 5/8 curve needles and place Kocher clamps on the 6 and 12 o'clock sutures for ease in identification later. I have found that placement of these sutures prior to complete urethral transection allows for the most accurate placement.

Following urethral suture placement, finger dissection on the posterior prostate is continued until the prostatic pedicles are encountered. These must be taken immediately adjacent to the prostate in order to avoid injury to the cavernous nerves. Vascular clips are usually satisfactory. The pedicles of the seminal vesicles are treated similarly.

The ureteral orifices can usually be seen easily after the bladder neck is transected and indigo carmine is only required when they are not seen readily. Single layer closure of the racquet handle using 2–0 chromic works well as long as the mucosa is opposed and good bites of muscle are taken. I agree with the advantages of the raquet-handle closure as described. I use a 16 french silicone foley catheter, being certain that the balloon has been tested and use gentle traction on the catheter to oppose the bladder neck and urethra while the anastomotic sutures are being tied. A suction drain is preferable but I remove it as soon as the drainage decreases to less than 75 cc per day (usually 3–4 days) and most often the patient is discharged with a leg bag on day 6 or 7 to return 1 week later for a urethrogram around the catheter. If no leak is observed, the catheter is then withdrawn.

I have recently been placing bulldog vascular clamps on the internal iliac arteries distal to the superior gluteal artery during the procedure as recently described by Dr. Walsh and have found the blood loss to average under 1100 cc utilizing this approach.

I too have been concerned about efficacy of the operation with respect to ablation of the cancer but now having done over 50 such operations, I am convinced that the potency-sparing approach does not compromise the cancer operation if one chooses patients carefully and does not persist with attempts to salvage potency in cases where the tumor nodule is excessively large or when the the bundles appear to be stuck to the prostate. I agree with Dr. Catalona that in my hands the modification does not result in a higher incidence of positive margins. The definitive proof that compromise has not occurred, however, awaits results of longitudinal follow-up of the local recurrence rate of these patients in the future.

The results in our patients thus far are that, of the patients potent preop who have been followed 6 months or more, 60% have erections sufficient for intercourse, while another 20% have only partial erections. Longer term follow-up will be required to determine actual potency rate with time; however, it was noted that as experience was gained it became apparent that of patients in whom potency was retained, erections most often occurred by three to six months after surgery.

It is also pertinent to note that we have attempted to salvage potency in 8 potent patients undergoing radical cystoprostatectomy and have been successful in 4 (50%), one of whom had a total urethrectomy in continuity. The same surgical principles described above were used in these patients in that the prostatic and cavernous nerve dissection was done prior to developing the plane posterior to the bladder and the lateral pedicles were then taken high well away from the prostate. The dissection on the urethra was carried close to the urethra through the pelvic diaphragm separating the neurovascular bundles laterally as they coursed toward the cavernous bodies. It should also be noted that ligation of the internal iliac arteries should be foregone if potency-sparing is attempted during cystectomy.

I am in full agreement with Dr. Catalona that the operation as he describes it, can preserve sexual function in the majority of patients but that it should be reserved for those with stage A or B disease.

References

1. Williams RD, Finkle AA: Sexual potency before and after radical prostatectomy. West J of Med 143: 474, Oct 1985
2. Walsh PC, Mastwin JL: Radical prostatectomy and cystoprostatectomy with preservation of potency. Results using a nerve-sparing technique. Br J of Urol 56: 964, 1984

3. Ureteroscopic resection of upper tract urothelial tumors

HARRY W. HERR and JEFFRY L. HUFFMAN

Introduction

Primary epithelial tumors of the upper urinary tract often present a diagnostic challenge and therapeutic dilemma. Considerable uncertainty exists regarding treatment of these uncommon neoplasms, especially with regard to the selection of patients who might benefit from conservative (kidney-sparing) surgery. Therapeutic guidelines have emanated largely from retrospective analysis of different surgical approaches, or from pathologic mapping of nephroureterectomy specimens, since accurate preoperative clinical staging could not always be obtained.

Recent advances in the design of endoscopic instrumentation, especially the rigid ureteropyeloscope, and refinements in the techniques of ureteral dilation for instrument passage, have opened the ureter and renal pelvis to routine endoscopic assessment [1, 2]. We have found the ureteropyeloscope to have uses similar to the cystoscope. These include: diagnosis of upper tract tumors, serveillance of urothelium following previous therapy, and primary endoscopic treatment of selected tumors [3].

Current treatment recommendations of bladder tumors are based upon tumor stage, grade, site and multicentricity. The ureteropyeloscope permits similar information to be obtained for upper tract tumors. One may biopsy directly, map, and occasionally completely resect tumor(s). The ureteropyeloscope is a valuable technical addition to the widely used indirect methods to assess upper tract lesions such as retrograde pyelography, lavage cytology and blind (or image-guided) brush biopsy. Just as it is inconceivable for the urologist to think of managing bladder tumors without cystoendoscopy, ureteropyeloscopy is rapidly evolving into an invaluable and indispensible method for assessing and managing urothelial tumors of the upper collecting system.

The present chapter reviews the authors' experience in managing upper tract urothelial neoplasms at the Memorial Sloan-Kettering Cancer Center (MSKCC) and the New York Hospital-Cornell University Medical Center.

Ratliff, T.L. and Catalona, W.J. (eds), Genitourinary Cancer. ISBN 0–89838–830–9
© *1987, Martinus Nijhoff Publishers, Boston. Printed in the Netherlands.*

Indications

The indications for ureteropyeloscopy include: (1) radiographic filling defect or obstruction (2) tumor found cystoscopically near (within 1 cm), at, or emerging from within the ureteral orifice(s), (3) unilateral upper tract hematuria, (4) upper tract positive urinary cytology, (5) surveillance of upper tracts after conservative treatment of a ureteral or renal pelvis tumor (6) surveillance of the juxtavesical ureters after intravesical therapy in the patient with a positive urinary cytology, and negative bladder and prostatic urethral biopsies, (7) differentiate between transitional cell and renal cell carcinoma in difficult cases, (8) help plan conservative surgical approach to tumors involving a solitary or ectopic kidney, (9) diagnosis and treatment of tumor recurrences after pyeloenterostomy (or ileal or colon conduit), (10) obtain tissue diagnosis of metastatic tumors to the upper collecting system (colon, cervix, breast, etc.), (11) facilitate safe and sure passage of an indwelling ureteral stent (and avoid open diversion or operation) in patients with neoplastic obstruction of the ureters, (12) provide access to the upper urinary tract for the delivery of topical therapeutic agents and (13) evaluate response of primary tumors to systemic or topical chemotherapy.

These are currently the common uses of ureteropyeloscopy at MSKCC. Other uses undoubtedly will become apparent as we gain experience, and is consistent with the trend toward conservative management of urothelial neoplams in general.

Techniques

Ureteropyeloscopy is performed in the operating room under general anesthesia. The initial step is cystoendoscopy and a bulb (occlusive) retrograde ureteropyelogram (may be omitted on repeat procedure if the anatomy is well-known to the operator). If a tumor(s) is found within the bladder, the ureteropyeloscopic procedure is postponed because of the potential risk of upper tract tumor seeding (may be more of a theoretical rather than a real risk). A retrograde study is done to document the course of the ureter and its distensibility and allows the endoscopist to anticipate any problems that may be encountered in passing the instrument owing to tortuosity or narrowing of the ureter.

The ureteral orifice and intramural ureter are then dilated to at least 13.5 French (F) using oliveshaped metal bougies passed over a previously placed guide-wire through an accommodating cystoscope sheath (23.5 or 25 F). Under direct vision, a 9.5 F. ureteropyeloscope with a 5 F working channel, is inserted into the ureter and passed to the level of the filling defect, obstruction, or renal pelvis if no lesion is identified. If a suspicious lesion is found, it is biopsied using flexible cup forceps and fulgurated, or preferably resected, using the 11 or 11.5 F ureteroresectoscope (working elements similar to the pediatric resectoscope). Care must be taken to maintain strict hemostasis and to retain the resected tissue within the loop and remove it from the ureteroscopic sheath after each bite inorder to avoid washing (and perhaps losing) the specimen proximally into the renal pelvis. Restricted operative space makes biopsy and resection of extensive tumor tedious, but which care, ample tumor tissue and ureteral muscle (important for staging) can be excised for thorough pathologic evaluation.

After resection or fulguration of a tumor(s), the entire urothelium is mapped visually and diagrammatically. In cases of tumor believed too extensive to completely resect, only biopsy is performed. However, if the tumor appears papillary and low-grade, complete removal with fulguration of the base is performed, the coagulation and cutting current being set to the effective minimum. Superficial and deep portions of the tumor are submitted separately for pathology. Tumor size, bleeding, reduced vision, low flow (1.16cc/sec, reduced to 0.60cc/sec with 4F catheter in channel) may prelude a complete and safe resection of some tumors. Similar to eradicating mutiple papillary bladder tumors, several operative procedures may be required inorder to completely control multifocal tumors within the upper collecting system.

Following the procedure, a ureteral catheter is left in place for 12–48 hours (unnecessary after diagnostic ureteropyeloscopy with fulguration and may be omitted if therapeutic manipulation has been minimal). Several additional urine samples are collected for cytology. Antibiotic prophylaxis is not routinely used. Patients are usually discharged one or two days after the procedure.

Complications

The ureteropyeloscopic procedure was unsuccessful in 5 patients (in over 150 procedures). This was due to an inability to dilate a normal-appearing orifice in two, to reach the renal pelvis in two (narrow, delicate ureter in one female patient, and a crossed-fused ectopic ureter draining a pelvic kidney in the other), and to negotiate a stenotic, previously-resected and tumor-involved ureteral orifice and intramural ureter in one (serial ureteropyeloscopies were accomplished successfully after distal ureterectomy and reimplant). We anticipate ureteropyeloscopy will be successful for diagnostic purposes in over 90% of patients, including those with tumor involvement, or after segmental ureterectomy (but in the latter case, subsequent examinations may prove difficult, or even impossible, with time).

We have had no serious complications of urosepsis, recognized perforation during the procedure or other problems requiring immediate operative intervention. Two patients experienced moderate lower abdominal and flank pain for 48 hours (ureteral catheters were not placed), associated with minor radiographic extravasation, after extensive endoscopic resection of ureteral tumors. Both recovered without incident (and without ureteral drainage) and have subsequently had ureteropyeloscopic procedures on several occasions with normal appearing mucosa. Delayed stricture or stenosis are potential long-term complications of ureteropyeloscopy.

The ureter and renal pelvis are remarkably forgiving, and with proper care, patience and respect, endoscopic manipulation and surgery in these areas can be accomplished safely

Results

We have now assessed and/or managed 43 patients with primary tumors of the upper urinary tract. Of these, 6 subsequently underwent nephroureterectomy, 4 had segmental ureterectomy, and 33 were managed by endoscopic resection and/or fulguration alone.

Patients who undergo open surgical resection after ureteropyeloscopic staging present an important opportunity to correlate T-category with P-catgegory and thus define the accuracy (and limits) of clinical staging of upper tract tumors. Table 1 shows our results. Of the 10 mapped nephroureterectomy or segmental ureterectomy specimens (over 130 slides of each specimen examined), 3 of 4 renal pelvic tumors were understaged (T < P) whereas an accurate stage (T = P) was made preoperatively in 5 of the 6 primary ureteral tumors. Extent of tumor within the renal pelvis, poor visualization and low flow of irrigating fluid, inability to biopsy base of the lesion or to gain access to tumors involving the lower pole calyx, collectively contributed to an often indequate endoscopic assessment of renal pelvis tumors. At the present time, we recommend primary endoscopic resection (in the patient with two kidneys) only of those renal pelvic tumors that are small (less than 2 cm), papillary, low-grade (negative urine cytology), non-invasive, located in an accessible extra renal pelvis, and associated with no other mucosal abnormalities on biopsy.

Of the 33 patients selected for primary endoscopic treatment, 30 had localized, low-grade appearing papillary tumors or focal flat high-grade carcinoma insitu of the ureter, and 3 patients had noninvasive papillary renal pelvic tumors. Following biopsy, these patients had ureteroscopic resection and/or fulguration. Endoscopic, cytologic and radiographic followup was done at 2–3 month intervals. Thus far, 71 surveillance procedures (one or more) have been done in 25 patients. With an average followup of 18 months, 16 recurrences have been biopsied, fulgurated or resected (2 had flat in situ carcinoma near the site of the original ureteral tumor). One patient died of a myocardial infarction (unrelated); the other 24 are alive with no apparent evidence of local or systemic disease. The longest patient available for followup has had 14 procedures over 75 months with local control of 6 recurrent tumors.

Clinico-pathologic features of upper collecting system tumors

It is necessary to consider this preliminary experience in light of the known natural history of upper tract tumors, although the information regarding recurrence rates and ureteropyelocalyceal urothelial polychronotopism after various surgical procedures is admittedly imcomplete. This is nonetheless important since a conservative endoscopic approach to such tumors requires: (1) knowledge of the probability of complete, reliable control of the primary tumor(s); (2) accessibility to the upper tract for regular surveillance; (3) prompt recognition, and treatment, of recurrent tumors prior to their dissemination.

Regarding upper collecting system tumors in general, clinical multicentricity is associated twice as often with papillary (30%) than nonpapillary (15%) tumors, increases with garde (21% for grade I to 37% for grade IV), and is more frequent with renal pelvic tumors (29%) than ureteral tumors (8%). 20 to 30% are benign (papilloma) or grade I papillary carcinoma [4]. Bilateral tumors are seen in 1–5% of patients.

Three features discourage routine conservative (kidney-sparing) management of renal pelvic and pyelocalyceal tumors: (1) in patients having nephrouretectomy for renal pelvic neoplasms, increased abnormalities are found in adjacent and remote urothelium as the stage and grade of the extant tumor increase. With a high-grade, infiltrating cancer, moderate to severe mucosal atypia occurs in 62%, unsuspected renal papillary carcinoma in 26% and multifocal carcinoma in situ in 26% [5]; (2) locoregional failures after open (conservative) surgical excision of renal pelvic tumors are high as shown in Table 2. Whether such 'recurrences' are the result of failure to control the primary tumor or to new tumor occurences is uncertain; (3) operative facility for complete excision of pyelocalyceal tumor(s),

Table 1. Correlation of clinical and pathological assessment of surgical specimens

Pt. No.	Ureteroscopy	Pathology	Tumor site
	(Nephroureterectomy)		
1.	Bx, G III, T2	G III, CIS	Pelvis/calyx*
2.	Bx, G III, T2	G III, P2	Pelvis
3.	Papilloma	G II, P2+CIS	Pelvis
4.	Papilloma, CIS	Papilloma, CIS	Pelvis
5.	Papilloma	Papilloma	Mid-ureter
6.	G II, T2	G III, P3	Mid-ureter
	(Segmental ureterectomy)		
1.	Papilloma	Papilloma	Distal ureter
2.	Pap Ca. – T1	T1	Distal ureter
3.	Papilloma	Inverted Papilloma	Distal ureter
4.	Pap Ca. – Ta	Ta	Distal ureter

accurate staging, adequate surveillance and control of recurrences is not always optimum when compared with ureteral tumors.

Small, papillary, low-grade and noninfiltrating tumor(s) arising in a renal pelvis that anatomically provides good access for resection and followup may be managed endoscopically. However, inability to fulfill the strict criteria for conservative management listed above, suggest that kidneysacrificing (nephroureterectomy) surgery may be prudent in the patient witha normal opposite kidney.

On the otherhand, multicentricitys much less frequent with tumors involving the distal one-third of the ureter. Survival and local urothelial recurrences are similar for distal ureteral tumors after nephroureterectomy versus segmental ureterectomy. Recurrence rates with conservative surgery increase progressively with higher locations of the primary tumor. This is consistent both with the concept that polychronotopism is more a centrifugal than a centripetal phenomenon and with the better accessibility of ureteral lesions than pelvocaliceal lesions to 'good' conservative treatment [8].

Surveillance of the juxtavesical ureters is becoming increasingly important in patients with multifocal carcinoma in situ (CIS) of the bladder treated conservatively since the risk of relapse involving the distal ureters may be as high as 35% (39/105 cystectomy patients with primary invasive bladder cancer plus diffuse bladder CIS had insitu carcinoma of the distal ureter). Moreover, of 66 patients with multifocal bladder CIS who achieved a complete response to topical BCG for more than one year, 15 (23%) had CIS detected in one or both distal ureters after 13–30 months (7 patients had distal ureterectomy and reimplant and 8 were treated by ureteroscopic resection and fulguration). These data suggest that regular ureteroscopic surveillance and treatment may be of value in patients at high risk forureteral polychronotopism. In the past one year, 24 patients with multifocal bladder CIS treated and sterilized with intravesical BCG had uretreroscopy on one [8] or more than one [16] occasion (14 patients had 'routine' examination and 10 were evaluated because of a positive urine cytology and negative bladder biopsy). Of the 14 'routine' ureteroscopies, ureteral CIS was found in only 1 (7%), whereas 3/10 (30%) clinically suspect patients had ureteral CIS. All were treated by biopsy and fulguration. Followup ureteroscopy (at 3 month intervals) has documented recurrent or persistent CIS in 4 patients (endo-

Table 2. Recurrences after local excision of renal pelvic tumors

Series	No.	Urothelial recurrences	Local pelvic failures
Mazeman [4]	23	15	8
Wallace [6]	7	4	3
Mayo [7]	17	12	10
Totals	47	31 (64%)	21 (42%)

scopically treated). This ongoing preliminary experience suggests routine ureteropyeloscopy in patient with CIS of the bladder responding to conservative management may be nonproductive, but it is of value in such patients with conversion of a negative to positive urine cytology, especially in the absence of documented recurrent CIS of the bladder or urethra.

Summary

The ureteropyeloscopic procedure in our hands has proved to be a safe and reliable technique. Endoscopic diagnosis and better presurgical staging appears to be the greatest advantage afforded by this method. Although followup is short, selected patients with localized, superficial and low-grade tumors may be amenable to ureteropyeloscopic treatment. The role of topical prohylactic or therapeutic chemotherapy or immunotherapy is yet to be determined. However, the ability to obtain routine access to the upper urinary tract makes this approach feasible. Endoscopic surveillance has been accomplished safely on a regular basis, even after segmental ureterectomy. Longitudinal studies of the results of this and other experiences will indicate the ultimate place of ureteropyeloscopy in the management of upper collecting system urothelial neoplasms.

References

1. Huffman JL, Bagley DH, Lyon ES: Extending cystoscopic techniques into the ureter and renal pelvis – experience with ureteroscopy and pyeloscopy. JAMA 250: 2002–2005, 1983
2. Perez-Castro EE, Martinez-Pineiro JA: Transurethral ureteroscopy – a current urlogical procedure. Arch Esp Urol 33: 445–460, 1980
3. Huffman JL, Morse MJ, Bagley DH, Herr HW, Lyon ES, Whitmore Jr WF: Endoscopic diagnosis and treatment of upper tract urothelial tumors – A preliminary report. Cancer 55: 1422–1428, 1985
4. Mazeman E: Les tumeurs de la voie excretrice urinaire superievre calices, bassinet, uretere. Association Francaise D'Urologie, Paris, 25–29, Sept 1972
5. McCarron JP, Mills C, Vaughan Jr ED: Tumors of the renal pelvis and ureter: Current concepts and management. Semina in Urol 1: 75–81, 1983
6. Wallace DMA, Wallace DM, Whitfield HN, Hendry WF, Wickham JEA: The late results of conservative surgery for upper tract urothelial carcinomas. Brit J Urol 53: 537–541, 1981
7. Zincke H, Neves RJ: Feasibility of conservative surgery for transitional cell cancer of the upper urinry tract. Urol Clin N Amer II: 717–724, 1984
8. Whitmore Jr WF: Management of urothelial tumors of the upper collectiny system. In: Urological Cancer, Skinner DG (ed). Grune and Stratton, New York 181–198, 1983

42

Editorial Comment

EDWARD S. LYON

The authors present an unusually clear, concise, and thorough assessment of the current state-of-the-art for the role of ureteroscopic procedures in upper tract urothelial neoplasia. Although much of urologist's expertise with urothelial disease in the bladder can be readily transposed to the upper urinary tract through ureteroscopic techniques there exist important differences brought out by the authors: the procedures are not 100%, one should avoid potential seeding of tumors, the effect of topical chemotherapy is yet to be evaluated, the techniques and studies are preliminary and evolving currently.

The one criticism I have of their report relates to their inference from two cases mentioned in the discussion of complications. The cases were managed without ureteral drainage catheters in the presence of ureteral extravasation after tumor resection. Both patients recovered satisfactorily and would be tallied as having only a minor complication. I feel it is necessary to drain the upper tract with an internal catheter for 48 hours when extravasation has been demonstrated in such a circumstance and impose that requirement on my own practice.

This excellent series is well under way and will be a major contribution to our basic understanding and management of disease most of us see infrequently. I greatly admire and value the authors objectivity and candor in their presentation of the material.

4. Growth factors in urology

STEPHEN C. JACOBS and MICHAEL T. STORY

Introduction

Growth factors are non-nutritive substances or hormones that regulate cell growth or cell proliferation, but do not take part in cell biosynthesis, metabolism or catabolism [1]. Hormones are similarly non-nutritive substances that travel through body fluids and produce their effect on cells distant from where they were synthesized. Many growth factors may prove to be hormones, but their in vivo function is not known yet. The growth factors are proteins produced by a cell which are capable of stimulating cell growth or cell division. When a growth factor stimulates cell division it is called a mitogen.

Most growth factors have been studied in cell culture systems. DNA synthesis in the target cells has been measured by the uptake of radiolabeled DNA precursors in response to exposure to the growth factor. A true mitogen will not only cause incorporation of radiolabeled nucleotides into DNA, but will also increase cell number. While the cell culture systems employed make isolation of growth factors much easier, they yield little information on the physiologic importance of the growth factors in the living organism.

Growth factors are manufactured by the protein synthesis machinery of the cell. They are then released and ultimately attach to a specific receptor on the cell membrane. If the growth factor producing cell is distant from the receiving cell, and travel through the bloodstream is involved in getting the growth factor to its target, then the process is referred to as endocrine. If the growth factor travels only a short distance to an adjacent cell, then the process is called paracrine. If the growth factor producing cell is also the receptor containing cell, the stimulation is said to be autocrine [2].

There are numerous known or suspected growth factors. Many of these may prove to be the same or to belong to the same class of growth factors after further characterization. Table 1 lists some of the better characterized growth factors and cites review articles where more information about the growth factors may be obtained.

Ratliff, T.L. and Catalona, W.J. (eds), Genitourinary Cancer. ISBN 0–89838–830–9
© *1987, Martinus Nijhoff Publishers, Boston. Printed in the Netherlands.*

This review will emphasize growth factors and oncogene products that have largely contributed to our current understanding of how extracellular signals regulate cell division. We have used examples from urologic studies where sufficient information has accumlated in hopes of appealing to the reader in this speciality of medicine.

EGF as a model

We would to like to describe briefly epidermal growth factor (EGF), the best characterized of the growth factors, in order that a model may be established to compare to less well studied growth factors such as prostatic growth factors.

EGF was first isolated from the mouse submaxillary gland by Stanley Cohen in 1962 [22]. Since then, numerous papers concerning EGF have been published. These studies have provided the frame work for understanding how extracellular signals regulate cellular events.

EGF is a 53 amino acid single polypeptide chain with a molecular weight of 6045. The protein has three intramolecular disulfide linkages that are essential for biological activity. The tertiary structure of the protein is very stable to acid and boiling [5].

In homogenates of the submaxillary gland prepared at neutral pH, EGF is found as a component of a higher molecular weight complex. The complex has a molecular weight of 74,000 and is composed of two molecules of EGF and two molecules of binding protein. The binding protein has arginime specific peptidase activity. Frey et al [23] have isolated a precursor of EGF with a molecular weight of 9,000. This pre-EGF is converted to EGF by the esteropeptidase found in the high molecular weight EGF complex. Interestingly, mRNA encoding the precur-

Table 1. Some of the better characterized growth factors

Growth factor	References
EGF/Urogastrone, epidermal growth factor	3–6
TGF, Transforming growth factor, at least 3 types described	2,7–9
FGF, Fibroblast growth factor, basic and acetic forms described	10,11
NGF, Nerve growth factor	12–14
PDGF, Platelet-derived growth factor	15,16
Somatomedin, a class of growth hormone-dependent proteins	17–18
Hemopoietic colony stimulating factors, at least 5 types described	19,20
PrGF, Prostate growth factor, possibly a member of the heparin-binding growth factors	21

sor to mouse submaxillary gland EGF is unexpectively large. It consist of 4750 nucleotide bases and predicts the sequence of prepro EGF, a protein of 1217 amino acids with a molecular weight of 133,000. The amino terminal segment of 976 amino acids contains seven peptides with sequences that are similar, but not identical to EGF. The sequence of the EGF-binding protein is not contained in the prepro EGF sequence. Thus, the function of much of the molecule remains to be determined [24].

A human counterpart of mouse EGF (mEGF) was isolated from urine by Gregory [25]. The peptide is very similar, but not identical to mEGF with respect to its physical and chemical properties. Of the 53 amino acid residues comprising each of the two polypeptides, 37 are common to both molecules, and the three disulfide bonds occur in the same relative positions. Sixteen variable residues occur at intervals along the polypeptide chain, of these, 14 could result from single base changes in the triplet code and most of the changes are conservative replacements. Furthermore, human EGF (hEGF) and mEGF elicit nearly identical biological responses. Human EGF occurs in various fluids as follows: urine, 100 ng/ml; milk, 80 ng/ml; plasma, 2 ng/ml; saliva, 12 ng/ml; aminotic fluid 1/ng/ml. The quantities of hEGF in tissues are exceedingly low compared to the daily urinary excretion of the growth factor (50–60 µg) [3].

Unlike the mouse submaxillary gland where one can obtain up to 1.0 g of EGF/gram of tissue, the human submaxillary gland contains only 1 to 2 ng of EGF per gram of tissue. Interestingly, EGF appears to be present in much higher levels in rat and guinea pig prostate than in human prostatic tissue [26–28].

EGF is synthesized in the mouse submaxillary gland and stored in secretory granules in the tubular cells. The production of EGF is under androgen control. Adult male mice have about 1 µ g/mg tissue compared to 70 ng/mg tissue in the female. Castration reduces the level of EGF ten-fold and testosterone-treated females have EGF levels that are comparable to these in intact males.

Release of EGF into the bloodstream and particularly into the saliva is under alpha adrenergic control [29].

The number of biologic activities of EGF is widely varied. EGF enhances epidermal growth and keratinization by increasing mitosis in the basal epidermal cells [30]. In the corneal epithelum EGF causes hyperplasia and speeds wound healing [31]. In the GI tract EGF accelerates healing of experimentally induced ulcers and reduces gastric acid secretion [32]. All responses to EGF in the intact animal appear to be limited to epithelial cells.

The regulation of cell proliferation by EGF has been extensively studied using cultured human foreskin fibroblasts as a model system. These cells are considered 'normal' as they maintain a diploid chromosome number and their growth is well regulated by mechanisms such as density-dependent inhibition of growth, a high serum requirement, and anchorage-dependent growth. Cells grown in the continuous presence of EGF (ng quantities) continue to proliferate when the culture becomes confluent, forming a multilayered cell population, and reaching population densities four-to-six fold higher than the controls. Also, when fibroplasts are incubated in media containing low serum (1%), cell proliferation in normally restricted, but supplementation of these media with EGF yields cell growth equal to that obtained in the presence of optimal serum concentrations (10%) [33]. The apparent loss of sensitivity to these growth-regulating mechanisms by cells cultured in the presence of EGF bears some resemblance to the behaviour of 'transformed' cells *in vitro*. Transformed cells are frequently characterized by their insensitivity to normal growth-controlling mechanisms. Transformed cells in culture are heteroploid, are not contact inhibited, have a lower serum requirement for growth, and exhibit anchorage-idenpendent growth. Thus, EGF, while not transforming cells, does have the effect, under cell culture conditions, of creating an imbalance of homeostatic signals favoring cell proliferation.

Cell replication is the end result of a complex series of biochemical and morphologic events following exposure to growth factors. These events outlined in Table 2 are similar regardless of the cell type or the mitogenic agents.

In order for cells to respond to EGF, cell surface receptors must be present. A single fibroplast cell has 40,000 to 100,000 high affinity (10^{-9} to 10^{-10}M) binding sites for EGF on its surface.

The membrane receptor for EGF plays a key role in the transduction

Table 2. Components of the mitogenic response

Event	Time
1. Biological response at the membrane	minutes
a) Binding to receptor	
b) Receptor phosphorylation (Tyr specific)	
c) Phosphorylation of other proteins	
d) Increased transport amino acids, sugar, ions, polyamines	
2. Responses in the cytoplasm	2–12 hours
a) Activation of glycolysis	
b) Synthesis of extracellular macromolecules (glycosaminoglycans, hyaluronic acid)	
c) Activation of RNA, protein synthesis	
d) Activation of ornithine decarboxylase	
3. Nuclear events	
a) Stimulation of DNA synthesis	12 hours
b) Mitosis	24 hours

of the signals mediated by EGF leading to cell proliferation. Monoclonal antibody has been produced against the EGF receptor. In some cases, antibody blocks the binding of EGF to EGF receptors. It also induces EGF-like activity: the phosphorylation of membrane proteins, activation of ornithine decarboxylase, and the stimulation of DNA synthesis and cell division [34]. These findings support the notion that the EGF receptor, rather than EGF itself, is the active moiety and that the role of the growth factor is to perturb the receptor which then stimulates the many cellular responses.

Carpenter, Cohen and co-workers discovered that EGF induces a rapid, cyclic nucleotide-independent and tyrosine-specific phosphorylation of a number of membrane proteins when added to purified plasma membranes from human epidermoid carcinoma cells (A-431). Several proteins of molecular weights corresponding to 170,000, 150,000, 80,000 and 22,000 are phosphorylated. The major phosphorylated proteins with molecular weight of 170,000 to 150,000 daltons were identified as EGF receptor. Both ATP and GTP can act as the phosphate donor of the phosphorylation reaction and either Mn^{+2} or Mg^{+2} is required for optimal activity of the protein kinase. The kinase activity is copurified with EGF-binding activity by EGF affinity-chromatography. This finding together with the fact that the phosphorylation is very rapid, even at $0°C$, suggests a close proximity between the receptor and the kinase. In fact, Cohen provided strong evidence that the protein kinase is an integral part of EGF receptor by photoaffinity label of an ATP binding on the receptor molecule [35].

In the past year, complementary DNA (cDNA) to the EGF receptor mRNA has been cloned [36]. From the amino acid sequence, predicted from the nucleotide sequence of cDNA clones covering the entire coding region, the following picture of the EGF receptor has emerged. A signal peptide of 24 amino acids is cleaved from a precursor molecule to yield a mature protein of 1,186 amino acids. The receptor can be divided into an amino-terminal EGF-binding domain of 621 amino acids, a 26 hydophobic amino acid membrane spanning domain, and a c-terminal domain of 542 amino acids having the protein kinase catalytic activity. The c-terminal region also shows considerable homology to the catalytic domains of other protein kinases, and as will be discussed is homologous with the acute transforming virus, erb B, oncogene product. The final 240 amino acids at the c-terminas shows no homology with known proteins.

Following binding of EGF to its receptor the growth factor-receptor complex is internalized within 10–30 minutes. EGF is eventually degraded by the lysosomal enzymes and new receptors are manufacturated or old receptors are released in a process that requires new protein synthesis.

EGF induces many cellular changes by interacting with its receptor. An increase in ruffling of the cell membrane and extension of filipodia on the surface is seen within minutes of exposure to EGF. Fluid phase pinocytosis is enhanced leading to increased cellular uptake of a number of substances: active transport of ions and nutrients occurs rapidly.

In contrast to these rapid changes that require only a small content of EGF, stimulation of DNA synthesis requires 6–12 hours of a relatively high dose of EGF exposure. If 25% of EGF receptors are bound, then enhanced DNA synthesis will occur at 12 hours. EGF stimulates glycolysis, the synthesis of protein and glycoprotein, and the activation of the enzyme ornithine decarboxylase [37].

Although much has been learned from studies of EGF, it is as yet not possible to explain the biochemical basis by which growth factors regulate cellular processes.

Transforming growth factors

Transforming growth factors (TGFs) are a class of polypeptides of MW 5,000–20,000. Physiochemically they are acid stable and contain disulfide bonds important to their biologic activity. TGFs are secreted by transformed cells; these cells have lost the requirement that growth be controlled by hormones and growth factors. Malignant cells or virally infected cells are examples of transformed cells that have escaped from normal growth controls and do not seem the require the same amounts of growth factors and hormones to proliferate. TGFs appear to be secreted by the transformed cell and they act on the same cell and its neighbors. Thus, if the producing cell also has TGF receptors the secretion of TGF produces an autocrine stimulation [38]. TGF may also affect neighboring cells with TGF receptor resulting in paracrine regulation. TGF s stimulate mitogenesis and cause anchorage independent growth of cells; a property in cell structure that correlates best with tumorigenicity *in vivo* [39]. One type of TGF, called α- or type 1 TGF, completes for EGF receptor binding [38]. Transformed cells that produce α-TGF have a diminished number of EGF receptors compared to their nontransformed counterpart. Fewer available receptors appears to result from internalization of the growth factor-receptor-complex leaving fewer receptors on the cell surface; a phenomenon known as receptor down regulation.

The amino acid sequence of rat α-TGF is a single-chain polypeptide consisting of 50 amino acids and has a molecular weight of 5616. The protein shows 33 and 44% sequence homology with mEGF and hEGF, respectively. Like EGF, rat α-TGF has 3 intramolecular disulfide bridges which would lie in the same location as those in EGF except for a single amino acid deletion. The sequence for this α-TGF is not coded for in the prepro-EGF transcript previously described for mEGF.

Bladder cancer cells produce TGFs. Messing et al [41] found >5,000 MW TGF produced by human transitional cell carcinoma cell line 647V that stimulated mitosis when applied to the same 647V cells. They not only demonstrated that autocrine secretion and stimulation was operative in these cells, but also demonstrated that the secreted TGF transformed normal rat renal fibroblasts to grow in an anchorage-independent fashion.

The TGF from bladder carcinoma cell line 647V did not compete with EGF for EGF receptors on the bladder cancer cell surfaces. EGF, however, was capable of stimulating normal rat bladder cells and bladder tumor cell lines that had EGF receptors. Neal et al [42] have reported that bladder cancers that are invasive are more likely to have EGF receptors than non-invasive bladder tumors and that normal transitional epithelium does not contain EGF receptors.

Lin and Fay [43] looked at three TGFs produced by bladder cancer cell line MGF-U1. They found a MW 30,000 peak that transformed kidney cells in culture and two smaller TGFs (MW 15,000 and 9,000) that competed with EGF. The three TGFs when added together were synergistic in producing transformation.

Prostatic growth factor

Two areas of prostatic research show promise for investigation of the role of a prostatic tissue growth factor. In both the area of prostatic cancer metastases and the area of BPH, protein growth factors may be important in the genesis of the disease state.

Osteoblastic metastases

Human prostatic cancer is unique in that it is the only cancer that consistently produces osteoblastic metastases in bone. Greater than 90% of bone lesions due to prostatic cancer are osteoblastic, rather than osteolytic. Breast cancer is the second most common cancer to induce osteoblastic metastases, but does so only 8% of the time. The malignant prostatic epithelial cells spread to the red marrow spaces of cancellous bone. New bone formation then follows surrounding the nests of malignant prostatic cells (Fig. 1). Osteoblasts become more numerous on the trabecular surfaces. New bone is layed down by the osteoblasts in the vicinity of the malignant prostatic cells. In normal bone remodeling, osteoclastic bone resorption must precede osteoblast activity. In the juxta-metastatic modeling of prostatic cancer, osteoclastic resorption does not preceed osteoblastic differentiation. Using histomorphometric analysis of bone metastases, Charhon et al [44] concluded that a local trophic factor released by the cancer cells could be responsible for the histologic picture.

In 1979 we reported our first growth factor experiments involving prostatic tissue [45]. We found that tissue extracts of prostatic tissue, normal and benign or malignant, stimulated mitogenesis in fetal rat calvarial-derived osteoblasts. The osteoblasts responded to the prostatic tissue extracts in a dose dependent and time dependent fashion. While the osteoblasts stimulated mitogenesis maximally at 24 hours, protein synthesis was only modestly stimulated [46].

Cultured osteoblasts still produced primarily Type I collagen (unpublished

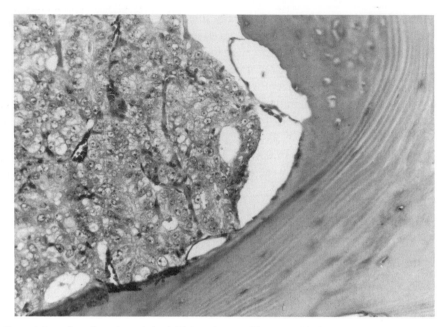

Figure 1. Lamellae of new bone being laid down by osteoblasts possibily in response to a local trophic growth factor being produced by malignant prostatic epithelial cells within the marrow space.

observations), the basis for *in vivo* new bone matrix. In the prostatic cancer patient, the new bone matrix avidly binds calcium leading to low serum calcium and phosphorus. Secondary hyperparathyroidism and increased 1,25 $(OH)_2$ vitamin D levels follow and patients develop osteomalacia in the uninvolved bones as well as the osteoblastic changes aound the prostatic cancer metastases [47]. Once the growth factor is purified, it will be important to determine if the factor can mimic *in vitro* the response of bone to prostatic metastases.

Benign prostatic hyperplasia

The genesis of BPH in man and the dog has been a very perplexing problem to generations of researchers. It is accepted that androgens are required to maintain growth and morphology of the epithelial cells of the normal prostate, but the role of steroids in the genesis of prostatic hyperplasia is not established.

In the developing prostate Cunha et al [48, 49] have shown there is an interaction between the mesenchymal or stromal portions of the prostate gland and the epithelial cells that will line the ducts and acini. In development of the prostate the stroma appears to dictate to the epithelium to differentiate into prostatic epithelium. Furthermore, quiescent adult prostatic epithelium can be induced to proliferate again by embryonic urogenital sinus mesenchyme.

Bartsch has done extensive stereological analyses of BPH and shown that there is a significant increase in the fibrostromal volume over the glandular volume when compared to the normal gland of the young adult male [50, 51]. Many researchers have suggested that the BPH may begin as fibrostromal nodules which then induce the ingrowth of adjacent epithelial elements [52–55]. McNeal has described a transition zone in the prostate from which he believes BPH begins and suggests that a local stromal inductive effect may account for early fibrostromal nodule formation. He further states that the histogenesis involves three distinct processes: early diffuse gland growth, small nodule proliferation, and later nodule enlargement [56].

Paracrine secretion of PrGF as a possible model for the etiology of BPH

In our laboratory in collaboration with Dr. Russell Lawson, we have identified and partially purified a growth factor from BPH tissue that we have termed prostatic growth factor (PrGF). This growth factor stimulates a number of different cells in culture to divide.

Tackett et al [57] found that mitogenic activity was present in human prostatic secretions. While they found several large MW fractions in BPH tissue, they found a 30,000 daltons MW species in prostatic secretions that stimulated ^{3}H-thymidine incorporation by 3T3 fibroblasts. These studies markedly strengthen the concept that PrGF is produced by the epithelial cells of the prostate and is secreted into the prostatic fluid. Lawson et al [58] separated BPH into acinar-enriched and stromal-enriched homogenates. Acinar-enriched preparations demonstrated more PrGF activity than stromal-enriched preparations. This points again to the prostatic epithelial cell as the source of PrGF.

The stromal cells may well be the responding target cell for PrGF in BPH. Lawson et al [58] also grew prostatic fibroblasts in culture and found that PrGF from the same prostate gland stimulated mitogenesis in these prostatic fibroblasts. Furthermore, prostate did not respond to PrGF as well as BPH derived prostatic fibroblasts, suggesting that there may be a change in the stromal fibroblasts with aging.

At the recent NIADDK symposium on BPH, Maxhinney [59] suggested that stroma and collagen were very important in the genesis of BPH, but that they may be stimulated by prostatic fluid growth factors. Figure 2 illustrates a theoretical model for what might be happening in the development of BPH (Fig. 2).

The bioassay for PrGF employs newborn human foreskin fibroblasts as the test cell culture system [21]. These foreskin fibroblasts are grown in culture medium with 10% newborn calf serum and, then, nutritionally downshifted for 24 hours to only 0.5% newborn calf serum. These conditions are throught to inhibit cell growth in the G_0 phase of the cell cycle [60]. Test samples of growth factor are then applied to the quiescent cells and their uptake of ^{3}H-thymidine is measured

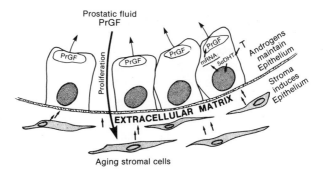

Figure 2. Possible Model for Genesis of BPH
Prostatic stroma induces growth and differentiation of prostatic epthelium. Testosterone maintains growth and protein synthesis by epithelial cells. PrGF is secreted into acinar lumen probably under autonomic nervous system control. Some PrGF enters the extracellular matrix where it stimulates mitogenesis by aging stromal cells. The fibrostromal nodule begins and induces ingrowth of more epithelial cells.

after 24 hours. The stimulation of ^{3}H-thymidine uptake as a measure of DNA synthesis is compared to a standard, the stimulation caused by the addition of 10% serum. One unit is defined as the amount of the growth factor that gives a response equal to 10% serum.

PrGF stimulates a number of cell types to undergo mitosis. Besides human foreskin fibroblasts, other responding cells include rat calvarial osteoblasts, rat shin fibroblasts, and fibroblastic cell lines BUD 8 and 3T3. The stimulation of ^{3}H-thymidine incorporations by fibroblasts is detectable by 12 hours, reaches a peak at 18–24 hours, and disappears by 36 hours after the addition of PrGF [45, 46]. Autoradiographic studies have shown that PrGF causes a 15 fold increase in labeled mitoses 36 hours after addition [61]. The enhanced mitotic activity observed at 36 hours is consistent with the increase in ^{3}H-thymidine incorporation occuring at 18–30 hours and is indicative of cells completing S phase and traversing G2 before entering Mitosis. By 65 hours after exposure to PrGF 100% of fibroblast nuclei are labeled, compared to only 33% of control culture nuclei. PrGF causes a 194% increase in absolute cell number. Furthermore, cell protein increases 152% if exposed to PrGF for 3 days. These studies indicate that nearly the entire confluent fibroblast population participates in the proliferate process as a result of stimulation by PrGF.

Isolation and physiochemical characteristics of prostatic growth factor

Homogenization
BPH tissue was obtained at open prostatectomy or by transurethral resection

(TURP). The tissue was stored at $-80c$ prior to use. Pathology was performed on all speciemens to confirm BPH, but it cannot be ruled out that specimens were entirely free of prostatitis or carcinoma. All steps in preparing homogenates and isolating PrGF were at 0–4C. The tissue was rinsed in saline and cut into small cubes. The pieces of tissue were homogenized in an equal volume of homogenization buffer. When tissue obtained at open prostatectomy was homogenized in high ionic strenght buffer, 3 to 6 times more activity was recovered per gram of tissue. Tissue obtained by TURP has also been used as a source of the growth factor. However, extracts prepared from TURP specimens yielded fewer units of growth factor than did extracts prepared from glands obtained by the open procedure as shown in Table 3.

Lipid extraction of BPH extracts
To determine if the growth factor activity in BPH extract was due to a component in the lipid fraction, preparations were extracted with ether (not shown) or dichloromethane (Table 4). PrGF was recovered in the aqueous phase. Lipid affiliated protein was removed without affecting growth factor activity.

The BPH extract was mixed with an equal volume of dichloromethane in a selratory funnel. After phase separation, the aqueous phase was extracted a second time. The aqueous phase was centrifuged and a portion of the supernatant was dialyzed vs. Tris buffer (0.05M Tris, 0.05M NaCl, pH 7.6) and tested for growth factor activity.

Ammonium sulfate precipitation and concentration
An average of 56.4% (range 52–64%, $n=5$) of the growth factor in BPH extracts was precipitated between 33 and 67% saturation with ammonium sulfate, pH 7.6.

Table 3. Growth factor activity of BPH homogenates prepared in low and high ionic strenght buffer

Source of BPH tissue	Extraction condition	Units/mg of protein	Units/gr net weigth of tissue
Open Prostatectomy[a]	Low ionic strenght[c]	20 (10–47)	420 (300–890)
Open Prostatectomy[a]	High ionic strength[d]	143 (112–165)	2949 2758–3086)
TURP[b]	Low ionic strength[c]	32	458
TURP[b]	High ionic strength[d]	96	927

[a] Four pools of at least 100 g of BPH tissue per pool
[b] Pool of 116 gr of TURP tissue
[c] Tris 0.05 M with o.05 M NaCl, pH 7.6 (Tris buffer)
[d] Tris 0.05 M with 1.55 M NaCl, pH 7.6 with EDTA (10 mM), Phenylmethylsulfonyl fluoride (1 mM), L-1-tosylamide-2-phenylethyl-chloromethyl ketone (0.03 mM), ethylamalemide (0.05 mM), soybean trypsin inhibitor (10 mg/1), (TSI buffer)

The specific activity of precipitates was increased by only about 2-fold. Eighteen precent of the PrGF was recovered at 33% ammonium sulfate and 8% remained in the supernatant at 67% ammonium sulfate.

Influence of heat, acid, pH, and dissociating agents
The stability of crude (138 units/mg) and highly purified PrGF (236, 250 units/mg) was compared at 56C and 100C. The crude preparation retained full activity after 40 min at 56C but lost 90% activity when boiled for 5 min. Highly purified PrGF lost 60% activity after 40 min at 56C and all activity when boiled for 5 min. This confirmed earlier observations that PrGF was heat labile [45] and suggested that the activity in crude preparations was partially protected by other proteins.

The activity of crude extracts of BPH was irreversibly inactivated at acid pH. Reducing the pH from 7.3 to 4.6 decreased activity by 30–40% and at pH 1.5 only about 20% of activity remained. Highly purified PrGF (236,250 units/mg) was even more susceptible to acid denaturation. An 80–85% loss in activity was seen at pH 4.6 and no activity could be found in preparation brought to pH 2.5. On the other hand, growth factor activity appeared stable in alkaline solutions (pH 8.8).

More than 50% of the growth factor activity was lost after dialyses with 6M urea or 6M guanidine-HC1, pH.6. Growth factor activity was recovered after exposure to 2-mercaptoethanol, but was lost in the presence of the reducing agent and 1% sodium dodecyl sulfate.

Fractionation of BPH homogenates
PrGF has been subjected to a variety of fractionation techniques. The details of this work have been published [21] so only a summary of our findings are described in this section. All of these studies used BPH homogenates that had been precipitated with ammonium sulfate between 33 and 67% saturation as starting material.

Table 4. Dichloromethane extraction of crude BPH homogenates

Study no.	Unextracted		Extracted	
	Protein (mg/ml)	Activity (units/mg)	Protein (mg/ml)	Activity (units/mg)
1	4.5	28	1.9	55
2	7.5	152	6.3	353
3	7.5	165	6.3	295
4	10.4	112	5.6	144

Gel filtration chromatography. The elution position of growth factor activity from gel filtration columns was markedly different when performed in low *vs.* high ionic strength buffers. In low ionic strength solution the activity was distributed in the MW region ranging from 17,000 to 100,000. Over 70% of the activity was in fractions eluting with an apparent MW of >67,000. When fractionated in high ionic strength buffer the predominant growth factor was found at MW 17,000 [12]. The different behaviors of PrGF in low and high ionic strength solutions is most likely a result of growth factor interaction with other proteins. Low ionic strength conditions are known to promote protein-protein interaction.

A number of other growth factors are known to interact with proteins in a manner resembling PrGF. Endothelium-derived growth factor behaves like a protein with a MW > 150,000 in 25 mM Tris or in isotonic phosphate buffer. When exposed to detergent or high concentrates of chaotropic ions the growth factor activity was predominantly found in 14,000 to 24,000 MW fractions. Platelet-derived growth factor exhibited similar gel filtration properties. This growth factor acitivity was distributed in several MW regions ranging from 10,000 to >100,000 in borate buffer. However, gel filtration in 6M guanidine-HCl produced a more discrete active fraction corresponding to a MW of 12,000 to 24,000 [62, 63]. Since PrGF was inactivated by 6M guanidine or 6M urea, it was necessary to use buffers of neutral to alkaline pH containing high concentrations of salt to achieve dissociation of PrGF from other proteins and to discourage self aggregation. Other growth factors such as epidermal growth factor (EGF), multiplication-stimulating activity, and nerve growth factor are known to possess specific carrier proteins of considerably larger MW than the active growth factor [64–66]. It has not been determined if a specific binding protein exists for PrGF.

Ion exchange chromatography. In low ionic strength buffer about 50% of the protein and 80% of the activity bound to DEAE-cellulose [21]. The activity was recovered by increasing the ionic strength to 0.35M NaCl. About 20% of the activity did not bind to the anion-exchanger under these conditions. Subsequent studies showed that the activity that did not bind to DEAE eluted as a large MW component on gel filtration chromatography in high ionic strength buffer (unpublished observations)

Con A-Sepharose chromatography. Growth factor did not bind to Con A suggesting that PrGF is not a member of the class of glycoproteins that bind to this lectin.

Preparative electrofocusing
The predominate activity electrofocused between pH 4.7 and 5.3. Only 15% of the applied activity was recovered from the gel; presumably due to inactivation

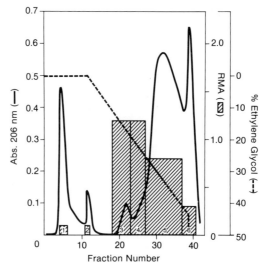

Figure 3. Phenyl-Sepharose adsorption chromatography
Ammonium sulfate precipitated BPH extract was brought to 30% ammonium sulfate in Tris with 1.55M NaCl, pH 7.6 (TS buffer). After centrifugation the sample was run over a 1.6 × 15 cm column of Phenyl-Sepharose equilibrated with 30% ammonium sulfate in TS buffer. After washing the column of unbound material, a linear gradient (formed from starting buffer and Tris buffer with 50% ethylene glycol was started to elute bound material. Fractions were pooled and concentrated as indicated by the bars, dialyzed and tested for growth factor activity.

of growth factor at acid pH. As electrofocusing was conducted in low ionic strength solution, it is possible that the PI of purified PrGF may significantly differ from the observed value.

Hydrophobic chromatography
Growth factor in 0.05M Tris with 0.05M or 1.55M NaCl, pH 7.6, does not bind the phenyl-Sepharose (Pharmacia) or octyl-Sepharose (not shown). However, if the sample was brought to 30% ammonium sulfate, activity bound to the adsorbents. About 65% of the activity applied to a column of phenyl-Sepharose was recovered in fractions 3 and 4 following elution with a 0 to 50% ethylene glycol gradient (Fig. 3). PrGF appears therefore to be weakly hydrophobic.

Isolation scheme

Steps:
1. Homogenization in high ionic strength buffer with protease inhibitors.
2. Dichloromethane extraction (aqueous phase).
3. Ammonium sulfate precipitation, 30% saturation (supernatant).
4. Phenyl-Sepharose (gradient elution with ethylene glycol).

5. Ultrafiltration.
6. G-75, low ionic strength buffer.
7. DEAE (elution with high ionic strength buffer).
8. Ultrafiltration.
9. fdG-75, high ionic strength buffer.
10. Con A-Sepharose (unbound fraction).
11. Ultrafiltration.
12. P-150, high ionic strength buffer.
13. Ultrafiltration.

The isolation scheme has been used to partially purify PrGF from three different pools of BPH tissue (Table 5).

Purity of a >200,000 units/mg preparation was assessed by SDS-PAGE under reduced conditions (Fig. 4). Silver staining bands with apparent molecular weights (X 10-3) of 24.8, 21.2, 16.6, 14.6, 13.1, and 11.2 were observed. If was not possible to determine which band(s) was PrGF as the conditions used to prepare the sample inactivates the growth factor.

The recovery of PrGF (1 to 14%) may appear low, but compares favorably with a 6% yield reported for PDGF [67] and a recovery of 3–5% originally reported for human EGF [68]. It should also be noted that the biological activity of the starting material, on which the calculation of recovery was based, included a large MW component(s) that was not dissociated into the 17,000 MW growth factor and consequently was not isolated by this procedure. Recently, we have found that the growth factor binds to heparin-Sepharose (Pharmacia) and such fractionation as an early step may well speed the purification and increase the recovery of PrGF.

Table 6 compares the properties of PrGF and some of the better characterized growth factors. It is apparent that PrGF differs from EGF, TGF's, FGF (basic form), PDGF, somatomedin (SM-C), and NGF, but appears similar to endothelial cell growth factor (ECGF) and seminiferous growth factor (SGF) which is described on page 62.

Table 5. Application of the isolation scheme to three BPH preparations

Study No.	Gr of BPH tissue	Fold increase in activity	Final Growth factor activity (units/mg)	Percent recovery
1	103	1400	236,250 (4ng = 1 unit)	1
2	101	1000	55,143 (18ng = 1 unit)	6
3	100	500	55,000 (18ng = 1 unit)	14

Table 6. Properties of PrGF and some other growth factors

Properties	Growth factors									
	EGF	TGF2	TGF B	FGF[a]	PDGF	SM-C	NGF	ECGF	SGF	PrGF
Prostate location	+[b]	NR	NR	NR	NR	NR	+[c]	NR	NR	+
Carrier protein	+	−	−	−	+[d]	+	+	NR	NR	NR
MW ($\times 10^{-3}$)	6	5.6	25	16	28–31	7.6	26	18.5, 19.3	15.7	17
PI	4.6	Neutral	Neutral	9.6	9.8–10.2	8.2–8.4	9.3–10	5.2	4.5–5.5	4.7–5.3
Number of peptides	1	1	2	1	2	1	2	1	1	1
Stable to:										
Heat	+	+	+	−	+	−	−	−	−	−
Acid	+	+	+	−	+	+	+	−	−	−
Urea	+	+	NR	NR	+	NR	+	NR	−	−
Reduction	−	−	NR	−	−	−	+	NR	+	+
Hydrophobicity	NR	NR	NR	NR	NR	NR	NR	NR	Low	Low
Heparin binding	−	NR	NR	+	+[e]	NR	NR	+	NR	+

[a] bovine pituitary
[b] rat, guinea pig
[c] several species, not human
[d] α-2-macroglobulin
[e] low affinity cationic exchange property

NR, not reported

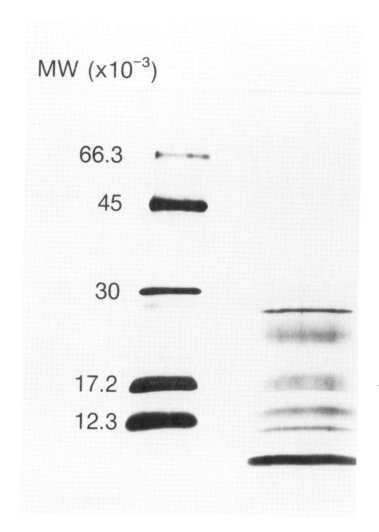

Figure 4. Reduced SDS-PAGE of PrGF (>200,000 U/mg)
One μg of PrGF (t200,000 u/mg) was applied to a SDS-PAGE gradient gel (10 to 22.5% acrylamide) using Laemmli buffers. Molecular weight markers were applied to an adjacent lane. Electrophoresis was performed in a vertical slab gel apparatus (LKB) at constant current. The gel was silver stained to visualize proteins.

Species variations of PrGF

Our laboratory has identified PrGF activity in homogenates of prostatic tissue from the human, gorilla, dog, and rat. There are differences between the human, dog, and rat in the PrGF activity on gel filtration chromatography (Fig. 5).

In human prostatic homogenates, as indicated above, the growth factor elutes in high molecular weight fractions when chromatographed in low ionic strength solutions. In contrast the growth factor activity in dog prostate elutes as two

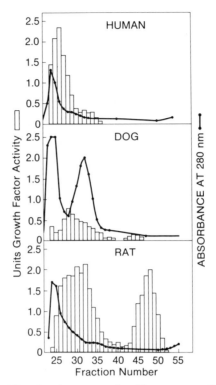

Figure 5. Sephadex G-75 gel filtration chromatography of homogenates of human fog, and rat ventral prostate.

intermediate molecular weight species of approximately 40,000 and 20,000 daltons. The amount of growth factor activity per weight of the prostate appears to be lower in the dog than in human or rat prostates.

The growth factor activity of homogenates of rat ventral prostate also elutes from the gel filtration as two distinct species. Further studies showed that the lower molecular weight species, approximately 6,000, is probably EGF [27]. This conclusion was based on the observaton that it competed with mEGF binding to fibroblast receptor and for antiserum to mEGF and is both heat and acid stable.

By exposing crude rat ventral prostate homogenates to 100°C it was determined that approximately one half of the growth factor activity in the rat ventral prostate is due to EGF. The larger MW growth factor is about 58,000 daltons and is heat labile.

Rat PrGF appears to be a product of the prostatic epithelial cell and is present in prostatic fluid. Several tumors of the rat prostate are derived from the prostatic epithelial cell. Heston et al [69] found, and we have confirmed, growth factor activity in homogenates of the Dunning R2237 tumor in the Copenhagen rat. We have also found activity in both androgen dependent and androgen independent forms of the Nb tumor carried in the Nb rat [70].

We instituted studies to determine the androgen dependence of the growth factors in the rat prostate [27]. There were no differences seen in the levels of growth factor activity in prostatic homogenates from rats 3, 6, or 12 months of age. Orchiectomy produced a marked decrease in the weight of the rat ventral prostate over the course of 10 days. In parallel to this decrease, growth factor activity and tissue acid phosphatase levels also decreased. Testosterone replacement maintained prostatic weight, growth factor activity, and tissue acid phosphatase levels. The differentiated secretory epithelial cells of the rat ventral prostate are androgen dependent. The proteins produced by these differentiated secretory epithelial cells are, thus, also androgen dependent. After castrate induced prostatic involution, restoration of the proteins produced by prostatic epithelial cells occurs with exogenous testosterone administration. Androgens can have a specific effect on some protein produces of prostatic cells, causing a more rapid decrease with androgen removal or rise with androgen restoration when compared to total prostatic weight [71]. However, tissue growth factor activity in the rat appears to be affected by the total decrease in prostatic weight and cellular metabolism rather than by specific androgen dependence.

Future directions in the study of PrGF

Prostatic epithelial cells secrete protein growth factors. The rat prostate produces both EGF and a second growth factor that shares several properties with the growth factor produced by the human prostate. EGF is not produced in large amounts by the human prostate. It is safe to assume that PrGF has not been produced and preserved evolutionarily merely for the purpose of giving BPH to the elderly human male. Nor is its primary purpose to stimulate the growth of bone around prostatic cancer metastases. Its purpose may be in maintaining the lower genitourinary tract, but more likely physiologic actions will be found in fertility or the lower female genital tract.

The immediate need is to purify PrGF to homogeneity and in high yield from BPH tissue. Once purified its sequence can be compared to other growth factors and oncogene products.

Purified material will permit receptor identification, receptor number and binding affinity can be correlated with patient's age, and degree of BPH or prostatic disease. Production of antibody to the growth factor will markedly improved quantitation and permit studies on factors controlling synthesis and growth factor levels in prostatic disease. Tagged antibody can be used to localize the growth factor is tissue sections.

Further development of the dog and rat models for PrGF will permit manipulation of the hormoral milieu, studies not easily accomplished in man, to understand mechanisms regulating growth factor synthesis.

Seminiferous growth factor (SGF)

The production of spermatozoa by the mammalian testis is a complex process. Mitosis must be regulated by an intricate mechanisms that can produce millions of mature spermatozoa daily, but not exhaust stem cells. LH and FSH are required hormones, but do not seem to directly regulate germ cell proliferation. Bellve and collaborators [72] found that homogenates of mouse testis stimulated DNA synthesis in quiescent 3T3 cell cultures, thus suggesting that spermatogenesis may be controlled within the testis itself. Prepuberal tissue had twice the activity of adult tissue. The growth promoting activity was located in the seminiferous tubules with the highest activity found in the sertoli cells. This suggests that the sertoli cells may regulate the cell division of spermatogonia by the paracrine secretion of SGF. Growth factor activity was also found in the seminiferous tubules of the mouse, rat, guinea pig, and calf suggesting the activity may be ubiquitous to mammals.

Purification proceeded on the calf (SGF) because of the ease in obtaining large amounts of fresh tissue. SGF was found to be a polypeptide which was denatured by heat and extreme acidic or basic conditions. The molecule was not inactivated by reducing agents. SGF appeared to be bound to other proteins under low salt conditions and had a strong tendency to aggregate. However, in the presence of high salt it dissociated and appears as a 15,700 MW protein. Isoelectric focusing showed the pl to be 4.5–5.5.

SGF appear similar to both PrGF and endothelial growth factor isolated from bovine brain (Table 6) [73]. The three growth factors may ultimately prove to be members of the same class of growth factors or may be identical. Further progress is expected as soon as a monoclonal antibody is produced against the factors.

Transformation and oncogenes

Thus far, we have discussed several growth factors that promote cell replication. We have seen that the initial events that lead to cell proliferation involve binding of the growth factor to a cell surface receptor. This in turn leads to phosphorylation of the receptor by protein kinase that is itself a part of the receptor. By mechanisms poorly understoof this leads to cell replication. Another group of agents that profoundly influence cell growth and differentiation are the viruses that induce tumors in laboratory animals and acutely transform cells in culture.

Tumor viruses are members of the family of viruses known as retroviruses. When the retrovirus infects a mammalian cell, the viral RNA is copied into DNA by the enzyme reverse transcriptase, which is supplied by the virus. The DNA becomes integrated into the host cell's DNA. When the host DNA is transcribed into RNA, by cellular enzymes, the viral DNA is also transcribed. Some of the viral DNA provides copies of the viral genome for new virus particles and some of it is processed into mRNA. Some of the mRNA is translated into viral proteins such as reverse transcriptase and envelop material. In addition, if the retrovirus carries an oncogene its encoded protein is also transcribed. The oncogenes of retroviruses are not required for viral replication and their protein product is not a component of the virus. Oncogenes are the carrier of genetic information for cellular transformation and tumorigenesis in animals and for *in vitro* transformation of cells in culture [74].

From molecular hybridization studies, it appears that retrovirus oncogenes are derived from cellular genes (Proto-oncogenes). Hybridization experiments showed evidence for the presence of DNA and RNA related to viral oncogenes in each family of vertebrates examined including human. From these analyses, it appears that vertebrates possess and express genes that are closely related to oncogenes. The strong evolutionary conservation of these genes, and the observation that they were found to be expressed in every tissue and every species, suggests an essential function of these genes in cellular metabolism.

Of the 24 oncogenes listed in Table 7, half code for proteins that either have tyrosine-specific protein kinase activity or are related to these proteins. As we have already discussed, growth factors regulate normal cell division by processes involving phosphorylation of tyrosine.

The erb B oncogene appears to be derived from the cellular gene coding for a portion of the EGF receptor [76]. Amino acids 557–1154 of the EGF receptor shows an overall homology of 85% with the erb B gene product which rises to 97% in the protein kinase domain [36]. The similarity is especially remarkable since erb B was identified in the Avian Erythroblastosis virus, presumably originating in the chicken, and the EGF receptor was of human origin. This suggests a very conserved gene sequence. Thus, normal stimulants of cell division (growth factors) and the oncogene protein products responsible for tumorigenesis are mechanistically linked. The implication is that tyrosine phosphorylation has a role in regulating the growth of cells.

In 1984, two groups of investigators showed that the protein product of the sis oncogene and one of the peptide of PDGF (PDGF-2) were derived from the same or closely related cellular gene [76, 77]. Their conclusion was based on the demonstration of extensive sequence similarity between P28v-sis, the putative transforming protein of the Simian sarcoma virus (SSV), and the published partial amino acid sequence of PDGF. Eighty-seven percent of the 70 amino acids in the known sequence of PDGF-2 matched those predicted for the sis gene product. Based on current information, it seems that SSV-transformed cells produce a growth factor that is identical with PDGF in mitogenic dose responses, in radioimmunoassay, and in specific mitogenic activity [78]. Furthermore, the secreted transforming protein P28v-sis of SSV appears to stimulate the autocrine growth of SSV-transformed cells through the PDGF receptor [80].

Recently Siefert et al [80] reported that 1 to 18 day old rat aortic smooth muscle cells secrete a growth factor that completes whith authentic PDGF for binding to fibroblast receptors, reacts with antibody to PDGF, and is mitogenic for cultured cells. This cellular PDGF-like material is not secreted by adult aortic smooth muscle, suggesting that the PDGF-like material is developmentally regulated and may play a role in growth and morphogenesis. The suggestion is that embryonic-derived growth factors function normally in autocrine control. If this is so, why is PDGF a normal regulator of cell division and differentiation when released from platelets and a transforming agent when transmitted by the retrovirus? Three explanations have emmerged to account for the transplantation of normal cells by viral genes. 1) The mutational hypothesis proposes that the viral

Table 7. The oncogenes

Name	Virus and alleged species of origin	Function of oncogene protein
src	Rous Sarcoma Virus (chicken)	
yes	Y73 Sarcoma Virus (chicken)	Tyrosine-specific
fgr	Gardner-Rasheed feline Sarcome Virus (cat)	protein kinase
alb	Abelson Murine leukemia virus (mouse)	
fps	Fujinami Sarcoma Virus (chicken)	
fes	ST feline Sarcoma Virus (cat)	
ros	UR II Avian Sarcoma Virus (chicken)	
erb B	Avian Erythroblastosis Virus (chicken)	EGF receptor cytoplasmic Tyrosine-specific Protein kinase domain
fms	McDonough Feline Sarcoma Virus (cat)	possible cytoplasmic domain of a growth factor receptor
mil	MH2 Virus (chicken)	Tyrosine kinase
raf	3611 Murine Sarcoma Virus (mouse)	related proteins
mos	Avian Myeloblastosis Virus (chicken)	
sis	Simian Sarcoma Virus (woolly monkey)	PDGF
Ha-ras	Harvey Murine Sarcoma Virus (rat)	
Ki-ras	Kirsten Murine Sarcoma Virus (rat)	GTP-binding
N-ras	? (human neuroblastoma)	proteins
myc	MC29 Myelocytomatosis Virus (chicken)	DNA-binding protein
fos	FBJ Osteosarcoma Virus (mouse)	
myb	Avian Myeloblastosis Virus (chicken)	Nuclear location,
ski	Avian SKV770 Virus (chicken)	unknown function
B-lym	? (chicken lymphoma)	
rel	Reticuloendotheliosis Virus (turkey)	function and
erb-A	Avian erythroblastosis Virus (chicken)	location unknown
ets	E26 Virus (chicken)	

oncogenes differ from their cellular progenitor in subtle, but important, ways as a result of mutations introduced when the cellular genes were incorporated into the retrovirus genome. For example, the apparently similar enzymatic activities of the tyrosine-specific protein kinase of the viral src gene product and the cellular proto-oncogene might actually have different targets for phosphorylation thus having different effects on cellular behavior. 2) The alternative dosage hypothesis suggests that retrovirus oncogenes act by overburdening cells with too much of what are essentially normal cellular proteins. 3) Finally, it is possible that the proteins are no longer normally regulated in the cell cycle, but are inappropriately expressed by the action of a viral promotor gene. At the present time it is not possible to choose between these possibilities, and in fact all three mechanisms may be operable.

Many investigators have found elevated levels of oncogene product in viral transformed cells. In addition, DNA mediated gene transfer techniques have now made it possible to identify oncogenes in a variety of human tumors. More than 15 different human oncogenes have been identified in fresh human tumors, representing 20 different tumor types. One study involving tumors from 54 patients [81] reported that more than one cellular oncogene was transcriptionally active in all of the tumors examined. It is interesting that unlike some established cell lines that can be transformed by introducing a single oncogene, more than one oncogene also appears to be needed to transform normal primary embryo fibroblasts [82]. In some patients, it was possible to study normal and malignant tissue from the same organ. In many of these patients, the activity of certain oncogenes was greater in the malignant than the normal tissue. It will be important to determine if elevated expression of specific oncogenes is a specific finding in all tumors, or at least in certain types of tumor, or if differences simply reflect methodological difficulties inherent in these types of studies.

The concept that an aberrant oncogene may be required for transformation is illustrated by the EJ (T24) bladder carcinoma model. In the T24 cell line, the cellular ras^{HA} gene has a single point mutation of guanosine to thymidine, resulting in the incorporation of valine instead of glycine at the 12th position in the 21,000 dalton encoded protein [83]. Analyses of the flanking regions of the gene showed no discernable change in the transcription initiation or termination sites. Thus, a single point mutation seems to be a crucial step in conferring transforming potential to an otherwise normal cellular gene. However, analysis of then primary bladder carcinomas failed to show a similar mutational event, suggesting that the T24 cell line is not representative of human bladder carcinoma *in vivo* [84].

The availability of cloned DNA probes for a number of cellular genes, including several of the proto-oncogenes, has made it possible to examine the nuclear events following stimulation of quiescent cells with growth factors. Kelly et al [85] found that myc mRNA was expressed following the addition of PDGF to 3T3 cells. Further studies by Greenberg and Ziff [86] showed that transcription of the fos proto-oncogene was increased within minutes after growth factor addition. Studies by Muller and co-workers [87, 88] showed that oncogenes may have an important role in embryonic development; since specific oncogenes were expressed in a time-related and tissue-specific pattern. These studies suggest that proto-oncogenes are involved in cell cycle control and in the regulation of normal development. It is not difficult to envision that subsequent induction of cellular oncogene expression by carcinogenic agents, such as, radiation, chemical or viruses, could be responsible for the conversion of normal cells to the transformed phenotype.

Conclusions

The growth factors and proto-oncogene encoded proteins play a major role in the regulation of cellular differentiation. These factors appear to function in cell to cell communication over short distances by autocrine of paracrine mechanisms. These regulatory proteins may be in rather high concentrations in very small locales, but in very low concentrations when attempts are made to isolate them from whole tissues. During development growth factors and cellular oncogene proteins may be episodically produced during only a brief period in the life of the organism and the encoding genes then switched off. Switching errors in adult life might manifest themselves as proliferative disorders such as hyperplasia or neoplasia.

This chapter has only scratched the surface of the potential role of growth factors in urology. Over the next few years, researchers will be finding substantially more out about the basic mechanisms by which cells communicate.

References

1. Ham RG: Survival and growth requirements of nontransformed cells. In: Tissue Growth Factors, Baserga R (ed). Springer-Verlag, New York, 13–88, 1981
2. Todaro GJ, DeLarco JE, Fryling C, Johnson PA, Sporn MB: Transforming growth factors (TGFs): Properties and possible mechanisms of action. J Supramol Struct Cell Biochem 15: 287–301, 1981
3. Carpenter G: Epidermal growth factor. In: Tissue Growth Factors, Baserga R (ed). Springer-Verlag, New York, 89–132, 1981
4. Das M: Epidermal growth factor: Mechanisms of action. Inter Rev Cytology 78: 233–256, 1982
5. Carpenter G, Cohen S: Epidermal growth factor. Ann Rev Biochem 48: 193–216, 1979
6. Schlessinger J, Schreiber AB, Levi A, Lax I, Libermann T, Yarden Y: Regulation of cell proliferation by epidermal growth factor. Crit Rev Biochem 14: 93–111, 1983
7. Todaro GJ, DeLarco JE, Fryling CM: Sarcoma growth factor and other transforming peptides produced by human cells: Interactions with membrane receptors. Federation Proc 41: 2996–3003, 1982

8. Roberts AB, Frolik CA, Anzano MA, Sporn MB: Transforming growth factors from neoplastic and nonneoplastic tissues. Federation Proc 42: 2621–2626, 1982

9. Sporn MB, Roberts AB: Autocrine growth factors and cancer. Nature 313: 745–747, 1985

10. Gospodarowicz D, Rudland, P, Lindstrom J, Benirschke K: Fibroblast growth factor: Its localization, purification, mode of action, and physiological significance. Adv Metab Disorder 8: 301–335, 1975

11. Gospodarowicz D, Rauber J-P: Growth factors and the extracellular matrix. Endocrine Reviews 1: 201–227, 1980

12. Varon S, Adler, R: Nerve growth factors and control of nerve growth. Cur Topics Dev Biol 16: 207–251, 1980

13. Yankner BA, Shooter EM: The biology and mechanisms of action of nerve growth factor. Ann Rev Biochem 51: 845–868, 1982

14. Calissano P, Cattaneo A, Biocca S, Aloe L, Mercant D, Levi-Montalcini R: The nerve growth factor. Exptl Cell Res 154: 1–9, 1984

15. Ross R: The platelet-derived growth factor. In: Tissue Growth Factors, Baserga R (ed). Springer-Verlag, Berlin Heidelberg New York, 133–159, 1981

16. Antoniades HN: Platelet-derived growth factor and malignant transformation. Biochem Phar 33: 2823–2828, 1984

17. Clemmons DR, Van Wyk JJ, Somatomedin: Physiological control and effects on cell proliferation. In: Tissue Growth Factors, Baserga R (ed). Springer-Verlag, New York, 161–208, 1981

18. Rothstein H: Regulation of the cell cycle by somatomedins. Inter Rev Cytol 78: 127–232, 1982

19. Metcalf D: Hemopoietic colony stimulating factors. In: Tissue Growth Factors, Baqerga R (ed). Springer-Verlag, New York, 343–384, 1981

20. Metcalf D: The granulocyte-macrophage colony-stimulating factors. Science 229: 16–22, 1985

21. Story MT, Jacobs SC, Lawson RK: Preliminary characterization and evaluation of techniques for the isolation of prostate-derived growth factor. In: New Approaches to the Study of Beningn Prostatic Hyperplasia. Alan R Liss Inc, New York, 197–216, 1984

22. Cohen S: Isolation of a mouse submaxillary gland protein accelerating incision eruption and eyelid opening in the new-born animal. J Biol Chem 237: 1555–1562, 1962

23. Frey P, Forand R, Maciag T, Shooter EM: The biosynthetic precursor of epidermal growth factor and the mechanism of its processing. Proc Natl Acad Sci USA 76: 6294–6298, 1979

24. Scott J, Urdea M, Quiroga M, Sanchez-Pescador R, Fong N, Selby M, Rutter WJ, Bell GI: Structure of a mouse submaxillary messenger RNA encoding epidermal growth factor and seven related proteins. Science 221: 236–240, 1983

25. Gregory H: Isolation and structure of urogastrone and its relationship to epidermal growth factor. Nature 257: 325–327, 1975

26. Harper GP, Barde YA, Burnstock G, Carstairs JR, Dennison ME, Suda K, Vernon CA: Guinea pig prostate is a rich source of nerve growth factor. Nature 279: 160–162, 1979

27. Jacobs SC, Story MT, Tebo T, Kearns C, Lawson RK: Androgen regulation of growth factor activity in rat ventral prostate (submitted manuscript)

28. Story MT, Jacobs SC, Lawson RK: Epidermal growth factor is not the major growth-promoting agent in extract of prostatic tissue. J Urol 130: 175–179, 1983

29. Byyny RL, Orth DN, Cohen S, Doyne ES: Epidermal growth factors: Effects of androgens and adrenergic agents. Endocrinology 90: 1261–1266, 1972

30. Cohen S, Elliott GA: The stimulation of epidermal keratinization by a protein isolated from the submaxillary gland of the mouse. J Invest Dermatol 40: 1–5, 1963

31. Frati L, Daniele S, Delogu A, Covelli I: Selective binding of the epidermal growth and its specific effects on the epithelial cells of the cornea. Exp Eye Res 14: 135–141, 1972

32. Bower JM, Camble R, Gregory H, Gerring EJ, Willshire IR: The inhibition of gastric acid secretion by epidermal growth factor. Experientia 31: 825–826, 1975

68

33. Carpenter G, Cohen S: Human epidermal growth factor and the proliferation of human fibroblasts. J Cell Physiol 88: 227–237, 1976
34. Schreiber AB, Lax I, Yarden Y, Eshhar Z, Schlessinger J: Monoclonal antibodies against receptor for epidermal growth factor induce early and delayed effects of epidermal growth factor. Proc Natl Acad Sci USA 78: 7535–7539, 1981
35. Cohen S, Carpenter G, Jr King L: Epidermal growth factor-receptor-protein kinase interactions. In: Control of Cellular Division and Development, Part A. Alan R Liss Inc, New York, 557–567, 1981
36. Ullrich A, Coussens L, Hayflick JS, Dull TJ, Gray A, Tam AW, Lee J, Yarden Y, Libermann TA, Schlessinger J, Downward J, Mayes ELV, Whittle N, Waterfield MO, Seeburg PH: Human epidermal growth factor receptor cDNA sequence and aberrant expression of the amplified gene in A431 epidermoid carcinoma cells. Nature 309: 418–425, 1984
37. Schlessinger J, Schreiber AB, Levi A, Lax I, Libermann T, Yarden Y: Regulation of cell proliferation by epidernal growth factor. Crit Rev Biochem 14: 93–111, 1983
38. Sporn MB, Todaro GJ: Autocrine secretion and malignant transformation of cells. New Engl; J Med 303: 878–880, 1980
39. Roberts AB, Frolik CA, Anzano MA, Spron MB: Transforming growth factors from neoplastic and non-neoplastic tissue. Fed Proc 42: 2621–2626, 1983
40. Marquardt H, Hukkapiller MW, Hood LE, Todaro GJ: Rat transforming growth factor type 1: Structure and relation to epidermal growth factor. Science 223: 1079–1082, 1984
41. Messing EM, Bubbers JE, DeKernion JB, Fahey JL: Growth stimulating activity produced by human bladder cancer cells. J Urol 132: 1230–1234, 1984
42. Heal DE, Bennett MK, Hall RR, Marsh C, Abel PD, Sainsbury JRC, Harris AL: Epidermal-growth-factor receptors in human bladder cancer: Comparision of invasive and superficial tumors. Lancet i: 366–368, 1985
43. Lin CW, Fay CA: Human Bladder tumor cells produce multiple synergistic interacting transforming growth factors. Proceedings American Association for Cancer Research, Toronto, Canada, 215, 1984 (abstract)
44. Charhon SA, Chapuy MC, Delvin EE, Valentin-Opran A, Edouard CM, Meunier PJ: Histomorphometric analysis of sclerotic bone metastases from prostatic carcinoma with special reference to osteomalacia. Cancer 51: 918–924, 1983
45. Jacobs SC, Pikna D, Lawson RK: Prostatic osteoblastic factor. Invest Urol 17: 195–198, 1979
46. Jacobs SC, Lawson RK: Mitogenic factor in human prostate extracts. Urology 16: 488–491, 1980
47. Charhon SA, Chapuy MC, Delvin EE, Meunier PJ: Parathyroid function and vitamin D status in patients with bone metastases of prostatic origin. Mineral Electrolyte Metab 11: 117–122, 1985
48. Cunha GR, Chung LWK, Shannon JM, Taguchi O, Fujii H: Hormone-induced morphogenesis and growth: Role of mesenchymal-epithelial interactions. Recent Progress Hormone Research 39: 559–598, 1983
49. Cunha G: Stromal factors in the development and control of growth in the prostate. 2nd NIADDK symposium on the study of Benign Prostatic Hyperplasia. DHEW publication (in press)
50. Bartsch G, Muller HR, Oberholzer M, Rohr HP: Light microscopic stereological analysis of the normal human prostate and of benign prostatic hyperplasia. J. Urol 122: 487–491, 1979
51. Bartsch G, Frick J, Ruegg I, Bucher M, Holliger O, Oberholzer M, Rohr HP: Election microscopic stereological analysis of the normal human prostate and of beningn prostatic hyperplasia. J Urol 122: 481–486, 1979
52. LeDuc LE: The anatomy of the prostate and the pathology of early benign hypertrophy. J Urol 42: 1217–1241, 1939
53. Moore RA: Benign hypertrophy of the prostate: A morphological study. J Urol 50: 680–710, 1943
54. Pradhan BK, Chandra K: Morphogenesis of nodular hyperplasia-prostate. J Urol 113: 210–213, 1975

55. Franks LM: Benign nodular hyperplasia of the prostate: a review. Ann Royal College of Surg Eng 14: 92–106, 1954

56. McNeal JE: Origin and evolution of benign prostatic enlargement. Invest Urol 15: 340–345, 1978

57. Tackett RE, Heston WDW, Parrish RF, Pletscher LS, Fair WR: Mitogenic factors in prostatic tissue and expressed prostatic secretion. J Urol 133: 45–48, 1985

58. Lawson RK, Story MT, Jacobs SC: Possible paracrine activity in human benign prostatic hyperplasia. The Prostate (in press)

59. Mawhinney M: The role of the stroma collagen in prostate growth. 2nd NIADDK Symposium on the study of Benign Prostatic Hyperplasia. DHEW publication (in press)

60. Pardee AB: A restriction point for control of normal animal cell proliferation. Proc Natl Acad Sci USA 71: 1286–1290, 1974

61. Lawson RK, Story MT, Jacobs SC: A growth factor in extracts of human prostatic tissue. In: The Prostatic Cell: Structure and Function, Part A. Alan R Liss Inc, New York, 325–336,

62. DiCorleto PE, Gajdusel DM, Schwartz SM, Ross R: Biochemical properties of the endothelium-derived growth factor. J Cell Phy 114: 339–345, 1983

63. Heldin CH, Westermark B, Wasteson A: Platelet-derived growth factor: Purification and partial characterization. Proc Natl Acad Sci USA 76: 3722–3726, 1979

64. Taylor JM, Cohen S, Mitchell WM: Epidermal growth factor: High and low molecular weight forms. Proc Natl Acad Sci USA 67: 164–171, 1970

65. Knauer DJ, Wayne FW, Smith GL: Purification and characterization of multiplication-stimulating activity (MSA) carrier protein. J Supramol Struct 15: 177–191, 1981

66. Varon S, Nomura J, Shooter EM: The isolation of the mouse nerve growth factor protein in a high molecular weight form. Biochemistry 6: 2202–2209, 1967

67. Heldin CH, Westermark J, Wasteson A: Platelet-derived growth factor. Biochem J 193: 907–913, 1981

68. Gregory H, Willshire IR: The isolation of the urogastrones-inhibitors of gastric acid secretion from lumen urine. Hoppe-Syler's E Physiol Chem 356: 1765–1774, 1975

69. Heston WDW, Parrish R, Tackett R, Pletscher S, Fiar WR: Fibroblast mitogenic activity of Copenhagen rat prostate and prostate derived tumors. Program of the American Urological Association Annual Meeting, New Orleans, LA, abstract, 1981

70. Drago JR, Goldman LB, Maurer RE: The Nb rat prostatic adenocarcinoma model system. In: Models for prostate cancer. Alan R Liss Inc, New York, 265–291, 1980

71. Heyns W, Peeters B, Mous J, Rombauts W, DeMoor P: Androgen-dependent synthesis of a prostatic binding protein by rat prostate. J Steroid Biochem 11: 209–213, 1979

72. Bellve AR, Feig LA: Cell proliferation in the mammalian testis: Biology of seminiferous growth factor (SGF). Recent Progress Hormone Research 40: 531–567, 1984

73. Maciag T, Hoover GA, Weinstein R: High and low molecular weight forms on endothelial cell growth factor. J Biol Chem 257: 5333–5336, 1982

74. Bishop JM: Oncogenes. Sci Am: 80–93, March 1982

75. Downward J, Yarden Y, Mayes E, Scrace G, Totty N, Stockwell P, Ullrich A, Schlessinger J, Waterfield MD: Close similarity of epidermal growth factor receptor and v-erb-B oncogene protein sequences. Nature 307: 521–527, 1984

76. Waterfield MD, Scrace GT, Whittle N, S Ttroobant P, Johnsson A, Wasteson A, Westermark B, Heldin CH, Huang JS, Deuel TF: Platelet-derived growth factor is structurally related to the putative transforming protein. p28[sis] of simian sarcoma virus. Nature 304: 35–39, 1983

77. Doolittle RF, Hunkapiller MW, Hood LE, DeVare SG, Robbins KC, Aaronson SA, Antoniades HN: Simian sarcoma virus oncogene, v-sis, is derived from the gene(s) encoding a platelet derived growth factor. Science 221: 275–277, 1983

78. Deuel TF, Huang JS, Huang SS, Stoobant P, Waterfield MD: Expression of a platelet-derived growth factor-like protein in simian sarcoma virus transformed cells. Science 221: 1348–1350, 1983

79. Deuel TF, Tong BD, Huang JS: Autocrine regulation of SSV-transformed cell growth by PDGF-like activity. In: Cancer Cells/3: Growth factors and transformation, Feramisco J, Ozanne B, Stiles C (eds). Cold Spring Harbor Laboratory, 167–173, 1985

80. Seifert RA, Schwartz SM, Bowen-pope DF: Developmentally regulated production of platelet-derived growth factor-like molecules. Nature 311: 669–671, 1984

81. Slamon DJ, Dekernion JB, verma IM, Cline MJ: Expression of cellular oncogenes in human malignancies. Science 224: 256–262, 1984

82. Land H, Parada LF, Weinberg RA: Tumorigenic conversion of primary embryo fibroblasts requires at least two cooperating oncogenes. Nature 304: 596–602, 1983

83. Reddy EP, Reynolds RK, Santos E, Barbacid M: A point mutation is responsible for the acquisition of transforming properties by the T24 human bladder carcinoma oncogene. Nature 300: 149–152, 1982

84. Feinberg AP, Vogelstein B, Stroller MJ, Baylin SB, Nelkin BN: Mutation affecting the 12th amino acid of the c-Ha-ras oncogene product occurs infrequently in human cancer. Science 220: 1175–1177, 1982

85. Kelly K, Cochran BH, Stiles CD, Leder P: Cell 35: 603–610, 1983

86. Greenberg ME, Ziff EB: Stimulation of 3T3 cells induces transcription of the c-fos proto-oncogene. Nature 311: 433–438, 1984

87. Muller R, Slalom DJ, Tremblay JM, Cline MJ, Verma IM: Differential expression of cellular oncogenes during pre and postnatal development of the mouse. Nature 299: 640–644, 1982

88. Muller R, Slamon DJ, Adamson ED, Tremblay JM, Muller D, Cline MJ, Verma IM: Transcription of c-onc genes c-raski and c-fms during mouse development. Mol Cell Biol 3: 1062–1069, 1983

Editorial Comment

WARREN D.W. HESTON, Muhammed A. BULBUL and WILLIAM R. FAIR

'*Growth Factors in urology*', by Drs. Jacob and Story represents a broad overview of a rapidly growing area in cell biology as it relates to urology. Their emphasis was on the peptide growth factors and oncogenes. It should be underscored that these peptide growth factor(s) are growth regulatory *in vivo* in concert with other modulatory factors such as steroids and neurotransmitter substances.

One urologic tissue which did not receive attention in their article was the kidney. In addition to being responsive to sex steroid hormones, the kidney is also responsive to growth factors, one of which is present in pituitary gland extract [1]. This growth factor has been termed renotropin and has been associated with kidney hyperplasia following unilateral nephrectomy [1–3]. It appears that androgens induce kidney hypertrophy and interfere with renotropin-induced hyperplasia [1]. The role of this pituitary factor in the growth of tumors of the kidney was investigated by Sufrin and co-workers [4, 5]. Using unilateral nephrectomy to induce renotropin induction and a transplantable Wilms tumor, they observed that the tumor responded with an increase in growth rate and tumor size following nephrectomy [4]. However, unilateral nephrectomy did not alter the take or growth rate of a rapidly growing renal adenocarcinoma in Balb/c mice [5]. Renotropin, a pituitary factor, and testosterone, a testicular factor, obviously are acting as endocrine factors. The nature of paracrine and autocrine factors in growth and differentiation of the normal and tumorous kidney still need to be elucidated.

One paracrine growth factor likely to be particularly associated with kidney carcinoma is tumor angiogenesis factor (TAF) [6]. Indeed the normal kidney was found to be the most responsive tissue when a number of tissues were screened for angiogenic responsiveness to salivary gland extracts [7]. Mydlo and associates have reported tumor angiogenesis factor to be present in extracts of kidney carcinoma [8]. Recently, a tumor angiogenic factor termed angiogenin has been isolated from human colon tumor cells by Dr. B. Vallee and colleagues [9–12]. They purified angiogenin to homogeneity with cation-exchange and high performance liquid chromatography. It is a single-chain protein consisting of 123 amino acids. Angiogenin is a very basic molecule having a isoelectric point greater than 9.5.Vallee and colleagues found HT-29 cells to produce 0.5 ng of angiogenin per liter of supernatant. As little as 35 femtomoles (10^{-15} M) produced significant angiogenesis in the chick embryo chorioallantoic membrane assay [10]. There was substantial homology between angiogenin and pancreatic ribonucleases, but angiogenin does not display ribonuclease activity. It remains to be determined whether it is the same factor responsible for the hypervascularity associated with renal cancer. If so, antibodies against TAF or TAF receptors or TAF antagonists may be useful in controlling the growth of these hypervascular tumors [6].

Metastatic renal cancer is an extremely deadly disease with no effective form of therapy currently available. Indeed renal cancer is notable for its resistance to chemotherapy. It is of interest that Meyers and Biedler have found an increase in EGF receptors in multiple drug-resistant cells [14]. Receptors for epidermal growth factor appear to be abundantly present on renal cancer cells relative to normal kidney cells [13]. It may be that manipulation of the epidermal growth factor receptor will increase the sensitivity of renal cancer to chemotherapy. Dr. Mendelsohn and co-workers have reported that they can inhibit the growth of human tumor cells in nude mice with the administration of monoclonal anti-EGF receptor antibodies [15]. Whether such antibodies will be useful in the treatment of renal cell cancers or other urologic cancers and what effect they will have on the proliferation of normal cells remains to be determined.

In their report Drs. Jacobs and Story bring us up to date on their progress on the purification of a growth factor from prostate tissue that stimulates the growth of fibroblasts and osteoblasts. Our findings agree with theirs on the presence and purification of a prostatic factor which stimulates fibroblasts. We are able to obtain as great a purification by heparin affinity chromatography combined with anion exchange chromatography. The role such a factor plays in the development of BPH requires further study [16]. While we have focused on the growth stimulatory properties of the prostate extract or of expressed prostatic secretion, it should be noted that it may be just as important to examine the presence of growth *inhibitory* substances. We have reported the presence of such inhibitory factors [16]. Whether these inhibitor(s) are the same or different from fibroblastic toxic compounds such as zinc and spermine normally present in high concentrations in the prostate is being investigated.

Koutsilieris, Bablini, and Goltzman have extracted peptides which are mitogenic for osteoblasts from human prostatic tissue [17]. These investigators reported that normal, cancerous and benign prostate stimulated the growth of osteoblasts and osteosarcoma cells *in vitro*. Extracts of BPH tissue consistently were mitogenic for fibroblasts but extracts of cancerous tissue were not mitogenic or only weakly mitogenic for fibroblast growth. This activity was associated with material that bound to a CM column and was considered to be the basic in nature. This basic peptide was not mitogenic towards 3T3 cells. This implies that there are at least two different growth factors present in the prostate. The acidic (Lawson & Jacob, and work in our lab) and the basic (Koutsilieris et al) factor coming from the same tissue, each of which has similar yet also different target cells, is remindful of the pituitary-derived anionic and basic forms of capillary endothelial cell growth factors [18].

It is interesting that the factor found by Koutsilieris et al is cationic, because the cationic polypeptide hormone relaxin also been reported to stimulate rat and human osteoblasts [19]. Further relaxin has been found in human semen and is thought to be of prostatic origin [20].

While these factors affect the growth of fibroblastic and osteoblastic cell types, they have not been reported to be active on the prostatic epithelial cells. The autocrine peptide factor for the epithelium has yet to be determined. Dr. L.W.K. Chung has found that transplants of rat prostatic tissue tend to lose markers of epithelial function unless they are supplemented with adrenergic neurotransmitter agents [21]. Adrenergic agents have also been found to increase ornthine decarboxylase activity and cyclic AMP levels in the rat prostate [22].

Dr. Donna Peehl has produced growth of epithelial cells from human prostatic BPH or cancer on a regular basis using a modified growth medium, a major component of which is cholera toxin [23]. This growth-promoting effect was not specific for cholera toxin but was produced by agents which would increase cyclic AMP. Of the agents examined, cholera toxin appeared to be the most active prostate epithelial cell growth-producing agent. The prostatic epithelium appears to be cyclic AMP responsive for proliferation in a fashion similar to that reported for other epithelial cells [24]. As cholera toxin is unlikely to be the endogenous mediator of prostatic epithelial cell growth and function, what is? Another possible agonist, which has been found in rat prostate in high concentration which binds to prostatic epithelial cells with high affinity and actively elevates cyclic AMP, is vasoactive intestinal polypeptide (VIP) [25, 26]. Whether VIP has growth-promoting activity in human prostatic epithelium remains to be determined.

In addition to cholera toxin, Dr. Peehl has found that the growth of adult human prostatic epithelial cells is further enhanced by the addition of epidermal growth factor, pituitary extract, hydrocortisone, insulin and selenium to PFM4 medium [27–29]. It is of interest that this supplementaion glucocorticoids but not androgens appear to be required for optimal growth *in vitro*. Whether factors will be found in the pituitary extract that will serve as andromedans *in vivo* in a fashion similar to that reported for enstromedans also requires further investigation [30, 31].

Because of many noted similarities, it may be that facts learned from established human breast carcinoma cell lines will have applicability to the human prostate. Dr. Marc Lippman has published a recent review article on the many factors considered to be relevant to the growth of normal and cancerous breast epithelium [32]. The long list of trophic hormones other than estrogen influencing the growth of these breast cells includes glucocorticoids, androgens, progestins, iodothyronins, vitamin D, retinoids, epidermal growth factor (EGF), insulin-like growth factor 1 (IGF-1), calcitonin and prolactin. A very similar list would be used to describe factors implicated in cancerous growth of the prostate.

These workers reported that breast cancer cell lines secrete transforming growth factor alpha (TGF α). TGF α binds to EGF receptors. Estrogen-independent lines secrete more than estrogen-dependent lines and estrogen-dependent, estrogen-supplemented lines secrete more TGF α than do estrogen-dependent, estrogen-deprived lines. TGF α is considered to be a progression factor, that is, once the cell has been primed (made competent) for division all that is required is the presence of an appropriate progression factor such as EGF or TGF α. Platelet-derived growth factor is a competence factor for appropriate cell types. All of the breast tumor lines produced a competency factor, the identity of which was under active investigation [32, 33].

TGF β which is considered to be a growth-promoting factor for some cell types was associated with inhibition of mammary tumor growth. TGF β production was increased by estrogen withdrawal in estrogen-dependent cells and decreased in estrogen-independent and estrogen-stimulated, estrogen-dependent cells [32].

Transfection with the ras oncogene of estrogen-dependent MCF-7 breast carcinoma cells produced cells with increased EGF receptor production, increased TGF-α production and estrogen-independent growth. The similarities and differences between prostatic carcinoma and breast carcinoma in these regards needs to be established.

In studies of the culturing of prostate epithelium, Dr. Peehl includes EGF in the tissue culture medium [27–28]. Dr. Smith has reported the presence of v-sis in a human prostate-derived tumor line [34, 35]. The v-sis oncogene is similar to PDGF. Usually PDGF is considered to be active on mesenchymal cells. Whether PDGF acts on stroma cells to produce growth factors for epithelial cells or acts directly to induce competence in the LNCaP cells need further investigation. That these growth factors are important in tumor cell growth is further underscored by the recent observed relationship between mouse mammary tumorigenesis and submandibular gland epidermal growth factor [34]. In the mouse, the submandibular gland is a major source of EGF. Surgical removal of the submandibular gland reduced mammary tumor incidence from 63% to 13% and delayed tumor latency by as much as 14 weeks. Sialyladenectomy of tumor-bearing mice caused a rapid and sustained cessation of tumor growth while injection of EGF restored that growth [34].

In conclusion, much has been written on possible endocrine factors which stimulate prostatic growth. Unfortunately, most of his work has been performed with impure material. It is only after the isolation of pure material and its addition to a totally defined medium [27] that a truly accurate assessment of the role of the growth stimulatory activity can be assessed. Jacobs and Story have performed that critical purification function on at least one growth factor present in the prostate. Following the total purification of their prostate-derived growth factor, we should soon know how similar or dissimilar it is to other known growth factors, which cells produce it, which cells it acts on, how it interacts with prostatic glycosaminoglycans [37], how it relates to the development of pathological states such as BPH and prostatic cancer, and potentially discover new therapeutic approaches to these pathological states.

Note added in proof: Other investigators have recently isolated from the prostate by heparin affinity chromatography a 'basic' fibroblast growth factor (Nishi et al., Biochem. Biophys. Res. Comm. 132: 1103, 1985), a heparin binding growth factor from the brain that is mitogenic for prostatic epithelial cells (Crabb et al., Biochem. Biophys. Res. Comm. 136: 1151, 1986) and purified to homogeneity an acidic growth factor for fibroblast from the rat ventral prostate (Maehama et al., Proc. Natl. Acad. Sci. 83: 8162, 1986 USA).

74

References

1. Nomura K, Demura H, Shizume K: Stimulation of renal deoxyribonucleic acid synthesis by a pituitary-derived renotropin and its inhibition by testosterone and thyroxine. Endocrin 116: 616–621, 1985
2. Malt RA: Humoral factors in regulation of compensatory renal hypertrophy. Kid Int'l 23: 611–615, 1983
3. Ogawa K, Nowinski WW: Mitosis stimulating factor in serum of unilaterally nephrectomized rats. Proc Soc Exp Biol Med 99: 350, 1958
4. Sufrin G, Green D, Pontes JE, Williams PD, Murphy GP: Effect of unilateral nephrectomy on growth of the Wistar/Furth Wilm's tumor. J Urol 131: 378–382, 1984
5. Murphy GP, Sufrin G, Williams PD: Effect of unilateral nephrectomy on tumor growth of the murine renal cell adenocarcinoma and neuroblastoma. Oncology 41: 417–419, 1984
6. Folkman J: Toward an understanding of angiogenesis: search and discovery. Perspect Biol Med 29: 10–36, 1985
7. McCauslan BR, Hofman H: Endothelial stimulating factor from Walker carcinoma cells. Relation to tumor angiogenic factor. Exp Cell Res 119: 181–190, 1979
8. Mydlo J, Bard R, Freed SZ: Deection of tumor angiogenesis factor in adenocarcinoma of the kidney: A preliminary study (in press).
9. Vallee BL, Riordan JF, Lobb RR, Higachi N, Fett JW, Crossley G, Buhler R, Budzik G, Breddam K, Bethune JL, Alderman EM: Tumor-derived angiogenesis factors from rat Walker 256 carcinoma: an experimental investigation and review. Experientia 41: 1–142, 1985
10. Fett JW, Strydom DJ, Lobb RR, Alderman EM, Bethune JL, Riordan JF, Vallee BL: Isolation and characterization of angiogenin, an angiogenic protein from human carcinoma cells. Biochem 24: 5480–5486, 1985
11. Strydom DL, Fett JW, Lobb RR, Alderman EM, Bethune JL, Riordan JF, Vallee BL: Amino acid sequence of human derived angiogenin. Biochem 24: 5486–5494, 1985
12. Karachi K, Davie EW, Strydom DJ, Riordan JF, Vallee BL: Sequence of the cDNA and gene for angiogenin, a human angiogenesis factor. Biochem 24: 5495–5499, 1985
13. Carlos Cordon-Cardo, Memorial Sloan-Kettering, Dept of Pathology, personal communication
14. Myers MB, Spengler BA, Biedler JL: Epidermal growth factor binding is increased in multidrug-resistant cells. Proc AM Assoc Cancer Res 26: 337, abstract #1328, 1985
15. Masai H, Kowamoto JD, Wolf B, Sato G, Mendelsohn J: Growth inhibition of human tumor cells in athymic mice by anti-epidermal growth factor receptor antibodies. Cancer Res 44: 1002-1007, 1984
16. Tackett RE, Heston WDW, Parrish RF, Pletscher LS, Fair WR: Mitogenic factors in prostatic tissue and expresses prostatic secretion. J Urol 133: 45–48, 1985
17. Koutsilieris M, Rabbani SA, Goltzman D: Extraction of peptides which are mitogenic for osteoblasts from human prostatic tissue. Proc Amer Soc Bone Min Res 7: abstract #197, 1985
18. Klagsburn M, Shing Y: Heparin affinity of anionic and cationic capillary endothelial cell growth factors: analysis of hypothalmus-derived growth factors and fibroblast growth factors. Proc Natl Acad Sci USA 82: 805–809, 1985
19. Brand JS, Puzas JE: Relaxin stimulates bone cell proliferation. Proc Am Soc Bone Min Res: abstract #76, 1985
20. Kemp BE, Niell HD: Relaxin. Vit and Horm 41: 79–0115, 1984
21. Chung LWK, Univ of Colorado, Sch of Pharmacy, Boulder, Colo, personal communication
22. Wombie JR, Russell DH: Catecholamine-stimulated β_2-receptors coupled to ornithine decarboxylase induction and to cellular hypertrophy and proliferation. Adv Polyamine Res 4: 549–562, 1983
23. Peehl DM, Stamey TA: Serial propagation of adult human prostatic epithelial cells with cholera toxin. In Vitro 20: 981–986, 1984

24. Green H: Cyclic AMP in relation to proliferation of epidermal cells: a new view. Cell 15: 801–811, 1978

25. Prieto J-C, Carmena MJ: Receptors for vasoactive intestinal peptide on isolated epithelial cells of rat ventral prostate. Biochem Biophys Acta 763: 408–413, 1983

26. Carmena M-J, Prietro J-C: Cyclic AMP-stimulating effect of vasoactive intestinal peptide in isolated epithelial cells of rat ventral prostate. Biochem Biophys Acta 763: 414–418, 1983

27. Peehl DM, Stamey TA: Serum-free growth of adult prostatic epithelial cells. In Vitro, 22: 82–90, 1986

28. Peehl DM, Stamey TA: Growth responses of normal, benign hyperplastic, and malignant human prostatic epithelial cells *in vitro* to cholera toxin, pituitary extract and hydrocortisone. Prostate, 1986

29. Peehl DM: Serial culture of adult human prostatic epithelial cells. J. Tissue Culture Meth 9: 53–60, 1985

30. Ikeda T, Danielpour D, Sirbasku DA: Characterization of a sheep pituitary-derived growth factor for rat and human mammary tumor cells. J Cell Biochem 25: 213–229, 1984

31. Danielpour D, Sirbasku DA: New perspectives in hormone-dependent (responsive) and autonomous mammary tumor growth: role of autostimulatory growth factors. In Vitro 20: 975–980, 1984

32. Lippman Me: Growth regulation of human breast cancer. Clin Res 33: 375–382, 1985

33. Rozengurt E, Sinnett J, Taylor-Papadimitriou J: Production of PDGF-like growth factor by breast cancer cell lines. Int J Cancer 36: 247–252, 1985

34. Syms AJ, Nag A, Smith R: Rearrangement of the C-515 proto-oncogene in a human prostatic carcinoma cell line (LNCaP). J Urol 133: 120A, 1985

35. Rijndert AWM, Vanderkorput JAGM, Van Steenburge GJ, Romijn JC, Trapman J: Expression of cellular oncogenes. In: Human Prostatic Carcinoma Cells. Biochem Biophys Res Commun 132: 548–554, 1985

36. Kurachi H., Okamoto S, Oka T: Evidence for the involvement of the submandibular gland epidermal growth factor in mouse mammary tumorigenesis. Proc Natl Acad Sci USA 82: 5940–5943, 1985

37. DeKlerk DP: The glycosaminoglycan of normal and hyperplastic prostate. Prostate 4: 73–81, 1983

5. Methods of detecting prostatic tumors

DOV KADMON

It has been estimated that in 1985, 25,500 patients will die of carcinoma of the prostate and 86,000 new cases will be diagnosed [1]. Currently, prostate cancer is the third most common cause of cancer death in American males and accounts for 10% of such deaths [1].

There is considerable evidence in the literature that the natural history of this disease can be influenced by curative therapy [2, 3]. The sine-qua-non, however, for achieving cures is tumor confined to the prostate [2]. No curative therapy is available for advanced disease [4].

A large number of patients with early stages of prostate cancer are totally asymptomatic [4]. The only clinical evidence of an early tumor may be a circumscribed area of induration on digital rectal examination of the prostate. However, in 10% to 24% of the patients, prostatic carcinoma is not suspected on rectal examination and is discovered postoperatively in enucleated prostatic tissue removed for presumed benign hyperplasia [4, 5]. A recent American College of Surgeons survey revealed that about 50% of the patients with newly diagnosed prostate cancer have either locally extensive disease (stage C) or evidence of distant metastases (stage D) [6].

The early diagnosis of prostate cancer, a highly desirable goal, remains a formidable challange. In the ensuing paragraphs we will review the current methods for detecting prostate cancer, analyzing their efficacy, advantages, disadvantages and relative clinical usefulness.

Biochemical and immunologic tumor markers

Intensive research for a substance potentially useful for early diagnosis of prostate carcinoma has failed to yield a satisfactory marker. Fluids that may contain tumor markers include serum, urine and prostatic secretions. Table 1 lists substances that have been investigated as possible markers. Many have shown early promise. Those that have generated the most enthusiasm will be discussed in detail.

Ratliff, T.L. and Catalona, W.J. (eds), Genitourinary Cancer. ISBN 0–89838–830–9
© *1987, Martinus Nijhoff Publishers, Boston. Printed in the Netherlands.*

Serum markers

Prostatic acid phosphatase (PAP)

Ever since the 1930's when Gutman and Gutman found elevated serum levels of this enzyme in the serum of patients with metastatic carcinoma of the prostate [7], acid phosphatase has been considered a valuable marker for prostate cancer. The enzymatic assay evolved through several stages, in order to improve its specificity for the prostatic isoenzyme. Perhaps the most popular assay at the present time is the catalytic method of Roy et al using thymolphthalein monophosphate as the substrate [8]. PAP detected by the enzymatic assay is found to be elevated in about 70% of patients with metastatic prostate cancer [9, 10]. However, the vast majority of patients with early stage disease have normal serum levels of enzymatically detectable PAP [9, 10]. Evidence has been accumulating for years that patients with clinical stage A or B disease and a persistently elevated PAP level may in fact have diffuse micrometastases and most of them will develop overt metastases within a short period of time [9, 11–13].

In the 1970's radioimmunoassay (RIA) techniques were developed for the detection of PAP [14–16]. In 1977 Foti et al claimed that an RIA determination of the serum PAP detected 33% of patients with stage A carcinoma of the prostate, 79% of stage B, 71% of stage C and 92% of stage D patients [14]. The false positive rate of patients with benign prostatic hyperplasia (BPH) was only 6%. Considerable hope was raised that this test, because of its improved sensitivity and specificity, could be used for screening the population at large for early detection of prostate cancer [17]. Several institutions, including our own, conducted large scale studies in an effort to confirm these results [18–20]. No one has been able to confirm or duplicate the results published by Foti et al. Table 2 summarizes the Washington University series and Table 3 is a compilation of some of the other reports including our own. There was no significant advantage to the RIA method over the enzymatic method in detecting early prostate cancer. In a follow-up study of the Washington University data, Fleischman et al observed

Table 1. Possible markers for prostatic carcinoma

1. Acid phosphatase	11. Transferrin
2. Creatine phosphokinase (CK-BB)	12. Ribounuclease (RNAse)
3. Prostate specific antigen	13. Alpha-fetoprotein (AFP)
4. Alkaline phosphatase	14. Carcinoembryonic antigen
5. Lactic dehydrogenase (LDH)	(CEA)
6. Total cholesterol	15. Human chorionic
7. Non-esterified cholesterol	gonadotropin (HCG)
8. Spermidine (a polyamine)	16. Seromucoid
9. Fibronectin	17. Hydroxyproline
10. Complement	18. Isoleucine

that for every single correct acid phosphatase elevation in patients with stage A or B carcinoma of the prostate, there were 24 patients with BPH who had a falsely elevated RIA-PAP [21].

There are scattered reports in the literature suggesting an increased sensitivity of the RIA-PAP test when compared to the enzymatic assay [22, 23]. A more recent study comparing four methods of PAP determination including RIA, counterimmunoelectrophoresis (CIEP), immunoenzymatic assay (IEA) and the enzymatic method concluded that there was little difference in the diagnostic accuracy of the four assays [24].

The consensus regarding the RIA-PAP assay appears to be that even if it has a slight sensitivity advantage over the enzymatic assay, this has not proved clinically helpful [4, 21, 25]. As a screening test for early prostate cancer, the RIA has limited usefulness because of its high false positive rate [26–28].

Creatine phosphokinase
Reports by Feld et al, Silverman et al and Forman [29–31] suggested that patients with prostatic carcinoma had an elevation in the BB band of the serum creatine phosphokinase (CK-BB). Our experience is given in Table 4 and indicates that CK-BB is elevated in only a small fraction of patients with stage A or B disease. It is therefore useless as a screening test for early prostate cancer.

Prostate specific antigen
In 1979, Wang, et al identified and characterized a prostate specific antigen (PSA), distinct from prostatic acid phosphatase [32]. Wang et al have subsequently demonstrated elevated serum levels of PSA in patients with prostatic carcinoma [33–35]. Table 5 lists their results. The problem is that while this antigen may be specific for the prostate, it certainly is not specific for carcinoma of the prostate. Ten percent of normal patients and at least two thirds of men with BPH also had elevations of their serum PSA level [33]. Consequently, this

Table 2. Acid phosphatase in untreated patients (Washington University series)

Stage	Number elevated assays (%)			
	Enzymatic		RIA-PAP	
A	1/16	(6.2)	1/16	(6.2)
B	1/27	(3.7)	2/29	(6.9)
C	10/31	(32.3)	13/31	(41.9)
D	16/21	(76.2)	16/22	(72.7)
Unstaged	3/18	(16.7)	3/20	(15.0)
Totals	31/113	(27.4)	35/118	(29.7)

marker's usefulness as a screening test for prostatic carcinoma is limited and is subject to the same lack of specificity as RIA-PAP.

Alkaline phosphatase
Alkaline phosphatase (AP) serum level may be elevated in up to 90% of patients with bone metastases from carcinoma of the prostate [36]. Most of the elevation in AP under these circumstances is due to the bone isoenzyme of AP [36]. Because of the mechanism of elevation of AP in patients with prostate cancer, this marker is obviously not a candidate for a screening test for early stage disease.

Lactic dehydrogenase
Dennis and Prout found elevated tissue levels of isoenzymes 4 and 5 of lactic dehydrogenase (LDH) in prostatic cancer tissue [37]. Prout et al found elevated serum levels of these isoenzymes in patients with advanced prostate cancer [38]. No clinical information is available about the usefulness of serum LDH isoenzymes in screening patients with early stage disease.

Polyamines
The erythrocyte polyamine levels were found to be elevated in patients with advanced carcinoma of the prostate [39]. Plasma spermidine levels (a basic polyamine) were also reported to be elevated in patients with prostate cancer [40, 41]. From the information available it appears that elevations of blood polyamine

Table 3. Comparison of percentage elevations of prostatic acid phosphatase to other series of patients with CAP or BPH (Commercial PAP-RIA kit, NEN – New England Nuclear, Boston, mass, Mallinck-Mallinckbrodt Inc, St Louis, Mo)

| | Disease | | | | |
| | BPH | CaP stage | | | |
Investigator		A	B	C	D
Foti et al[a]	6	33	79	71	92
Bruce et al[a]	3	14	29	25	89
Bruce – NEN	11	13	26	14	71
Griffiths – NEN	9	12	32	47	86
Bruce – Mallinck	27[b]	16	45	36	85
Bruce – Mallinck revised	11[c]	13	24	14	80
Wash Univ, Mallinck	7.5	6	9	35	65

[a] Investigators own antibody procedure
[b] Bruce data based on the 95.5th percentile of the normal male population. The critical value used was 1.9 ng/ml
[c] Bruce data revised by Bruce with the critical value raised to 2.5 ng/ml

levels are associated with advanced disease. These substances, therefore do not fulfill the requirements for early detection of carcinoma of the prostate.

Urine markers

Since the prostate empties its secretion directly into the urethra, it is conceptually very appealing that alterations in prostatic biochemistry, occasioned as the result of malignant change in the gland, would ultimately be reflected in the urinary concentrations of these substances. Logistically, a screening test that utilizes the urine, such as is done in screening studies for diabetes mellitus, would have far more patient appeal than a test involving a venipuncture. Table 6 lists the substances that have been investigated in urine as possible markers for carcinoma of the prostate. Despite a good deal of intensive study, no marker has been found in the urine that even approaches the serum acid phosphatase predictability. In 1975 Fair et al published their results with urinary polyamine determinations in patients with carcinoma of the prostate [42]. In these preliminary observations it appeared that the urinary excretion of the polyamine spermidine was increased in patients with carcinoma of the prostate compared to controls. However, subsequent investigations conducted at our institution, using a more sensitive technique for polyamine detection, have failed to confirm this finding. In conclusion, to date, no urinary screening test for carcinoma of the prostate exists, nor does one appear promising in the immediate future.

Prostatic fluid markers

Prout et al [38] and Belitsky et al [43] found that there was an alteration in the LDH isoenzyme pattern in the serum of patients with carinoma of the prostate as compared with normals. In the normal individual there was a much higher level of LDH 1 as compared to LDH 5, however, in patients with carcinoma of the prostate this finding was reversed. In subsequent years Grayhack et al [44] have done a detailed study of biochemical changes in the prostatic fluid of patients with

Table 4. CK-BB in untreated patients (Washington University series)

Stage	Number elevated assays	(%)
A	1/13	(7.7)
B	1/23	(4.3)
C	4/24	(16.7)
D	4/19	(21.1)
Ustaged	0/5	(0.0)
Totals	10/84	(11.9)

carcinoma of the prostate. Table 7 is a summation of their findings. It appears that the measurement of LDH 5/1 ratio, increased C3 levels and an elevation of transferrin values, are found in the prostatic fluid of patients with carcinoma of the prostate compared with normals or patients with BPH. One caveat is that in patients with increased number of white cells in the prostatic secretion, the LDH 5/1 was frequently found to be elevated. Hence, this ratio is of little value in separating patients with inflammatory disease of the prostate from those with carcinoma of the prostate.

Another factor that limits the usefulness of the prostatic secretion to make the diagnosis of prostatic carcinoma is the logistical problem that must be surmounted. Obviously, the patient must be referred to a physician who is skilled in the technique of prostatic massage so that the fluid can be obtained. Furthermore, in young patients, or some patients with carcinoma of the prostate, it is often not possible to obtain prostatic secretion despite vigorous massage.

Conclusions

There is currently no biochemical or immunologic tumor marker, detectable in blood, urine or prostatic fluid, that can fulfill the rigorous criteria required of a screening test for early detection of carcinoma of the prostate.

The interested reader is referred to a diligent review by Catalona and Menon assessing the quantitative potential of many of the markers outlined above in terms of their sensitivity, specificity and predictive value [45].

Imaging modalities

Radiologic imaging is the primary diagnostic modality in a substantial number of human malignancies – carcinoma of the lung, gastrointestinal tumors, intracra-

Table 5. Prostate antigen (PA) (Wang, et al. [42])

Group	No.	PA elevated	(%)
Normal females	17	0	
Normal males	51	5	(9.8)
BPH	19	13	(68.4)[a]
Stage A	8	5	(62.5)
Stage B	34	27	(79.4)
Stage C	56	43	(76.8)[a]
Stage D	344	296	(86.0)[a]

[a] $P = 0.01$

nial tumors – to name a few. Mammography is a classic example of a radiologic technique used in screening a high risk population for a common neoplasm.

Traditionally, imaging modalities have played no role whatsoever in the initial diagnosis of carcinoma of the prostate. However, with the advent of new imaging techniques this situation may be changing rapidly.

Plain film radiography and contrast radiography have no value in diagnosing early prostate cancer. Computed tomography (CT), magnetic resonance imaging (MRI) and sonography have been tried clinically and will be discussed. Radioimmunodetection and positron emission tommography (PET) scanning are experimental techniques that hold promise for the future and will be addressed.

Computed tomography (CT)

Because the attenuation values for prostate cancer overlap those of benign hyperplasia, CT scanning cannot diagnose carcinoma confined to the prostate [46]. In fact, a CT image of the prostate cannot outline any detailed features of the parechnyma of the gland – except for calcification [47]. A CT diagnosis of prostatic malignancy can only be based on the identification of secondary signs i.e. bladder base filtration, abnormalities of the seminal vesicles, and infiltration of tissue planes surrounding the prostate [47, 48]. These signs, when present, clearly represent advanced disease.

Magnetic resonance imaging (MRI)

This is a relatively new technological development that has generated a great deal of enthusiasm in the last three years. Briefly – MRI imaging is based on the response of hydrogen protons in tissues (mostly in tissue water) to applied radio-frequency pulses. By computer reconstruction an image reflecting the distribution of protons in transverse, sagittal or coronal planes of the body is obtained.

Clinical experience in the application of MRI to the diagnosis and staging of

Table 6. Possible urinary markers – carcinoma of the prostate

Polyamines (spermidine)
Cholesterol
Carcinoplacental antigen
Carcinembryonic antigen
Hydroxyproline
Isoleucine
Fibronectin

prostate cancer is limited at the present time. Preliminary work at our institution and at other centers suggests that prostatic carcinoma has a distinctive appearance on MRI images, that extension outside the capsule can be detected, and that lymph node involvement can be visualized as well [49–52].

Large scale clinical studies comparing the value of MRI to CT scanning and/or ultrasound for early detection of low stage prostate cancer are not available at the present time.

Prostatic ultrasonography

Most of the emphasis in recent years has been placed on ultrasonography for the diagnosis of prostatic pathology, including carcinoma of the prostate. This is reflected in the large number of publications on prostatic ultrasound imaging since the introduction of the transrectal approach by Watanabe et al in 1971 [53–69].

Ultrasonic images of the prostate can be obtained by transabdominal, transperineal, transurethral or transrectal routes. The transperineal route, however, is limited in its ability to adequately visualize the prostate and has been abandoned [47]. The transurethral approach requires the use of a sterile technique and general or regional anesthesia and therefore, has not been used extensively [47]. The transabdominal ultrasonogram can define general features like the size and shape of the prostate, however, it depicts only about 50% of the focal lesions seen on the transrectal image [65]. Consequently, transrectal ultrasound is the most sensitive and currently the most popular method for evaluation of the prostate [47, 58–60, 64–69].

The initial transrectal ultrasound intrumentation used a bistable display which enabled little more than a visualization of the prostatic capsule and a definition of the size and shape of the gland [53]. The introduction of gray-scale sonography constituted a major advance providing a better definition of the parenchymal echo texture as well as of the prostatic capsule [55, 56].

Current instrumentation for transrectal ultrasonography includes specialized rectal probes that use either a radially rotating (transverse images) or a linear array (longitudinal images) real-time transducer [47]. The earliest radial scan units

Table 7. Prostatic fluid values (Grayhack and Lee [44])

	Normals		BPH		Cancer	
Assay	No.	Mean	No.	Mean	No.	Mean
LDH5/LDH1	228	.69	117	2.01	92	5.91
C₃ Complement	58	1.82	67	3.63	60	17.86
Transferrin	56	6.46	66	11.45	58	42.73

incorporated a specially designed chair which the patient was required to sit in. The rectal probe covered by a rubber condom protruded through a central hole in the chair, and was inserted into the rectum as the patient was seated [47, 53]. More recently, commercially available radial scanners utilize a hand-held probe that can be inserted into the rectum with the patient in the lateral decubitus, lithotomy or knee-chest positions. The radial probe images the prostate in a transverse orientation and the examiner moves the probe superiorly and inferiorly at sequential intervals to achieve complete visualization of the prostate from the apex to the seminal vesicles and vice versa. The linear array real time transducer, introduced more recently is also mounted on a hand-held probe and displays a longitudinal orientation of the prostate. The probe has to be rotated clockwise and counterclockwise in order to encompass the entire gland.

Several questions need to be addressed, in order to evaluate the exact role of transrectal ultrasound in detection of prostatic malignancy: (1) What are the ultrasonic characteristics of prostatic carcinoma? (2) Are these characteristics specific enough to enable an accurate diagnosis? (3) Is transrectal ultrasound capable of depicting stage A lesions? (4) Is transrectal ultrasound superior to the digital examination for detecting stage B or C lesions? And finally, (5) Is transrectal ultrasound a potential screening tool for detection of early prostate cancer?

Advanced prostatic cancer displays a characteristic constellation of features on the sonographic image. The gland is usually enlarged in size with marked deformation and asymmetry, a distorted irregular capsule with interruptions in its continuity and a heterogenous internal echo pattern observed on occasions, to extend through the capsule into the periprostatic tissues or into the seminal vesicles [47, 57–60]. The sonographic pattern produced by smaller tumors confined to the capsule of the prostate is less clearly defined. Traditionally most authors considered the echo texture of prostatic cancer to be isoechoic or moderately hyperechoic in relation to the normal prostatic parenchyma [47, 57–60, 65–68]. Recently, Lee et. al examined 211 patients with transrectal ultrasound in both the longitudinal and transverse planes, and reported that all of the 33 histologically confirmed cancers were either purely hypoechoic or had mixed echogenicity [69]. These authors concluded that prostate cancers are hypoechoic in echotexture and that a heterogenous mixed echogenicity pattern resulted when the tumor infiltrated either adjacent normal parenchyma or benign adenomatous nodules. The only way, in my mind, to reconcile these divergent views is to conduct a large scale prospective study involving patients who undergo radical prostatectomy. By step-sectioning the surgical specimens and comparing them to preoperative prostatic sonograms, it should be possible to determine the exact echotexture associated with cancerous lesions.

Unfortunately, the ultrasonic characteristics of prostatic carcinoma are nonspecific. Heterogeneity of the internal echotexture can be produced by a variety of inflammatory conditions (bacterial and non-bacterial prostatitis, granulomatous prostatitis, tuberculous prostatitis) as well as by prostatic infarcts and surgical procedures. These entities can also cause asymmetry of the gland and distortion of the capsule [57–60].

Evidence is accumulating that some stage A tumors can be detected by transrectal ultrasound. Resnick diagnosed 10 histologically confirmed prostatic cancers on transrectal ultrasonograms of 621 patients with symptoms of bladder outlet obstruction and normal rectal examinations [58]. Four other patients in the same study who were eventually found to have stage A2 cancers, had false negative sonograms. Brooman et al have picked up 3 unsuspected cancers by prostatic ultrasound examination of 68 patients with presumed benign hyperplasia [59]. They had a 4% rate of false negative sonograms. In a subsequent study, Brooman et al reported that 11 out of a total of 13 cancers found among 156 patients with presumed benign hyperplasia were correctly diagnosed ultrasonographically [60]. Fritzsche et al found no cases of clinically unsuspected cancer in their series of 228 patients examined by transrectal ultrasound [64]. However, only half of their patients were subjected to prostatectomy, and the prostatic needle biopsies in the remaining patients were not performed under sonographic control. It has been shown that random biopsies of non-palpable prostatic lesions are of limited value [70]. Hastak et al have demonstrated the accuracy of ultrasonically guided prostatic biopsy [62]. Needle biopsy of the prostate under sonographic control may well be the only reliable method to confirm the diagnosis of a small stage A tumor.

The standard by which any diagnostic technique for prostate cancer should be measured is the digital rectal examination. In the study by Brooman et al, out of 186 urological patients evaluated by both prostatic ultrasound and a rectal examination, 70 cases of histologically confirmed cancer were identified [59]. The ultrasound examination diagnosed 30 out of 32 patients with clinical stage C disease. There was one false negative ultrasonic diagnosis and another patient was correctly identified as having chronic prostatitis rather than prostatic cancer. The digital examination correctly identified 31 cancer patients and one patient (with chronic prostatitis) had a false positive diagnosis of carcinoma, thus, transrectal ultrasound and the digital rectal examination were comparable in accuracy for the detection of stage C disease. Only 30 out of 60 patients, considered on rectal examination to have stage B disease, were actually found to have cancer histologically. This is similar to other studies evaluating the accuracy of the rectal examination in the diagnosis of prostatic nodules [71]. Transrectal ultrasound, by comparison, identified 28 of the 30 patients with cancer, and correctly diagnosed 19 additional patients as having benign disease. In this group, therefore, prostatic ultrasound improved on the accuracy of the rectal examination by correctly diagnosing 47 out of the 60 patients (78%). Two patients, however, had a false-negative ultrasonic diagnosis. Perhaps more significantly, 13 of the patients with clinical stage B disease had evidence of a capsular breach and thus were upstaged by the ultrasound examination. Several other studies confirmed the improved accuracy of transrectal ultrasound in staging prostate cancer [60, 66–68]. The rectal examination is notorious for understaging prostatic tumors, most likely because an extension of the tumor through the anterior or anterolateral aspects of the capsule cannot possibly be detected by the palpating finger [59].

Watanabe et al initiated mass screening for prostate cancer by transrectal ultrasound and calculated that the examination could be performed within 15 minutes at a cost of $5 per patient [54]. In a subsequent study, these authors examined 1741 male patients by transrectal ultrasound [57]. This is the largest series of prostatic ultrasounds published to date. Several caveats need to be stressed. First, the study population comprised of patients visiting the urology clinic, in whom prostatic disease was suspected clinically. Secondly, the study was not double blinded, the rectal examination findings were taken into consideration when interpreting the ultrasonograms. Thirdly, the study was performed in Japan. The occurrence of prostate cancer is known to be significantly lower in a Japanese population in comparison to Western countries [54, 72, 73]. A histologic diagnosis of prostate cancer was eventually made in 68 patients. The diagnosis was made by ultrasound in 66 cases. Two cancers were missed by the ultrasonogram. The clinical stage of the tumors detected was not specified. An important aspect of this study is that prostatic cancer was suspected in 383 patietns (22% of the total patient population) and eventually confirmed in only 66, reflecting a considerable number of false positive diagnoses (for every patient diagnosed as having prostate cancer, 5 additional patients underwent an unnecessary biopsy).

In conclusion, transrectal gray scale prostatic ultrasonography is a tool of high sensitivity, but rather low specificity for the primary diagnosis of prostate cancer. Available data suggest that it is capable of detecting some clinically unsuspected (stage A) cancers and that it is superior to the rectal examination in the local staging of this disease. Meticulously conducted studies are still required to define the exact echotexture of prostatic tumors. Mass screening of an asymptomatic population with prostatic ultrasound for early detection of prostate cancer is probably impractical at the present time. Prostatic ultrasound, however, is here to stay. With additional experience and technological advances, its role in the diagnosis, staging and management of prostate cancer is certain to expand.

Radioimmunodetection

The idea of producing radiolabeled antibodies that target antigens on human tumors for tumor localization with nuclear medicine techniques is not new. Pressman is credited with some of the pioneer studies in animals using radiolabeled antibodies for tumor detection [74]. Goldenberg, DeLand and their associates were also among the pioneers in this field [75], and with time, studies in humans have demonstrated the ability of this technique to visualize human tumor metastases [76].

In recent years, efforts to apply this technique to prostatic carcinoma have concentrated on the natural marker of this tumor – prostatic acid phosphatase. Metastatic deposits of prostate cancer have been visualized using IgG antibodies against prostatic acid phosphatase labeled with I–131 [77]. This work is still in its infancy and it is premature to determine whether this method will be useful for early detection of prostatic carcinoma. Based on theoretical considerations – it seems unlikely that such a radiolabeled antibody will be able to distinguish a prostatic cancer from normal or hyperplastic prostatic tissue which also manufacture and secrete prostatic acid phosphatase. Furthermore, the extent to which monoclonal antibodies or the utilization of other antigens might enhance the sensitivity and specificity of clinical immunodiagnosis of prostate cancer is at present, still undetermined.

Position emission tomography (PET) imaging

The PET scanner utilizes positron emitting radionuclides. Positron decay involves the simultaneous emission of two photons at 180∘. The PET scanner is composed of circumferentially arranged individual pairs of detectors. Each member of a pair is situated on a ring in a diametrically opposed position to its mate. Events are accepted only when two photons are detected simultaneously by both members of a pair of detectors (termed 'annihilation coincidence detection'). A computer reconstructs the distribution of activity in a cross section of the body to create an image superficially resembling a CT scan [78]. This arrangement results in a resolution superior to that of conventional nuclear medicine equipment which utilizes single photon emitting radionuclides. Changes in amounts of radioactivity as small as 10% can be reliably quantitated between regions of $1.5\,cm^2$ on individual tomographic slices with 95% accuracy [79].

PET scanning has been applied clinically by neurologists and cardiologists with spectacular results [79–81]. The PET scanner has been exploited by Fair et al in 1977 to image the dog prostate with a positron-emitting putrescine analog which was preferentially taken up by the prostate [82]. Since then, no further work has been done with this imaging device in urology. However, studies have been published suggesting the potential usefulness of this instrument for imaging of brain and other tumors [83]. Given the proper tracer, the PET scanner could possibly be used in the future for detection of prostatic cancer.

Conclusion

Magnetic resonance imaging, radioimmunodetection and the PET scanner hold future promise for detection of prostatic carcinoma. However, of all the new imaging modalities, transrectal ultrasound has engendered the greatest expectations for early diagnosis, staging and follow-up of this disease.

Digital rectal examination

The rectal examination remains a keystone for early detection of prostate cancer. While, by definition, it cannot pick up any stage A lesion, about 50% of patients with a palpable abnormality of the prostate have subsequent histological confirmation of prostatic malignancy [71]. Guinan et al compared the relative accuracy of 10 diagnostic procedures for detection of prostate cancer in 300 elderly patients with symptoms of urinary obstruction [84]. They concluded that the rectal examination was the most efficient test superseding acid phosphatase determination (enzymatic, RIA or CIEP), urinary and prostatic secretion cytology, aspiration cytology, LDH V/I ratio or leukocyte adherence inhibition test.

Some reports have attested to the efficiency of routine rectal examination in detecting early prostate cancer, and have demonstrated an increase in the percentage of tumors diagnosed while still confined to the prostate [85, 86]. Several more recent series have shown that rectal examination screening for carcinoma of the prostate detected the disease in 1.0%–1.7% of an unselected male population over the age of 50 years [87, 88, 89]. Overall, prostate cancer was confirmed histologically in 26%–29% of patients with palpable prostatic abnormalities [87, 88]. This, perhaps, reflects a higher index of suspicion by the examining physicians than in previous studies [71].

Conclusion

It appears that screening an elderly population for carcinoma of the prostate by the digital rectal examination can be cost-effective and fairly sensitive. Although the sensitivity could be enhanced by transrectal prostatic ultrasound (to include some stage A tumors), this test would result in a considerably higher proportion of unnecessary prostate biopsies. The value of other new imaging modalities for early detection of prostate cancer remains to be determined. There is currently no biochemical or immunologic tumor marker that fulfills the rigorous criteria of sensitivity and specificity required of a screening test for early diagnosis of carcinoma of the prostate.

References

1. Silverberg E: Cancer Statistics–1985. CA35: 19–35, 1985
2. Walsh PC, Jewett HJ: Radical surgery for prostatic cancer. Cancer 45: 1906–1911, 1980
3. Hodges CV, Pearse HD, Stille L: Radical prostatectomy fot carcinoma: 30–year experience and 15–year survivals. J Urol 122: 180–182, 1979
4. Catalona WJ, Scott WW: Carcinoma of the prostate. In: Campbell's Urology, Walsh PC, Gittes RF, Perlmutter AD, Stamey tA (eds). 5th Edition. WB Saunders Company, Philadelphia, 1463–1534, 1986
5. Sheldon CA, Williams RD, Fraley EE: Incidental carcinoma of the prostate: A review of the literature and critical reappraisal of classification. J Urol 124: 626–630, 1980
6. Murphy GP, Natarajan N, Pontes RL et al.: The national survey of prostate cancer in the United States by the American College of Surgeons, J Urol 127: 928–934, 1982
7. Gutman AB, Gutman EB: 'Acid' phosphatase occurring in the serum of patients with metastasizing carcinoma of the prostate gland. J Clin Invest 17: 473, 1938
8. Roy AV, Brower ME, Hayden JE: Sodium thymolphthalein monophosphate: A new acid phosphatase substrate with greater specificity for the prostatic enzyme in serum. Clin Chem 17: 1093–1102, 1971
9. Nesbit RM, Baum WB: Serum phosphatase determination in diagnosis of prostatic cancer; a review of 1,150 cases. JAMA 145: 1321–1324, 1951
10. Murphy GP, Reynoso G, Kenny GM et al.: Comparison of total and prostatic fraction serum acid phosphatase levels in patients with differentiated and undifferentiated prostatic carcinoma. Cancer 23: 1309–1314, 1969
11. Ganem EJ: The prognostic significance of an elevated serum acid phosphatase level in advanced prostatic carcinoma. J Urol 76: 179–181, 1956
12. Byar DP, Corle DK, VACURG: VACURG randomized trial of radical prostatectomy for stages I and II prostate cancer. Urology 17(4) suppl.: 7–11, 1981
13. Whitesel JA, Donohue RE, Mani JH et al.: Acid phosphatase: Its influence on the management of carcinoma of the prostate. J Urol 131: 70–72, 1984
14. Foti AG, Cooper JF, Herschman H et al.: Detection of prostate cancer by solid-phase radioimmunoassay of serum prostatic acid phosphatase. N Engl J Med 297: 1357–1361, 1977
15. Chu TM, Wang MC, Scott WW, et al.: Immunochemical detection of serum prostatic acid phosphatase. Methodology and clinical evaluation. Invest Urol 15: 319–323, 1978
16. Vihko P, Sajatni E, Janne O, et al.: Serum prostate-specific acid phosphatase: development and validation of a specific radioimmunoassay. Clin Chem 24: 1915–1919, 1978
17. Gittes RF: Acid phosphatase reappraised. N Engl J Med 297: 1398–1399, 1977
18. Bruce AW, Mahan DE, Sullivan LD, et al.: The significance of prostatic acid phosphatase in adenocarcinoma of the prostate. J Urol 125: 357–360, 1981
19. Griffiths JD: Prostate-specific acid phosphatase: re-evaluation of radioimmunoassay in diagnosing prostatic disease. Clin Chem 26: 433–436, 1980
20. Fair WR, Heston WDW, Kadmon D, et al.: Prostatic cancer, acid phosphatase, creatine kinase-BB and race: a prospective study. J Urol 128: 735–738, 1982
21. Fleischmann J, Catalona WJ, Fair WR, et al.: Lack of value of radioimmunoassay for prostatic acid phosphatase as a screening test for prostatic cancer in patients with obstructive prostatic hyperplasia. J Urol 129: 312–314, 1983
22. Vihko P, Kontturi M, Lukkarinen O, et al. Immunoreactive prostatic acid phosphatase in prostatic cancer: diagnosis and follow-up of patients. J Urol 133: 979–982, 1985
23. Lindholm GR, Stirton MS, Liedtke RJ, et al.: Prostatic acid phosphatase bu radioimmunoassay JAMA 244: 2071–2073, 1980
24. Carson JL, Eisenberg JM, Shaw LM. et al.: Diagnostic accuracy of four assays of prostatic acid phosphatase. JAMA 253: 665–669, 1985

25. Pontes EJ: Biological markers in prostate cancer. K Urol 130: 1037–1047, 1983

26. Quinones GR, Rohner Jr TJ, Drago et al.: Will prostatic acid phosphatase of early prostatic cancer? J Urol 125: 361–364, 1981

27. Watson RA, Tang DB: The predictive value of prostatic acid phosphatase as a screening test for prostatic cancer. N Engl J Med 303: 497–499, 1980

28. Kiesling VJJr, Watson RA: A closer look at serum prostatic acid phosphatase as a screening test. Urology 16: 242–244, 1980

29. Feld R, Witte D: Presence of creatine kinase BB isoenzyme in some patients with prostatic cancer. Clin Chem 23: 1930–1932, 1977

30. Silverman L, Chapman J, Jones M, et al.: Creatine kinase BB and other markers of prostatic carcinoma. Prostate 2: 109–119, 1981

31. Forman DT: The significance of creatine kinase (CKBB) in metastatic cancer of the prostate. Ann Clin Lab Sci 9: 333–337, 1979

32. Wang NC, Valenzuela LA, Murphy GP, et al.: Purification of a human prostate specific antigen. Invest Urol 17: 159–163, 1979

33. Wang MC, Papsidero LD, Kuriyama M, et al.: Prostate antigen: a new potential marker ofr prostatic cancer. Prostate 2: 89–96, 1981

34. Kuriyama M, Wang MC, Lee CI, et al.: Use of human prostate-specific antigen in monitoring prostate cancer. Cancer Res 41: 3874–3876, 1981

35. Pontes JE, Chu TM, Slack N, et al.: Serum prostatic antigen measurement in localized prostatic cancer: correlation with clinical course. J Urol 128: 1216–1218, 1982

36. Wajsman Z, Chu JM, Bross D, et al.: Clinical significance of serum alkaline phosphatase isoenzymes in advanced prostate carcinoma. J Urol 119: 244–246, 1978

37. Denis LJ, Prout Jr GR: Lactic dehydrogenase in prostatic cancer. Incest Urol 1: 101–111, 1963

38. Prout GRJr, Macalalaf Jr EV, Fenis LJ, et al.: Alterations in serum lactate dehydrogenase and its fourth and fifth isozymes in patients with prostatic cancer. J Urol 94: 451–461, 1965

39. Killian CS, Vargas FP, Beckley, et al.: Analysis of serial erthrocyte polyamines by automated reverse-phase liquid chromatography (HPLC). Clin Chem abstract 122, 26: 983, 1980

40. Chiasiri P. Harper M, Blamey R, et al.: Plasma spermidine concentrations in patients with tumors of the breast or prostate or testis. Clin Chem Acta 104: 367–375, 1980

41. Durie BOM, Salmon SE, Russell DH: Polyamines as markers of response and disease activity in cancer chemotherapy. Cancer Res 37: 214–221, 1977

42. Fair WR, Wehner N, Bronson U: Urinary polyamine levels in the diagnosis of carcinoma of the prostate. J Urol 114: 88–92, 1975

43. Belitsky P, Elhilali MM, Oliver JA, et al.: Serum lactate dehydrogenase isoenzyme changes in carcinoma of the prostate. J Urol 103: 770–773, 1970

44. Grayhack JT, Lee C: Evaluation of prostatic fluid in prostatic pathology. In: The prostatic cell structure and function, Murphy GP, Sandberg AA, Karr JP (eds). Liss New York, 231, 1981

45. Catalona WJ, Menon M: New screening and diagnostic tests for prostate cancer and immunologic assessment. Urology 17(3) suppl. 61–65, 1981

46. Levitt RG, Sagel SS, Stanley RJ, et al.: Computed tomography of the pelvis. Semin Roentgenol 13: 192–200, 1978

47. Rifkin MD: The prostate and seminal vesicles, in Rifkin MD (ed): Diagnostic imaging of the lower genitourinary tract. Raven Press, New York, 122–208, 1985

48. Rickards D, Gowland M, Brooman P, et al.: computed tomography and transrectal ultrasound in the diagnosis of prostatic disease – a comparative study. Br J Urol 55: 726–732, 1983

49. Hricak H, Williams RD, Spring DB et al.: Anatomy and pathology of the male pelvis by magnetic resonance imaging. AJR 141: 1101–1110, 1983

50. Bryan PJ, Butler HE, LiPuma Jp: Magnetic resonance imaging of the pelvis. Radiol Clin of North Am 22: 897–915, 1984

51. Dooms GC, Hricak H, Crooks Higgins CB: Magnetic resonance imaging of the lymph nodes: comparison with CT. Radiology 153: 719–728, 1984

52. Lee JKT, Heiken JP, Ling D, et al.: Magnetic resonance imaging of abdominal and pelvis lymphadenopathy. Radiolgy 153: 181–188, 1984

53. Watanabe H, Kaiho H, Tonaka M, et al.: Diagnostic application of ultrasonotomography to the prostate. Invest Urol 8: 548–559, 1971

54. Watanabe H, Saitoh M, Mishina T, et al.: Mass screening program for prostatic diseases with transrectal ultrasonotomography. J Urol 117: 746–748, 1977

55. Harada K, Tanashashi Y, Igari D, et al.: Clinical evaluation of inside echo patterns in gray scale prostatic echography. J Urol 124: 216–220, 1980

56. Gammelgaard J, Holm HH: Transurethral and transrectal ultrasonic scanning in urology. J Urol 124: 863–868, 1980

57. Watanabe H, Date S, Ohe H, et al.: A survey of 3,000 examinations by transrectal ultrasonotomography. Prostate 1: 271–278, 1980

58. Resnick MI: Evaluation of prostatic carcinoma: noninvasive and preoperative techniques. Prostate 1:311–320, 1980

59. Brooman PJC, Griffiths GJ, Roberts E, et al.: Per rectal ultrasound in the investigation of prostatic disease. Clin Radiol 32: 669–676, 1981

60. Brooman PJC, Peeling WB, Griffiths GJ, et al.: A comparison between digital examination and per-rectal ultrasound in the evaluation of the prostate. Br J Urol 53: 617–620, 1981

61. Hastak SM, Gammelgaard J, holm HH: Transrectal ultrasonic volume determination of the prostate – a preoperative and postoperative study. J Urol 127: 1115–1118, 1982

62. Hastak SM, Gammelgaard J, Holm HH: Ultrasonically guided transperineal biopsy in the diagnosis of prostatic carcinoma. J Urol 128: 69–71, 1982

63. Peeling WB, Griffiths GJ: Imaging of the prostate by ultrasound. J Urol 132: 217–224, 1984

64. Fritzsche PJ, Axford PD, Ching VJ, et al.: Correlation of transrectal sonographic findings in patients with suspected and unsuspected prostatic disease. J Urol 130: 272–273, 1983

65. Rifkin MD, Kurtz AB, Choi HY, et al.: Endoscopic ultrasonic evaluation of the prostate using a transrectal probe: prospective evaluation and acoustic characitrization. Radiology 149: 264–271, 1983

66. Pontes EJ, Ohe H, Watanabe H, et al.: Transrectal ultrasonography of the prostate. Cancer 53: 1369–1372, 1984

67. Pontes ej, Eisenkraft S, Watanabe H, et al.: Preoperative evaluation of localized prostatic carcinoma by transrectal ultrasonography. J Urol 134: 289–291, 1985

68. Fujina A, Scardino PT: Transrectal ultrasonography for prostatic cancer: its value in staging and monitoring the response to radiotherapy and chemotherapy. J Urol 133: 806–810, 1985

69. Lee F, Gray JM, McLeary RD, et al.: Transrectal ultrasound in the diagnosis of prostate cancer: location echogenicity, histopathology and staging. Prostate 7: 117–129, 1985

70. Catalona WJ: Yield from routine prostatic needle biopsy in patients more than 50 years old referred for urologic evaluation: A preliminary report. J Urol 124: 844–846, 1980

71. Grayhack JT, Bockrath JM: Diagnosis of carcinoma of the prostate. Urology 17(3) Suppl: 54–60, 1981

72. Silverberg E, Lubera JA: A review of American Cancer society estimates of cancer cases and deaths. CA 33: 2–25, 1983

73. Hutchison GB: Incidence and etiology of prostate cancer. Urology 17(3) Suppl: 4–10, 1981

74. Pressman D, Korngold L: The in vivo localization of anti-Wagner osteogenic sarcoma antibodies. Cancer 6: 7619–7623, 1953

75. Goldenberg DM, DeLand FH, Kim EE, et al.: Use of radiolabeled antibodies to carcinoembryonic antigen for the detection and localization of diverse cancers by external photoscanning. N Engl J Med 298: 1384–1386, 1978

76. larson SM, carrasquillo Ja, Krohn KA, McGuffin RW, Hellstrom I, Hellstrom KE, Lyster D:

Diagnostic imaging of malignant melanoma with radiolabeled anti-tumor antiboedies. JAMA 249: 811–812, 1983

77. Goldenberg DM, DeLand FH, Bennett SJ, et al.: Radioimmunodetection of prostatic cancer: In vivo use of radioactive antibodies against prostatic acid phosphatase for diagnosis and detection of prostatic cancer by nuclear imaging. JAMA 250: 630–635, 1983

78. Ter-Pogossian M, Phelps ME, Hoffman EJ, et al.: A positron emission transaxial tomography for nuclear imaging (PETT). Radiology 114: 89–98, 1975

79. Phelps ME, Kuhl DE, Mazziotta JC: Metabolic mapping of the brain's response to visual stimulation: studies in humans. Science 211: 1445–1448, 1981

80. Phelps ME, Mazziotta JC: Positron emission tomography: Human brain function and biochemistry. Science 228: 799–809, 1985

81. Schelbert HR: Blood flow and substrate use in normal and diseased myocardium pp. 342–348: In Phelps Me, Moderator. Positron computed tomography for studies of myocardial and cerebral function. Ann Intern Med 98: 339–359, 1983

82. Fair WR, Miller TR, Siegel BA et al.: Radionuclide imaging of dog prostate. Urology 12: 575–578, 1978

83. Beaney RP: Position emission tomography in the study of human tumors. Semin Nucl Med 14: 324–341, 1984

84. Guinan P, Bush I, Ray V, et al.: The accuracy of the rectal examination in the diagnosis of prostate carcinoma. N Engl J Med 303: 499–503, 1980

85. Gilbertson VA: Cancer of the prostate gland: results of early diagnosis and therapy undertaken for cure of the disease. JAMA 215: 81–84, 1971

86. Donohue RE, Fauver HE, Whitesel JA et al.: Staging prostatic cancer: a different distribution. J Urol 122: 327–329, 1979

87. Thompson IA, Ernst JJ, Gangai MP, et al.: Adenocarcinoma of the prostate: results of routine urological screening. J Urol 132: 690–692, 1984

88. Chodak GW, Schoenberg HW: Early detection of prostate cancer by routine screening. JAMA 252: 3261–3264, 1984

89. Vihko P, Kontturi M, Lukkarinen O, et al.: Screening for carcinoma of the prostate. Cancer 56: 173–177, 1985

Editorial Comment

MARTIN I. RESNICK

Webster's Unabridged Dictionary defines editorial as: 'An article in a newspaper, magazine, etc. explicitly stating opinions of the editor or publisher' [1]. In defining opinion the same reference states: 'A belief not based on absolute certainty or positive knowledge but on what seems true, valid or probable to one's own mind.' I will attempt to exercise the perogatives of an editor and express my thoughts as defined in Webster's and hopefully clearly state *my opinion* as to the effectiveness and practicality of many of the studies and examinations described most amply by Dr. Kadmon.

Statistical terms

Many of the studies described by Dr. Kadmon are available to most practicing urologists but their value and usefulness has not been fully clarified. All too often a new test is described, the statistics as to its effectiveness reported and its universal application extolled. Unfortunately, the limitations of the test are infrequently reported, the costs rarely mentioned and its practical usefulness in the 'real world' never discussed. Statisticians have defined guidelines that are useful in assisting clinicians in evaluating the effectiveness of these new tests. A discussion of these statistical guidelines would therefore be useful in providing background information that will allow one to make an independent evaluation of a particular study. For purposes of discussion specific diagnostic tests will be described with the consideration that they be used for the purpose of screening a specified population in an attempt to diagnose early and potentially curable prostatic carcinoma.

It is important to have an understanding of several terms that are often used in reports of both diagnostic laboratory and imaging studies. These include: specificity, sensitivity, positive predictive value and negative predictive value. Oftentimes the effectiveness of the diagnostic study are reported in terms of false positive and false negative rates but more valid terms as will be described should be used more uniformly.

Sensitivity can be mathematically expressed as:

$$\frac{\text{number of patients with true positive study}}{\text{number of patients with positive histology}} \times 100$$

The term refers to the number of patients who actual have the disease and test positive divided by the total number of patients with the disease.

Specificity can be mathematically expressed as:

$$\frac{\text{number of patients with true negative study}}{\text{number of patients with negative histology}} \times 100$$

This term refers to the number of patients who actual do not have the disease and test negative divided by the total number of patients without the disease.

When relating studies to disease prevalence in a particular population the valid statistical terms to use include positive predictive value and negative predictive value. Utilizing data on sensitivity (Se), specificity (Sp) and prevalence or proportion of the population having the disease (P) positive predictive value can be expressed as [2, 3]:

$$\frac{(Se) \times (P)}{(Se)(P) + (1 - Sp)(1 - P)} \times 100$$

Utilizing similar terms negative predictive values can be expressed as:

$$\frac{(Sp) \times (1 - P)}{(Sp)(1 - P) + (P)(1 - Se)} \times 100$$

Similarly utilizing the terms true positive false positive, true negative and false negative when the proportion of the population having the disease is known the positive predictive value can be expressed as:

$$\frac{\text{number of true positives}}{\text{number of true positives plus number of false positives}} \times 100$$

and the negative predictive value can be expressed as:

$$\frac{\text{number of true negatives}}{\text{number of true negatives plus number of false negatives}} \times 100$$

Positive predictive value is the probability that the disease is in fact present given a positive result and similarly the negative predictive value is the probability the disease is absent given a negative result. Since these calculations are based on sensitivity, specificity and prevalence of the disease in a specific population they are helpful is assessing a test's value from a statistical standpoint. In that neither specificity or sensitivity relates to the prevalence of a specific disease in the population being studied, oftentimes misinformation can result when these terms are used alone in that the data cannot properly interpreted. This has been clearly emphasized by Sheps and Schechter who have shown both the misuse and lack of use of these terms in their medical literature [4].

In many reports the prevalence of the disease in the study population does not necessarily represent the true prevalence of the disease in the general population. If for example, 11 patients with a disease and 22 patients without the disease were studied and the sensitivity and specificity were 100 percent (11/11) and 91 percent (20/22) respectively, the prevalence of the disease in the population studied would be 11/33 or 33 percent. However, if the *true* prevalence of the same disease in the general population is 1/2000 (0.0005) the positive and negative predictive values would calculate to be 0.6 percent and 100 percent respectively. A negative test the chance the disease is absent, reliably excludes the disease but an abnormal test labels 9 percent (2/22) of individuals without the disease and 100 percent (11/11) with the disease as positive and is associated with an actual chance of having the disease of only 0.6%. The finding of a positive test would therefore cause much anxiety to the family and patient even though the chance of that individual having the disease is remote. It must be remembered that in this example the specificity and sensitivity are quite high.

Another example that has been cited relates to the misuse of these terms. In a recent report studying the value of rectal examination for the screening of a population in an attempts to detect carcinoma of the prostate the authors use the term specificity when they are referring to predictive value [5]. Recalculation of these data in fact shows the true predictive value to be lower than had originally been appreciated [6].

The ideal test

Prior to discussing specific studies it may be useful to speculate as to what whould be the ideal test that could be used to screen a specific population for prostate cancer. Initially most would agree that ideally a non-invasive test, preferably on an easily obtainable body fluid such as serum or urine would be preferable. It would also be desirable if a test not only was highly specific and sensitive but also very reliable in predicting either the presence or absence of the disease in a specific population. Finally, the test should not only identify patients with the disease but also differentiate those individuals whose disease is potentially progressive and lethal in contrast to those having indolent or dormant tumors that will not progress and therefore not be life threatening. Obviously those patients in the former category require further evaluation and therapy and those in the latter would neither benefit from nor require other therapeutic approaches.

Carcinoma of the prostate presents many problems when considering these ideals. The disease has a high prevalence rate in the American male population so that a highly sensitive and specific test would likely identify all patients with the disease. On first impression this concept seems advantageous but most clinicians recognize that many of these patients particularly those over 75 or 80 years of age often have non-progressive disease which is not likely to be life threatening. Jewett and associates and Whitmore have both reported that not all patients with discrete localized prostatic nodules will progress to more advanced stages but unfortunately clinical studies do not exist that will reliably permit separation of these two populations, i.e. those who will and those who will not progress [7, 8]. McNeal and associates recently reported the results of an autopsy and surgical series which showed that tumors with a volume of less than 1 cm were not associated with metastases and thus suggested that the ability to metastasize was associated with further growth and the development of poor differentiation by the tumor [9]. These authors believe that a tumor volume of 1 cm is the critical size that must be detected in the population if screening studies are to be of value. Therefore diagnostic or screening studies must be so refined that this entity can be reliably detected. As of this date, existing laboratory and imaging studies (CT, ultrasound, MRI) do not have this capability. Though we are all searching for the ideal test there is not a unanimity of opinion as to what is needed [10]. This must be remembered when one reviews and analyzes a specific 'screening' study.

Based on the above it may be useful to review several of the studies described by Dr. Kadmon. Enough data exists so they can be analyzed utilizing the statistical studies discussed and thus their true value may be more properly assessed. Because of the limitations of space only three studies will be reviewed: Rectal examination (physical finding); transrectal ultrasonography (imaging study); and serum acid phosphatase (laboratory study).

Rectal examination

Rectal palpation is probably the single most important step in the physical examination for the detection of carcinoma of the prostate and it is well recognised that there is an increased incidence of early disease detection when it is done routinely [11, 12]. Although small nodular areas in the prostate may be readily palpable the differentiation between benign and non-malignant lesions cannot be made by physical examination alone [13, 14, 15]. Interestingly, the value of the routine rectal examination in attempting to screen an asymptomatic population is somewhat controversial and its value and frequency has yet to be clearly established [5, 6, 15, 16, 17].

Calculated sensitivity and specificity from different studies indicate that for rectal examination they vary from 55–69 percent and 89–97 percent respectively. Based on varying prevalence rates the positive predictive values and negative predictive values range from 11–26 percent and 85–96 percent respectively. These date suggest that if one has a negative rectal examination the chances of having prostatic carcinoma are highly unlikely. The converse is not necessarily true in that one or two of every ten men with positive rectal examinations will be found to have prostatic carcinoma. Obviously the data is somewhat dependent on the skill of the individual performing the examination. It has also been inferred that the follow-up rectal examination is very important in surveilance because tumors detected in this manner rather than those detected on the initial examination tend to be associated with a higher rate of survival [18].

Transrectal ultrasonography

Transrectal ultrasonography is a relatively new imaging technique that has been utilized in a variety of applications [19, 20, 21]. Though the study has value in the total staging of prostatic carcinoma and can be used to measure prostatic size and subsequent changes in size following institution of endocrine therapy probably no area has been as controversial as that related to its use as a screening study. Watanabe and associates have been proponents of its use in this manner but others including this author have not advocated its use in this regard [22, 23]. The problem with the use of the technique for screening purposes is that its low sensitivity and specificity is an impediment to this concept. Studies indicate that stage A2 carcinomas connot be imaged with reliability and many benign conditions such as prostatic calculi, beningn prostatic hyperplasia and chronic prostatitis will mimic the echo changes observed in carcinoma [24, 25]. Utilizing the data in these reports the sensitivity and specificity for transrectal ultrasonography has been reported to be 71.4% and 85.8% respectively. Assuming a disease prevalence of 10% [26, 27, 28] the positive and negative values are 35.8% and 96.4% respectively. Utilizing the sensitivity and specificity data on rectal examination that were discussed previously (60% and 85% respectively) but assuming a 10% prevalence rate the positive and negative predictive values for this study are 30.7% and 95% respectively. Though the positive predictive value of transrectal ultrasonography is slightly higher the negative values are essentially the same. Based on these calculations most would agree that the added gain from screening a population with transrectal ultrasonography is not worth the time and expense because the additional useful information is minimal to non-existent. It must also be remembered that in all likelihood a significant number of patients with abnormal ultrasound examinations will also have positive rectal examinations.

Prostatic acid phosphatase

Prostatic acid phosphatase has been used since the 1940s in the evaluation and follow-up of patients with metastatic prostatic carcinoma. It certainly can be classified as the first 'tumor marker'. With the development of new radioimmunoassays for the enzyme Foti and associates in 1971 suggested that the study would be useful in detecting the disease while localized to the prostate [29]. Subsequently it was demonstrated that the test was positive in 6% of men with benign prostatic hyperplasia and furthermore the test would not accurately predict all patients with stage A disease [30, 31]. Based on this data and that reported by others sensitivity and specificity of the tests have been reported to be approximately 70% and 95% respectively [15]. As with previous calculations, assuming a disease prevalence rate of 10% the positive and negative values of this study are 60.8% and 96.6% respectively. Watson and Tang [2] emphasized that a proportion of patients with a positive test and prostatic carcinoma would likely have palpable prostatic nodules and they therefore have calculated that the positive predictive value in patients with no evidence of a nodule falls within the range of approximately 30 percent. Again one can conclude that because of the low predictive value of the test in individuals without prostatic nodules that the use of the prostatic acid phosphatase as a screening test for the early detection of prostatic carcinoma is also not warranted. It can than be concluded that routine periodic rectal examination though far from perfect remains the most effective method for screening patients with carcinoma of the prostate.

98

Summary

In summary, an effort has been made to more clearly define those criteria that should be examined when evaluating a new test and in the development of an ideal one. The specific problem with carcinoma of the prostate, namely the high prevalence of the disease in the United States and its varied biological potential must be considered when attempting to develop a reliable method for identifying early and potentially aggressive disease. Though many tests have been reported as being excellent for screening, when judged critically they do not appear to adequately meet this goal. Therefore, from both a practical and cost effective viewpoint periodic digital rectal examination appears to be the preferred screening test in attempting to diagnose early carcinoma of the prostate in a specified population. Other studies are obviously needed and it is likely and anticipated that they will be developed. A plea is made, however, that they be evaluated in the manner described and also compared to 'the old standard' so that their proprer role in the diagnosis of this disease can be best appreciated.

References

1. Webster's Deluxe Unabridged Dictionary. 2nd edition. New World Dictionary, New York, 1985
2. Watson RA, Tang DB: The Predictive Value of Prostatic Acid Phosphatase as a Screening Test for Prostatic Cancer. NEJM 303: 497–499, 1980
3. Vecchio TJ: Predictive Value of a Single Diagnostic Test in Unselected populations. NEJM 274: 1171–1173, 1966
4. Sheps SB, Schechter MT: The Assessment of Diagnostic Tests. A Survey of Current Medical Research. JAMA 252: 2418–2422, 1984
5. Chodak GW, Schoenberg HW: Early Detection of Prostate Cancer by Routine Screening. JAMA 252: 3261–3264, 1984
6. Letters to the Editor: Problematic Prostatic Prediction. JAMA 254: 1171–1173, 1984
7. Jewett HJ, Eggleston JC, Yawn DH: Radical Prostatectomy in the Management of Carcinoma of the Prostate: Prostate Causes of Some Therapeutic Failures. J Urol 107: 1034–1039, 1972
8. Whitmore WF: Natural History and Staging of Prostatic Cancer. Urol Clin. NA 11: 205–220, 1984
9. McNeal JE, Kindrachuk RA, Freiha FS, Bostwick DG, Redwine EA, Stamey TA: Patterns of Progression in Prostate Cancer. Lancet 1: 60–63, 1986
10. Grayhack JT, Bockrath JM: Diagnosis of Carcinoma of Prostate. Urology 27 (Suppl. March): 54–60, 1981
11. Barnes RW: Carcinoma of the Prostate: A Comparative Study of Mode of Treatment. J Urol 44: 169–176, 1940
12. Kimbrough JC, Rowe RB: Carcinoma of the Prostate. J Urol 66: 373–378, 1951
13. Jewett HJ: Significance of the Palpable Prostatic Nodule. JAMA 160: 838–839, 1950
14. Grabstald H: Further Experience with Transrectal Biopsy of the Prostate. J Urol 74: 211–222, 1955
15. Vihko P, Kontturi M, Lukkarinen O, Errasti J, Vihko R: Screening for Carcinoma of the Prostate. Rectal Examination and Enzymatic and Radioemmunologic Measurements of Serum Acid Phosphatase Compared. Cancer 56: 173–177, 1985
16. Thomson IM, Ernst JJ, Gangai MP, Spense CR: Adenocarcinoma of the Prostate: Results of Routine Urological Screening. J Urol 132: 690–692
17. Guinan P, Bush I, Ray J, Vieth R, Rao R, Bratti R: The Accuracy of the Rectal Examination in the Diagnosis of Prostate Carcinoma. NEJM 303: 499–503, 1980
18. Jenson CB, Shahon DB, Wgensteen OH: Evaluation of Annual Examination in the Detection of Cancer. JAMA 174: 1783–1788, 1960

19. Bartsch G, Egender G, Hubscher H, Rohr H: Sonometrics of the Prostate. J Urol 127: 1119–1121, 1982

20. Holm HH, Juul N, Pedersen JF, Hansen H, Stroyer I: Transperineal ^{125}Iodine Seed Implantation in Prostatic Cancer Guided by Transrectal Ultrasonography. J Urol 130: 283–286, 1983

21. Pontes JE, Eisenkraft S, Watanabe H, Ohe M, Saitoh M, Murphy GP: Preoperative Evaluation of Localized Prostatic Carcinoma by Transrectal Ultrasonography. J Urol 134: 289–291, 1985

22. Watanabe H, Ohe H, Inabe T, Itakura Y, Saitoh M, Nakao M: A Mobile Mass Screening Unit for Prostatic Disease. Prostate 5: 559–565, 1984

23. Resnick MI: Use of Transrectal Ultrasound in Evaluating Prostatic Cancer. J Urol 134: 314, 1985

24. Resnick MI: Evaluation of Prostatic Carcinoma: Noninvasive and Preoperative Techniques. Prostate 1: 311–320, 1980

25. Resnick MI, Willard JW, Boyce WH: Ultrasonography in the Evaluation of Prostatic Cancer. J Urol 124: 482–484, 1980

26. Denton SE, Choy SH, Valk WL: Occult Prostatic Carcinoma Diagnosed by the Stop-Section Technique of the Surgical Specimen. J. Urol 93: 296–298, 1965

27. Edwards CN, Steinhorsson E, Nicholson D: An Autopsy Study of Latent-prostatic Cancer. Cancer 6: 531–554, 1953

28. Catalona WJ. In: Prostate Cancer. Grune and Stratton, Orlando, Florida, 1–14, 1984

29. Foti AG, Cooper JF, Herschman H, Malvaez RR: Detection of Prostatic Cancer by Solid-Phase Radioinnunoassay of Serum Prostatic Acid Phosphatase. NEJM 297: 1357–1361, 1977

30. Carroll BJ: Radioimmunoassay of Prostatic Acid Phosphatase in Carcinoma of the Prostate. NEJM 298: 912, 1978

31. Fleischmann J, Catalona WJ, Fair WR, Heston WDW, Memon M: Lack of Value of Radioimmunoassay for Prostatic Acid Phosphatase as a Screening Test for Prostatic Cancer in Patients with Obstructive Prostatic Hyperplasia. J Urol 129: 312–314, 1983

6. Oncogenes and genitourinary neoplasia

ALEXANDER KIRSCHENBAUM and MICHAEL J. DROLLER

Introduction

The concept of an association between genes and cancer is not a new one. Over a century ago Broca observed a hereditary pattern of cancer among members of his wife's family [1]. Although others also described a familial nature of certain conditions, this did not necessarily prove a genetic basis for disease. Indeed, the very concept of genes was unknown at the time. However, such observations stimulated intense interest in the causes of uncontrolled cell growth and the factors responsible for the formation of specific tumors.

In the decades that followed, much evidence was gathered from laboratory and clinical studies in support of a genetic basis of tumor development. Yet, the precise mechanism by which genes were responsibile for cancer development remained elusive, and this gradually dampened the intensity of research activity in this area.

Recent development in microbiology and genetic engineering have completely reversed this apathy. The identification and characterization of so-called 'oncogenes', genes presumeably involved in the regulation of cell growth and possibly in the loss of growth regulation, has refired intense study of genetic factors that may determine tumor development. The idea that understanding of the cancer process may be at hand has intensified a general interest and enthusiasm within the medical community and has stimulated the imagination of a more medically sophisticated general population.

The purpose of this communication is to review recent evidence that has enhanced our understanding of the genetic basis of cancer development, to describe current directions in which such work is leading, and to assess this work in the context of tumors of the genitourinary tract; in so doing, we shall attempt to describe the clinical relevance of these new and exciting advances to urologic oncology and possibly also to our approach in the treatment of urologic neoplasia.

Ratliff, T.L. and Catalona, W.J. (eds), Genitourinary Cancer. ISBN 0–89838–830–9
© *1987, Martinus Nijhoff Publishers, Boston. Printed in the Netherlands.*

Historical perspectives

The association between oncogenes and cancer is based upon the recent convergence of several independent lines of investigation through inquiry from different scientific disciplines. To truly appreciate these events, it is important to understand that they occurred as isolated observations rather than in related sequence, and that their relevance to the genetic basis of cancer as it is known today represents in many instances only a retrospective assessment.

The signal observation that ultimately spawned the concept of genes and cancer was described by Rous in 1911 when he reported that a cell-free filtrate from chicken sarcoma could induce new tumors [2], and that the active agent in the filtrate was a virus (the Rous sarcoma virus) [3]. This virus became the prototypical tumor virus, belonging to a distinct family of viruses that contained RNA rather than DNA in their genome [4–9].

The ensuing 50 years witnessed an explosion of information on mechanisms of viral biology and replication. The RNA viruses became known as retroviruses because of their unique means of replication within the host cell, first processing RNA 'backwards' into DNA rather than the usual processing of genetic information from DNA to RNA. The enzyme, 'reverse transcriptase,' responsible for this form of genetic transcription was found to be encoded by the viral genome soon after infection of the host cell [10–12]. Thus, retroviruses, unlike most viruses, did not usually destroy their host cell. Rather, the viral DNA became incorporated within the host genome and viral genes could actually be replicated and expressed using the host cells' machinery instead of its own [4–9].

The application of these observations in understanding the mechanism of carcinogenesis required a technique whereby the molecular aspects of genetic events could be studied in the laboratory rather than in intact but complex organisms. The development of such a technique was described by Dulbecco who found that when a small DNA polyoma virus was placed upon monolayers of hamster embryo fibroblasts, it led to the production of stacks of cells in selected foci [13]. These cells, when injected into rodent hosts, proliferated to form tumors; whereas cells not afflicted with virus did not proliferate. This technique came to be known as 'cell transformation,' and became the standard method by which in vitro induction of a malignant phenotype could be reproducibly accomplished.

Despite these advances, the application of observations from Rous' initial experiments as well as from subsequent studies in experimental animal models to human cancer systems remained unsuccessful. Moreover, such studies did not fully explain the variety of factors (both chemical and physical as well as viral) that had been implicated in carcinogenesis.

In this regard, a separate pathway of study had focused on the hereditary aspects of neoplasia and the intrinsic cellular or genetic predisposition to neoplastic transformation. Although Broca had implied this as a mechanism of carcinogenesis in the mid-nineteenth century [1], the concept of specific 'tumor genes' appears to have had its actual inception in 1928 when researchers observed the development of spontaneous melanomas from black spots in certain hybrids from two ornamental fish [14]. The development of tumors in this system appeared to follow Mendelian laws of heredity. The gene that appeared to mediate neoplastic transformation was designated by the term 'oncogene.' It was further suggested that 'oncogenes' might also be needed to maintain the cancerous state, and might actually be the common denominator upon which the multiple factors associated with tumor development acted in the genesis and perpetuation of a particular cancer.

Although many of the viruses with the capacity to transform cells in vitro were found to contain 'oncogenes,' and although some animal tumors were found to be associated with viruses, continued attempts to associate viruses as causative of human tumors were unsuccessful. Insight into concepts that might unify these apparent discordant observations, however, was provided by Huebner and Todaro who postulated that retroviral oncogenes might actually be a natural part of the genome of *all* vertebrate cells [15]. They further suggested that such oncogenes may have been incorporated into vertebrate DNA early in evolution as a result of viral infection, but would only induce tumors when stimulated by various carcinogens [16].

Subsequent advances in techniques for analysis of gene composition, viral manipulation, and cell culture have permitted intensive testing of this hypothesis. This has resulted in a greater understanding of those genetic mechanisms that may control cell growth. This has also prompted the impression that a realistic characterization of the mechanisms responsible for the cancer process may be at hand.

Retroviruses and oncogenes

New techniques in molecular biology first focused on the Rous sarcoma retrovirus as a prototype of a tumor-causing virus. In addition to the wild type virus, there were found to be two mutants which differed in their ability to transform cells. One was conditional upon temperature for transformation to occur while the other was non-conditional and unable to transform cells under any circumstance [17–20]. Using these mutants, it was found that the fragment of the viral genome responsible for transformation was localized to a single gene, designated 'v-*src*' [4]. It was also found that the non-conditional mutant had deletions in the region of the viral genome responsible for transformation when compared to the wild type virus and that the temperature sensitive mutant had changes in the same genomic region [18, 19].

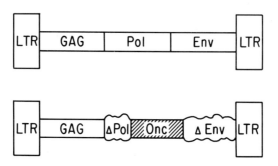

Figure 1. Schematic comparison between LL and AT viruses.
The LL (long latency) virus is composed of the viral genome flanked by two terminal repetitive nucleotide sequences called long terminal repeats (LTR's). LTR's contain the promotor-enhancer sequences that are responsible for the rate of transcription of the viral genome. The viral genome consists of sequences that code for the viral core (GAG), the enzyme reverse transcriptase (POL) and the viral coat (ENV). No oncogene is present in the LL virus.
The AT (acute transforming) virus is also composed of two long terminal repeats (LTR's) and portions of the viral genome derived from LL virus. It also contains an oncogene (ONC) derived from the host cellular chromosome. Note, however, that the AT virus is defective, with only fragments of the viral genome (POL, ENV).

Cellular oncogenes

A technique known as 'hybridization' was used in these studies to combine wild type DNA with mutant DNA, making use of the reverse transcriptase enzyme. This permitted isolation of the v-src oncogene, which was then used as a probe to locate corresponding loci on other DNA's. This then allowed direct testing of the Huebner-Todaro hypothesis to establish whether oncogenes were present primarily in the host cell or only secondarily, following viral insertion.

Thus, proof of this hypothesis was suggested by descriptions of a locus on mammalian DNA, complementary to the 'v-*src*' oncogene, and therefore designated as 'c-*src*' oncogene [21]. In addition, this locus was found to be part of the normal complement of cellular genes in several species.

Even more intriguing were subsequent studies demonstrating that the cellular src gene (c-*src*) was a more complex gene than the retrovirus gene (v-src) being composed of subunits called 'introns' and 'exons' [3]. Exons were found to be genomic areas that encoded for proteins and were separated from one another by introns, whose functions were thought to be regulatory of exon expression. When introns were removed from the cellular src gene, exons could be spliced together to form the v-*src* oncogene [3]. Since it seemed unlikely that the viral gene could be split in such order into the cellular genome, these findings suggested that the existence of the cellular gene had actually preceded that of the viral oncogene. The corollary was that the viral gene was a derivative of the cellular oncogene, having been incorporated into the virus during intracellular replication [22–27]. This prompted the designation of the cellular genome as a 'proto-oncogene' [28].

Proto-oncogenes, viral oncogenes, and cell transformation

These findings provided a basis for explaining some of the earlier observations on retroviruses. Retroviruses had been divided into two subgroups: 'long-latency' (LL) viruses, which induced tumors only after many months and were widely distributed in nature, and acute transforming' (AT) viruses, which induced tumors rapidly and were thought to be laboratory artifacts almost never transmitted in animal hosts [6, 29]. Subsequent studies showed that AT viruses originated when cells were infected with LL viruses as a result of the breakage of host cell DNA [29, 30]. The AT viruses also were found to contain a non-viral gene that had actually originated from the cellular chromosome. The portion of the LL virus that was incorporated into the AT virus was a long terminal sequence (LTR) needed for protein expression. Since the LL virus lacked an oncogene, the viral oncogene of the AT virus must have been derived from the cell chromosome [29]. It was therefore reasoned that the LTR sequence was responsible for activating the cell-derived oncogene, in turn leading to acute transformation of normal cells (Fig. 1).

The mechanism of viral oncogene formation and activation via incorporation of a mammalian proto-oncogene prompted a search for similar viral oncogenes in other systems. To date, more than 20 vertebrate proto-oncogenes have been identified in association with the oncogenes of retroviruses [31]. In addition, many proto-oncogenes were found in organisms that were phylogenetically disparate [21, 32–34]. This implied that proto-oncogenes had been conserved throughout evolution and further suggested that proto-oncogenes might also play a central role in normal cellular physiology.

As each new retrovirus was isolated, it served as a probe for corresponding new proto-oncogenes. However, searches with these new viruses all generally led to identification of the same limited number of proto-oncogenes [53]. This indicated that the number of proto-oncogenes was probably far less than the number of retroviral oncogenes. Another possibility was that the number of proto-oncogenes in mammalian cells was actually greater, with only a certain few being acquired by the retroviruses. Thus, proto-oncogenes that were not expressed in the cell, or that might be performing other functions, might be unavailable to the transforming retroviruses.

These results also implied that cell proto-oncogenes might not require the viral genome to become activated. Theoretically, other factors might activate the proto-oncogene. Observations of chemical and physical carcinogenesis could be explained by the presumption of such a mutational event without relying on the need for tumor induction by a viral genome.

If it was reasoned that the genetic material was the common demoninator of carcinogenesis, then it should be possible to transfer the appropriate genome of a cancer cell into a normal cell and induce transformation. This was demonstrated by a method known as transfection, in which DNA molecules, entrapped within a calcium phosphate crystal matrix, were engulfed by cells in culture, became integrated into the cells' chromosomes, and induced transformation [36]. Thus, DNA from a chemically-induced mouse fibroblast tumor was found to transform normal mouse fibroblasts in vitro, and when subsequently injected into normal mice, generated tumors [37]. When DNA from normal fibroblasts was used, no foci of transformed cells developed, and no tumors were induced.

In addition, the ability of DNA to transform cells was found to survive serial transfer in tissue cultures [38]. This implied that multiple genes were not responsible for transformation, since the long strands of DNA would have been repeatedly broken into progressively smaller fragments, and therefore gradually lose their cell-transforming capability. This was subsequently confirmed by demonstrations that only single cloned genes led to neoplastic transformation [38].

In many instances, cellular oncogenes or proto-oncogenes from tumors were found to be homologous if not identical to those that had been associated with viral oncogenes [39–44]. Thus, oncogenes from the bladder carcinoma cell lines, EJ and T24, could be traced to the c-oncogene that was associated with the v-oncogene of the Harvey murine sarcoma virus [45, 46]. Similarly, the oncogene from human lung and colon carcinoma could be traced to the proto-oncogene that had been associated with the viral oncogene of the Kirsten murine sarcoma virus [47, 48]. Moreover, the Harvey murine sarcoma virus and the Kirsten murine sarcoma virus were related evolutionarily as members of the same virus group [49]. This suggested not only that there were a relatively small number of cellular and viral proto-oncogenes but also that proto-oncogenes could be activated both by incorporation into acute transforming retroviruses as well as by genetic mutation without viral interaction.

Oncogene protein products and carcinogenesis

The critical question that remained unanswered was how oncogenes actually transformed cells. Antibody isolation techniques were used to identify the product of the v-src oncogene as a protein [50]. Since this protein was found to be a phosphoprotein of 60,000 daltons molecular weight, it was designated pp60v-src, for 'phosphoprotein 60,000 daltons molecular weight viral sarcoma gene product' [51].

However, whereas antibody against the v-src oncogene product formed an immunocomplex with the protein, radioactive phosphate, when added to the complex, tagged only the antibody band [52]. Thus, the protein product had actually acted as a protein kinase, attaching phosphate ions to the antibody.

Subsequent studies found that the pp60v-src protein attached phosphate ions specifically to the amino acid tyrosine [53]. The ability to phosphorylate tyrosine was highly unusual, since most protein kinases phosphorylated the amino acids serine and threonine. In fact, phosphotyrosine in normal cells represented only 0.03% of the phosphorylated amino acids, the remaining 99.97% being comprised of phosphoserine and phosphothreonine. In addition, when cells were transformed by the Rous sarcoma virus, the amount of phosphorylated tyrosine increased tenfold [53]. Taken together, it appeared that phosphorylation of tyrosine might be important in the oncogene-induced development of uncontrolled cell growth.

That other oncogene-encoded proteins (from Avian sarcoma virus, feline sarcoma virus, and Abelson murine leukemia virus) had similar phosphotyrosine activity was not surprising. Nor was the homologous sequence of their catalytic domain (the segment of the enzyme, which binds to the substrate) unexpected [54–57]. What this suggested was a common evolutionary origin of these oncogene proteins, a common role in cell transformation, and possibly a common function within normal cells.

In this context, it was predictable that tyrosine kinase activity could also be found in normal cells [58], In fact, the first tyrosine kinase identified in normal cells was found to be encoded by the c-src proto-oncogene [53].

Oncogenes and growth factors

The association between tyrosine kinases and blood-borne growth factors such as epidermal growth factor (EGF) and platelet derived growth factor (PDGF) provided additional clues to understanding cell transformation, cancer cell evasion of normal regulatory controls, and resultant unrestrained growth. These growth factors had been found to activate cells and stimulate their proliferation by binding to specific receptors located on the cell membrane [59–64]. Examination of the EGF receptor disclosed a protein which extended through the cell membrane. The portion of the protein outside the cell comprised the EGF binding site, while the portion within the cell was an enzyme that on subsequent analysis was found to be a tyrosine kinase [65, 66]. Moreover, the binding of EGF to the receptor was found to activate the catalytic domain of the enzyme, thereby unifying the concept of genetic control of cell growth and oncogene control of proliferation.

Additional confirmation of this concept was provided by the discovery that a segment of the EGF receptor had an amino acid sequence closely related to a sequence found within the oncogene protein product of the avian erythroblastosis virus (designated *erb*-B) [67, 68]. In fact, the *erb*-B protein was found to resemble or be identical to the EGF receptor without its binding site. Other studies reported that the EGF receptor was in fact encoded by oncogenes.

Similar observations were made for platelet derived growth factor (PDGF), a heat stable protein found within platelets and thought to function as a mitogen for connective tissue cells [69]. PDGF receptor was also found to be a tyrosine kinase [70, 71]. Moreover, PDGF was found to be nearly identical in structure to the protein product of the oncogene of the simian sarcoma, the so-called 'sis'-oncogene [72, 73]. Thus, when cells were infected with the simian sarcoma virus, they were found to secrete a growth factor much like PDGF [74]. In addition, the proto-oncogene associated with the sis-oncogene was found to be identical to the cellular gene that encodes for PDGF [72, 73]. The finding that PDGF and the EGF receptor are encoded by oncogenes appeared to be too closely associated to reflect mere coincidence or chance.

Oncogene protein products and cell membranes

A search for targets of these oncogene-encoded enzymes led to the identification of even more intriguing relationships. Because a transformed cell had an irregular shape which differs markedly from that of a normal cell, the cell cytoskeleton became a focus of such studies. In one report, vinculin, one of a number of cytoskeletal proteins, was found to contain twenty times more phosphotyrosine in cells transformed by the Rous sarcoma virus than in normal cells [75–77].

It was also learned that the pp60v-*src* protein is located along the inner surface of the plasma membrane, particularly at the site of adhesion plaques which are the same sites where the cytoskeleton is attached to the cell membrane [78, 79]. Since vinculin is an integral component of the adhesion plaque, the pp60v-src protein would be in a proximate position to phosphorylate the tyrosine residues of the vinculin. It was reasoned that an increase in phosphotyrosine might act to disrupt the adhesion plaque, thereby releasing actin filaments, and producing the cytoskeletal disorganization which characterizes transformed cells.

Further evidence in support of these hypotheses was obtained in experiments in which normal cells in culture were treated with radioactive phosphate and subjected to viral transformation by Rous sarcoma virus. Gel electrophoresis consistently revealed a protein band with a large amount of phosphotyrosine. This band, called P36 because of its 26,000 dalton molecular weight, was thought to be the major substrate for viral encoded tyrosine kinases [80–83]. Moreover, recent studies have shown that P36 is associated with the inner surface of the cell's plasma membrane, suggesting a structural function and possibly representing an effect on the cytoskeletal structure reminiscent of that of the pp60v-*src* protein [84, 85].

A separate but related line of investigation into the mechanism of action in oncogenesis concerned changes in plasma membrane phospholipids during neoplastic transformation. It was known that inositol lipid metabolism precedes cell proliferation. As this had been thought to signal the transmission of growth factors and hormones, it was postulated that certain oncogene enzymes might act via inositol lipid metabolism (essentially functioning as inositol lipid kinases) in promoting cell transformation.

The normal pathway of inositol lipid metabolism begins with the activation of cell membrane receptors and the subsequent breakdown of phosphatidyl inositol 4,5, di-phosphate into 1,2 diacylglycerol and inositol triphosphate [86, 87]. The latter acts to mobilize calcium ions from an intracellular depot, while the diacylglycerol activates protein kinase C [88]. Protein kinase C directs the phosphorylation of serine and threonine moieties in a variety of cell proteins which, in turn, control many normal cell functions including gene expression. This may have direct impact on the control of cell proliferation and growth. However, each of these factors has only been associated with the regulation of normal cell growth.

On the other hand, the substrate phosphatidyl inositol 4,5, di-phosphate, produced by the two-step phosphorylation of phosphatidyl inositol, first to phosphatidyl 4-phosphate and then to phosphatidyl 4,5, di-phosphate, has been reproduced in vitro by the src-gene product 'src tyrosine kinase,' [89]. If by simply increasing the availability of substrate, uncontrolled proliferation ensues, then a mechanism of oncogene—induced tumor growth may have been identified (Fig. 2).

Oncogenes and additional mechanisms of function

Other mechanisms of possible oncogene function have also been described. For example, not all products of transforming viral oncogenes are protein kinases. Harvey sarcoma virus, which has been implicated in the etiology of human cancers, has as the product of its oncogene a protein of 21,000 daltons molecular weight (ras-P21) which is situated along the inner surface of the plasma membrane and binds tightly to guanosine triphosphate (GTP) [90–93]. In normal cells, the cellular ras proto-oncogene product is a protein on the inner surface of the plasma membrane, which binds GTP, acts as a GTPase and assists in transmitting signals from the cell surface to its interior. It has been noted that when ras-P21 protein binds to GTP in the transformed cell, there is a concomitant decrease in GTPase activity. This has led to speculations that in the transformed cell, the ras-P21 protein has been changed and in its altered form may act as an unregulated perpetual transmitter [94].

In addition to these kinases, researchers have discovered a small group of nuclear transforming proteins. The product of the viral myc-oncogene of the avian myelocytomatosis virus, for example, has been found to bind to DNA [95, 96]. Since cellular myc-proto-oncogenes are active in growing cells just

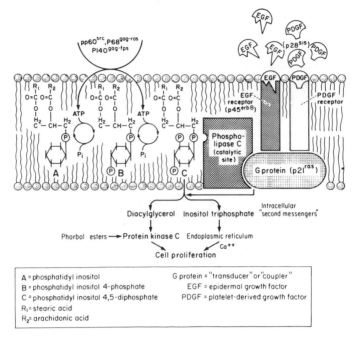

Figure 2. Proposed mechanism of inositol lipid metabolism in The regulation of cellular growth and transformation.

In the metabolism of inositol lipids, phosphatidyl inositol undergoes a two-step phosphorylation process to phosphatidyl inositol 4 phosphate and phosphatidyl inositol 4,5 diphosphate. This substrate is then broken down by the enzyme, phospholipase C into diacylglycerol and inositol triphosphate (both intracellular second messengers). The latter mobilizes Ca^{2+} from intracellular stores, while the former activates protein kinase C, both of which are needed for cellular proliferation to take place.

Phorbol di-esters, which are known tumor promoters, closely resemble diacylglycerol structurally and may also activate protein kinase C.

The protein products of several oncogenes (*src, ros, fps*) are tyrosine kinases which may be responsible for the formation of the substrate phosphatidyl inositol 4,5 diphosphate.

Epidermal growth factor, platelet-derived growth factor and their receptors and the coupling agent (G protein), may be needed to activate the enzyme phospholipase C.

Platelet-derived growth factor is encoded by the *sis* oncogene while epidermal growth factor receptor is the product of the *erb*-B oncogene. The protein is believed to be encoded by the *ras* oncogene.

These interrelationships are highly suggestive of an integral role of these factors in the determination and control of cell proliferation.

prior to DNA replication, some have suggested that these viral oncogene products may somehow bring about uninterrupted, continuous replication. Whether this also accounts for neoplastic transformation, however, remains to be determined. Table 1 presents listing of common oncogenes and their products.

Many questions remain unanswered but are central in attempting to understand the neoplastic process. Perhaps foremost is that which concerns the mechanisms whereby a gene changes from being an integral part of the normal cell into a cancer producing gene. Of related importance is the question of how viral and cellular oncogenes may interact. The structural similarities between cellular proto-oncogenes and viral oncogenes implies that the former, thought generally to be involved only in the regulation of normal cell functions, have the potential to be oncogenic. Furthermore, it has been observed that the retroviral genome is sandwiched between long terminal repetitive nucleotide sequences (LTR's) which signal initiation, promotion, enhancement, and termination of transcription [97–100]. Thus, if and when the retroviral genome is transposed in proximity to a mammalian proto-oncogene, malignant transformation might occur.

In additional studies, the cellular proto-oncogenes of the Moloney murine sarcome (c-mos) and the Harvey murine sarcoma (c-ras^{Ha}) were found to induce transformation of NIH 3T3 cells after being joined to retroviral terminal nucleotide sequences [101, 102]. Similarly, the avian leukemia virus (ALV) has been thought to act as a transcriptional promoter when inserted into the vertebrate genome adjacent to the proto-oncogene c-myc, resulting in malignant transformation [98].

A further possible mechanism of carcinogenesis has been suggested to involve oncogene translocation. In Burkitt's lymphoma, the c-myc oncogene was observed to be translocated from chromocome 8 to 14, bringing it into close association

Table 1. Current nomenclature of recognized oncogenes and their products

Type of tumor	Oncogene	Biochemical function of oncogene	
Sarcomas	src yes fps/fes ros fgr fms	TYR protein kinases	Kinase gene family
B-lymphoma	abl		
Erythroleukemias	erb-B	Truncated EGF receptor	
Sarcomas	raf/mil	SER/THR protein kinase	
Sarcomas	mos	Not known	
Erythroleukemia and Sarcoma	ras	GTP-binding/GTP-ase	
Carcinomas, sarcomas, myelocytic leukemia	myc		
Myeloblastic leukemia	myb	Nuclear proteins	
Osteosarcoma	fos		
Sarcomas	ski		
Sarcomas	sis	PDGF homology	
	rel	Not known	
	erb-A	Not known	

TYR, tyrosine; SER, serine; THR, theonine

with the heavy chain locus and resulting in a five-fold increase in c-*myc* messenger RNA production compared to normal controls [103–105]. In such instances the structural similarity of the c-*myc* oncogene product in both normal and malignant cells implied that the change was quantitative rather than qualitative.

Such mechanisms were consistent with a proposed 'dosage therory' of carcinogenesis in which an increased amount of the oncogene protein product, with or without a corresponding increase in its proto-oncogene, resulted in malignant transformation.

In contrast, the aberrant gene theory of carcinogenesis implicated qualitative changes in the oncogene product as the basis of carcinogenesis. This theory proposed that a structural change in the gene could change it from its normal state into a cancerous one. The model for this theory was the c-*ras* Harvey gene of the EJ and T24 bladder cell cancer lines, in which a single point mutation at amino acid 12 was postulated as being responsible for inducing tumor [106–109].

Thus far, point mutations have been observed to occur only with *ras* oncogenes, and only in approximately ten percent of those studies. Interestingly, these mutations have been found to occur solely at the amino acid 12 and 61. In addition, these mutations have not been observed within the proto-oncogenes of normal cells taken from the same patient, suggesting that the mutation was a somatic, or acquired, event. This further implied that the particular mutation was some how selected for by the tumor, and that activation of the *ras* oncogene directly contributed toward malignant transformation and was not a result of it.

Oncogenes and the stepwise process of carcinogenesis

As evidence in each of these areas has been accumulated, it has become apparent that carcinogenesis is a process that may proceed through a series of steps rather than as a precipitous solitary occurence. For example, the addition of the proto-oncogene c-*ras* to a cell culture system of rat embryo fibroblasts did not result in malignancy. However, when a second oncogene, such as the viral promoter *myc* or the adenovirus oncogene E1A, was added to the system, transformation occurred [110, 111]. In contrast, c-*ras* alone was able to transform cells of the NIH 3T3 line, a cell system of immortalized rodent fibroblasts, that had already undergone a preliminary step in transformation [112]. These studies seemed to indicate that multiple steps would be required to alter cell function. The oncogene alone could transform already altered cells of the 3T3 line, but two complimentary oncogenes were required to transform otherwise normal cells.

Oncogenes and genitourinary neoplasia

The association between oncogenes and genitourinary neoplasia is not simply based on the fact that oncogenes were first discovered in established cell lines derived from patients with bladder tumors. Indeed, it has been more difficult to document the presence of oncogenes in fresh bladder tumor tissue. What is more important, however, is the concept of oncogenes in the context of experimental observations taken together with what is known clinically of bladder cancer and other genitourinary neoplasias.

For example, in bladder cancer we seem to be dealing with a variety of pathways of tumor development. In the one, cell proliferation takes place and leads to the generation of papillary excrescences of low grade cancer cells in which recurrence after treatment is common, but progression is rare. In another pathway, cellular atypia and dysplasia occur with proliferation resulting in the infiltration of cells into the bladder wall, and beyond. This form of cancer appears to be more aggressive and ultimately leads in most instances to the patient's demise. Envisioning the role of oncogenes in these separate pathways is not difficult. Thus, the simple activation of an oncogene as a solitary event may result in cellular proliferation. In many instances, this is the only event that occurs. On the other hand, a sequence of oncogenes may be activated under the appropriate conditions leading to the genesis of the more aggressive type of tumor. Those physical and chemical influences to which the urothelium is exposed may be relevant to the type of oncogene activated and to the ultimate expression of the transitional cell cancer.

Analogous situations may be considered in renal cell carcinoma. Some of the tumors when initially diagnosed, even though quite large, have remained confined to the kidney and are eminently curable by surgery. In contrast, others are diagnosed in the presence of metastases, and in these cases the prognosis with any form of therapy is bleak. What determines the different biologic behavior of these tumors in unclear. However, if phenotypic expression is dependent upon the type and number of oncogenes activated for the development of a particular neoplasm, it is conceivable that only certain oncogenes lead to the development of tumors with more aggressive behavior.

Concept of initiation and promotion may also be factored into these considerations. The traditional definition of these processes to explain the influence of epidemiologic factors in the genesis of bladder cancer has indicated that initiation is an irreversible process occurring rapidly and resulting in the transformation of cells, while promotion is a reversible process occuring over time by repeated stimulations, and does not necessarily by itself generate a cancer but rather a proliferative tumor mass. The application of these principles to the different pathways of tumor development, such as in bladder or in kidney cancers as described above, supports the concept that more than one oncogene may be required to respond to stimuli in the environment and produce a malignant neoplasm. Clearly, however, much remains to be learned about these processes and their various possible interactions.

114

Conclusions

While the discovery and study of oncogenes has expanded understanding of carcinogenesis, the application of this knowledge in cancer treatment remains uncertain. Yet, tremendous strides in this direction have been made. That there are a limited number of oncogenes offers hope that the mechanisms for tumor formation can be elucidated and treatments therefore devised. However, since proto-oncogenes probably function in normal cell regulation, a simple treatment approach may be difficult to accomplish. At the present time, knowledge of how even the encoded proteins function remains obscure. Nonetheless, the detection of the various steps in carcinogenesis may enable the diagnosis of high risk patients and possibly lead to prevention and rational treatment.

References

1. Bishop JM: Cancer genes come of age. Cell 32: 1018–1020, 1983
2. Rous P: A sarcoma of the fowl transmissible by an agent separable from the tumor cells. J Exp Med 13: 397–411, 1911
3. Bishop JM: Oncogenes. Sci Amer 246: 80–93, 1982
4. Vogt PK: The genetics of RNA tumor viruses. In: Comprehensive Virology, Fraenkel-Conrat H, Wagner RR (eds). Plenum Press, Vol 9, New York, 341–455, 1977
5. Weiss RA, Teich NM, Varmus HE, Coffin JM (eds). In: RNA Tumor Viruses. The Molecular Biology of Tumor Viruses, edition 2. Cold Spring Harbor Laboratory, New York, 1982
6. Bishop JM: The molecular biology of RNA tumor viruses: A physicians' guide. N Engl J Med 303: 675–682, 1986
7. In: Oncogenic Urology, Klein G (ed). Raven Press, New York, 1980
8. In: Oncogene Studies, Advances in Viral Oncology, Klein G (ed). Raven Press, New York, Vol 1, 1982
9. Bishop JM: Retroviruses. Annu Rev Biochem 47: 35–88, 1978
10. Baltimore D: Viral RNA-dependent DNA polymerase. Nature 226: 1209–1211, 1970
11. Temin HM, Mizutani S: RNA dependent DNA polymerase in virions of Rous sarcoma virus. Nature 226: 1211–1213, 1970
12. Temin HM, Baltimore D: RNA-directed DNA synthesis and RNA viruses. Adv Virus Res 17: 129–186, 1972
13. Vogt M, Dulbecco R: Steps in the neoplastic transformation of Hamster embryo cells by polyoma virus. Proc Natl Acad Sci USA 49: 171–179, 1963
14. Anders F, Schartl M, Barnekow A, Anders A: Xiphophorous as an vivo model for studies on normal and defective control of oncogenes. In: Advances in cancer research vol 42. Klein G, Weinhouse (eds). Academic Press Inc, Orlando, Florida, 191–275, 1984
15. Huebner RJ, Todaro GJ: Oncogenes of RNA tumor viruses as determinants of cancer. Proc Natl Acad Sci USA 64: 1087–1094, 1969
16. Todaro GJ, Huebner RJ: The viral oncogene hypothesis: New Evidence. Proc Natl Acad Sci USA 69: 1009–1015, 1972
17. Toyoshima K, Vogt PK: Temperature-sensitive mutants of an avian sarcoma virus. Virology 6: 669–688, 1958
18. Martin GS: Rous sarcoma virus: A function required for the maintenance of the transformed state. Nature 227: 1021–1023, 1970

19. Wang LH, Duesberg P, Beemon K, Vogt PK: Mapping RNase T_1-resistant oligonucleotides of avian tumor virus RNA's: Sarcoma-specific oligonucleotides are near the poly (A) end and oligonucleotides common to sarcoma and transformation-defective viruses are at the poly (A) end. J Virol 16: 1051–1070, 1975

20. Vogt PK: Spontaneous segregation of non-transforming viruses from cloned sarcoma viruses. Virology 46: 947–952, 1971

21. Stehelin D, Varmus HE, Bishop JM, Vogt PK: DNA related to the transforming gene(s) of avian sarcoma viruses is present in normal avian DNA. Nature 260: 170–173, 1976

22. Hughes SH, Payvar F, Spector D, Schimke TR, Robinson LH, Payne SG, Bishop JM, Varmus EH: Heterogeneity of genetic loci in chickens: Analysis of endogenous viral and non-viral genes by cleavage of DNA with restriction endonucleases. Cell 18: 347–359, 1979

23. Padgett TG, Stubblefield E, Varmus HE: Chicken macrochromosomes contour on endogenous provirus and microchromosomes contain sequences related to the transforming gene of asv. Cell 10: 649–657, 1977

24. Spector PH, Baker B, Varmus HE, Bishop JM: Characteristics of cellular RNA related to the transforming gene of avian sarcoma viruses. Cell 13: 381–386, 1978b

25. Oppermann H, Levinson AD. Varmus HE, Levintow L, Bishop JM: Uninfected vertebrate cells contain a protein that is closely related to the product of the avian sarcoma virus transforming gene (src). Proc Natl Acad Sci USA 76: 1804–1808, 1979

26. Parker RC, Varmus HE, Bishop JM: Cellular homologue (c-src) of the transforming gene of Rous sarcoma virus: Isolation, mapping, and transcriptional analysis of c-src and flanking regions. Proc Natl Acad Sci USA 78: 5842–5846, 1981

27. Ta Keya T, Hanatusa H: Structure and sequence of the cellular gene homologous to the rsv src gene and the mechanism for generating the transforming virus. Cell 32: 881–890, 1983

28. Bishop JM: Cellular oncogenes and retroviruses. In: Annual Review of Biochemistry, Vol 52, Snell EE, Boyer PD, Meister A, Richardson CC (eds). Annual Revieuws Inc, Palo Alto 301–354, 1983

29. Androphy JE, Lowry RD: Tumor viruses, oncogenes and human cancer. J Amer Acad of Dermat 10: 125–141, 1984

30. Stehelin D, Varmus HE, Bishop JM: DNA related to transforming gene(s) of avian sarcoma viruses is present in normal avian DNA. Nature 260: 170–173, 1976

31. Bishop JM: Cellular oncogenes and retroviruses. Ann Rev Biochem 52: 301–354, 1984

32. Stehelim D, Guntaka RV, Varmus HE, Bishop JM: Purification of DNA complementary to nucleotide sequences required for neoplastic transformation of fibroblasts by avian sarcoma viruses. J Mol Biol 101: 349–365, 1976

33. Spector DH, Varmus HE, Bishop JM: Nucleotide sequences related to the transforming gene of avian sarcoma virus are present in the DNA of uninfected vertebrates. proc Natl Acad Sci USA 75: 4102–4106, 1978

34. Shilo BZ, Weinberg RA: Genes homologous to vertebrate oncogenes are conserved in Drosophila melanogaster. Proc Natl Acad Sci USA 78: 6789–6792, 1981

35. Weinberg AR: Fewer and fewer oncogenes. Cell 30: 3–4, 1982

36. Graham FL, Vander EBAJ: Transformation of rat cells by DNA of human adenovirus 5. Virology 52: 456–467, 1973

37. Shih C, Shilo BA, Goldfarb MP, Dannenbery A, Weinberg RA: Passage of phenotypes of chemically transformed cells via transfection of DNA and chromatin. Proc Natl Acad Sci USA 76: 5714–5718, 1979

38. Weinberg AR: A molecular basis of cancer. Sci Amer 249: 126–142, 1983

39. Shih C, Paghy LC, Murray M, Weinberg RA: Transforming genes of carcinomas and neuroblastomas introduced into mouse fibroblasts. Nature 290: 261–264, 1981

40. Krontiris TG, Cooper GM: Transforming activity of human tumor DNA's Proc Natl Acad Sci USA 78: 1181–1184, 1981

41. Krontiris TG: The emerging genetics of human cancer. N Engl J Med 309: 404–409, 1983
42. Perucho M, Goldfarb M, Shimizo K, Lama C, Fogh J, Wigler M: Human-tumor-derived cell lines contain common and different transforming genes. Cell 27: 467–476, 1981
43. Murray M, Shilo BZ, Shih C, Cowing D, Hsu HW, Weinberg RA: Three different human tumor cell lines contain different oncogenes. Cell 25: 355–361, 1981
44. Pulciani S, Santos, Lauver AV, Long LK, Aaronson SA, Barbaad M: Oncogenes in solid human tumors. Nature 300: 559–542, 1982
45. Pacada LF, Tabin CJ, Shih C, Weinberg RA: Human EJ bladder carcinoma oncogene is homologue of Harvey sarcoma virus ras gene. Nature 297: 474–478, 1982
46. Santos E, Tronick SR, Aaronson SA, Pulciani S, Barbaad M: T24 human bladder carcinoma oncogene is an activated form of the normal human homologue of BALB- and Harvey-MSV transforming genes. Nature 298: 343–347, 1982
47. Der CJ, Krontiris TG, Cooper GM: Transforming genes of human bladder and lung carcinoma cell lines are homologous to the ras genes of Harvey and Kirsten sarcoma viruses. Proc Natl Acad Sci USA 79: 3637–3640, 1982
48. Shimizu K, Goldfarb M, Suard V, Perucho M, li V, Kamata T, Feramisco J, Stavenzer E, Fogh J, Wigler HM: Three human transforming genes are related to the viral ras oncogenes. Proc Natl Acad Sci USA 80: 2112–2116, 1983
49. Shih TY, Weeks MO, Young HA, Skolnick EM: Identification of a sarcoma virus-coded phosphoprotein in non-producer cells transformed by Kirsten or Harvey murine sarcoma virus. Virology 96: 64–79, 1979
50. Brugge JS, Erikson RL: Identification of a transformationspecific antigen induced by an avian sarcoma virus. Nature 269: 346–348, 1977
51. Purchio AF, Erikson E, Brugge JS, Erikson RL: Identification of a polypeptide encoded by the avian sarcoma virus src gene. Proc Natl Acad Sci USA 75: 11567–1571, 1978
52. Collett MS, Erikson RL: Protein kinase activity associated with the avian sarcoma virus src gene product. Proc Natl Acad Sci USA 75: 2021–2024, 1978
53. Hunter T, Setton BM: The transforming gene product of Rous sarcoma virus phosphorylates tyrosine. Proc Natl Acad Sci USA 77: 1311–1315, 1980
54. Witte ON, Dasqupta A, Baltimore D: Abelson murine leukemia virus protein is phosphorylated in vitro to form phosphotyrosine. Nature 283: 826–831, 1980
55. Kawai S, Yoshida M, Segawa K, Sugiyama H, Ishizaki R, Toyoshima K: Characterization of Y7:3, an avian sarcoma virus: A unique transforming gene and its product, a phosphopolyprotein with protein kinase activity. Proc Natl Acad Sci USA 77: 6193–6203, 1980
56. Feldman AR, Karafusa T, Hanafusa H: Characterization of protein kinase activity associated with the transforming gene product of Fujinami sarcoma virus. Cell 22: 757–765, 1980
57. Hunter T: The proteins of oncogenes. Sci Amer 251: 70–79, 1984
58. Setton BM, HUnter T, Beemon K, Eckhart W: Evidence that the phosphorylation of tyrosine is essential for cellular transformation by Rous sarcoma virus. Cell 20: 807–816, 1980
59. Cohen S: Isolation of a mouse submaxillary gland protein accelerating incisor eruption and eyelid opening in the newborn animal. J Biol Chem 237: 1555–1562, 1962
60. Carpenter G, Cohen S: ^{125}I-labeled human epidermal growth factor. J Cell Biol 71: 159–171, 1976
61. Heldin EH, Westmart B, Wasteson A: Specific receptors for platelet-derived growth factor on cells derived from connective tissue and glia. Proc Natl Acad Sci USA 78: 3664–3668, 1981
62. Antoniades HN, Lewis LT: Human platelet-derived growth factor: Structure and function. Fed Proc 42: 2630–2634, 1983
63. Antoniades HN, Hunkapiller MW: Human platelet-derived growth factor (PDGF): Amino-terminal amino acid sequence. Science 222: 963–965, 1983
64. Carpenter G, King Jr L, Cohen D: Rapid enhancement of protein phosphorylation in A-431 cell membrane preparations by epidermal growth factor. J Biol Chem 254: 4884–4891, 1979

65. Cohen S, Carpenter G, King Jr L: Epidermal growth factor-receptor-protein kinase interactions. J Biol Chem 255: 4834–4842, 1980

66. Ushiro H, Cohen S: Identification of phosphotyrosine as a product of epidermal growth factor-activated protein kinase in A-431. J Biol Chem 255: 8363–8365, 1980

67. Downward J, Varden Y, Mayes E, Scrore G, Totty N, Stockwell P, Ullrich A, Schlessinger J, Waterfield MD: Close similarity of epidermal growth factor receptor and V-erb-B oncogene protein sequences. Nature 307: 521–527, 1984

68. Schechter LA, Stern FD, Vaidyanathan L, Decker JS, Deebin AJ, Green IM, Weinberg AR: The new oncogene: an erb-B-related gene encoding a 185,000—M$_r$ tumor antigen. Nature 312: 513–516, 1984

69. Westermark B, Heldin CH, EKB, Johasson A, Mellstrom K, Nister M, Wasteson A: Biochemistry and biology of platelet-derived growth factor. In: Growth and maturation factors, 1, Guroff G (ed). John Wiley and sons, New York, 73–115, 1983

70. EKB, Westermark B, Wasteson A, Heldin CH: Stimulation of tyrosine-specific phosphorylation by platelet-derived growth factor. Nature 295: 419–420, 1982

71. Nishimura J, Huang S, Deuel FT: Platelet-derived growth factor stimulates tyrosine-specific protein kinase activity in Swiss mouse 3T3 cell membranes. Proc Natl Acad Sci USA 79: 4303–4307, 1982

72. Doolittle RF, Hunkapiller MW, Hood LE, Devare SG, Robbins KC, Aaronson SA, Antoniades HN: Simian sarcoma virus one gene, v-sis, is derived from the gene (or genes) encoding a platelet-derived growth factor. Science 221: 275–277, 1983

73. Waterfield MD, Scrace GT, Whittle N, Stroobant P, Johnsson A, Wasterson A, Westermark B, Heldin CH, Huany JD, Deuel TF: Platelet-derived growth factor is structurally related to the putative transforming protein p28^{sis} of simian sarcoma virus. Nature 304: 35–39, 1983

74. Robbins KC, Devare SG, Reddy EP, Aaronson SA: In vivo identification of the transforming gene product of simiam sarcoma virus. Science 218: 1131–1133, 1982

75. Geiger B: A Bok protein from chicken gizzard: Its localization of the termini of microfilament bundles in cultures chickens cells. Cell 18: 193–205, 1979

76. Burridge K, Feramisco J: Microinjection and localization of a Bok protein in living fibroblasts. A relationship to actin and fibronectin. Cell 19: 587–595, 1980

77. Setton BM, Hunter T, Ball EH, Singer SJ: Vinculin: A cytoskeletal target of the transforming protein of Rous sarcoma virus. Cell 24: 165–174, 1981a

78. Courtneidge AS, Levinson DA, Bishop JM: The protein encoded by the transforming gene of avian sarcoma virus (pp60^{src}) and a homologous protein in normal cells (pp60$^{proto-src}$) are associated with the plasma membrane. Proc Natl Acad Sci USA 77: 3783–3787, 1980

79. Courtneidge AS, Bishop JM: Transit of pp60^{v-src} to the plasma membrane. Proc Natl Acad Sci USA 79: 7117–7121, 1982

80. Yih-Shyrun E, Chen BL: Detection of phosphotyrosine-containing 34,000-dalton protein in the framework of cells transformed with Rous sarcoma virus. Proc Natl Acad Sci USA 78: 2388–2392, 1981

81. Erikson E, Erikson RL: Identification of a cellular protein substrate phosphorylated by the avian sarcoma virus-transforming gene product. Cell 21: 829–836, 1980

82. Radke K, Martin GS: transformation by Rous sarcoma virus: Effects of src gene expression on the synthesis and phosphorylation of cellular polypeptides. Proc Natl Acad Sci USA 76: 5215–5216, 1979

83. Radke K, Gilmore T, Martin GS: Transformation by Rous sarcoma virus: A cellular substrate for transformation-specific protein phosphorylation contains phosphotyrosine. Cell 21:821–828, 1980

84. Amini S, Kaji A: Association of pp36, a phosphorylated form of the presumed target protein for the src protein of Rous sarcoma virus, with the membrane of chicken cells transformed by Rous sarcoma virus. Proc Natl Acad Sci USA 80: 960–964, 1983

85. Courtneidge SA, Ralston R, Alitalo K, Bishop JM: Subcellular location of an abundant substrate (p36) for tyrosine-specific protein kinases. Mol Cell Biol 3: 340–350, 1983
86. Berridge JM: Rapid accumulation of inositol triphosphate reveals that agonists hydrolyse polyphosphoinositides instead of phosphatidylinositol. Biochem J 212: 849–858, 1983
87. Berridge JM, Irvine FR: Inositol triphosphate, a novel second messenger in cellular signal transduction. Nature 312: 315–321, 1984
88. Nishizuka Y: The role of protein kinase C in cell surface signal transduction and tumour promotion. Nature 308: 693–698, 1984
89. Sugimoto Y, Whitman M, Cantley CL, Erikson LR: Evidence that the Rous sarcoma virus transforming gene product phosphorylates phosphatidylinositol and diacylglycerol. Proc Natl Acad Sci USA 81: 2117–2121, 1984
90. Shih TY, Weeks MO, Young HA, Scolnick EM: Identification of a sarcoma virus-encoded phosphoprotein in non-producer cells transformed by Harvey or Kirsten murine sarcoma virus. Virology 96: 64–79, 1979
91. Willingham M, Pastan I, Shih TY, Scolnick EM: Localization of the src gene product of the Harvey strain of murine sarcoma virus to the plasma membrane of transformed cells by electron microscopic immunocytochemistry. Cell 19: 1005–1014, 1980
92. Scolnick EM, Papageorge AG, Shih TY: Guanine nucleotide-binding activity as an assay for the src protein of rat-derived murine sarcoma viruses. proc Natl Acad Sci USA 76: 5355–5359, 1979
93. Shih TY, Papageaorge EG, Stokes PE, Weeks MO, Scolnic EM: Guanine nucleotide-binding and autophosphorylation activities associated with p21^{src} protein of Harvey murine sarcoma virus. Nature 287: 686–691, 1980
94. Sweet WR, Yokoyama S, Kamata T, feramisco RJ, Rosenberg M, Gross M: The product of ras is a GTPase and mutant is deficient in this activity. Nature 311: 273–275, 1984
95. Donner P, Griser-Wilke I, Moelling K: Nuclear localization and DNA binding of the transforming gene product of avian myelocytomatosis. Nature 296: 262–266, 1982
96. Alitalo K, Ramsay G, Bishop JM, Ohlsson Pfiefer S, Colby WW, Levinson AD: Identification of nuclear proteins encoded by viral and cellular myc oncogenes. Nature 306: 274–277, 1983b
97. Varmus HE: Recent evidence for oncogeneses by insertion mutagenesis and gene activation. Cancer Surv 2: 301–319, 1982
98. Hayward WS, Neel BJ, Astrin SM: Activation of a cellular oncogene by promoter insertion in ALV-induced lymphoid leukosis. Nature 209: 475–479, 1981
99. Nusse R, Van Oogen A, Cox P, Fung YK, Varmus HE: Mode of proviral activation of a putative mammary oncogene (int-1) on mouse chromosome 15. Nature 307: 131–136, 1984
100. Dickson C, Smith R, Brookes S, Peters G: Tumorigenesis by mouse mammary tumor virus: Proviral activation of a cellular gene in the common integration region int-2. Cell 37: 529–536, 1984
101. Blair DG, Oskarsson M, Wood TG, McClements WL, Fischinger PJ, Vande Woude GG: Activation of the transforming potential of a normal cell sequence: A molecular model for oncogenesis. Science 212: 941–942, 198
102. DeFeo D, Gouda AM, Young AH, Chang HE, Loury RD, Scolnick ME, Ellis WR: Analysis of two divergent rat genomic clones homologous to the transforming gene of Harvey murine sarcoma virus. Proc Natl Acad USA 78: 3328–3332, 1981
103. Taub R, Kirsch I, Morton C, Lenoir G, Swan D, Tronick S, Aaronson SA, Leder P: Translocation of the c-myc gene into the immunoglobulin heavy chain locus in human Burkitt lymphoma and murine plasmacytoma cells. Proc Natl Acad Sci USA 79: 7837–7841, 1982
104. Ar-Rushdi A, Nishikura F, Erikson J, Watt R, Rovera G, Groce CM: Differential expression of the translocated and the untranslocated c-myc oncogene in Burkitt lymphoma. Science 222: 390–393, 1983
105. Eva A, Robbins KC, Andersen PR, Srinivasan A, Tronick SR, Reddy P, Ellmore NW, Galen

AT, Lautenberger JA, Papas TS, Westin EH, Wong-Staal F, Gallo RC, Aaronson SA: Cellular genes analogous to retroviral oncogenes are transcribed in human tumour cells. Nature 295: 116–119, 1982

106. Reddy EP, Reynolds RK, Santos E, Barbaad M: A point mutation is responsible for the acquisition of transforming properties by the T24 human bladder carcinoma oncogene. Nature 300: 149–152, 1982

107. Tabin CJ, Bradley SM, Bargmann CI, Weinberg RA, Papageorge AG, Scolnick EM, Dhar R, Lang Dr, Chang EM: Mechanism of activator of a human oncogene. Nature 300: 143–149, 1982

108. Taparowsky W, Suard Y, Fasano O, Shimizu K, Goldfarb M, Wigler M. Nature 300: 762–765, 1982

109. Capon DJ, Chen EY, Levinson AD, Seeburg PH, Goeddel DV: Complete nucleotide sequences of the T24 human bladder carcinoma oncogene and its normal homologue. Nature 302: 33–37, 1983

110. Land H, Parada LF, Weinberg RA: Tumorigenic conversion of primary embryo fibroblasts requires at least two cooperating oncogenes. Nature 304: 596–602, 1983

111. Ruley HE: Adenovirus early region 1A enables viral and cellular transforming genes to transform primary cells in culture. Nature 304: 602–606, 1983

112. Newbold FR, Overell WR: Fibroblast immortality is a prerequisite for transformation by E5 c-Ha-ras oncogene. Nature 304: 648–652, 1983

Editorial Comment

DONALD S. COFFEY

The authors have provided the reader with a very lucid and informative overview of the historical development of many of the important concepts in the rapidly developing area of the oncogene. This chapter brings out the important issues without submerging the reader into minutia and confusion. It now appears that proto-oncogenes are essential to the development and normal growth and as such they function as any growth regulatory substance. Many oncogene functions are expressed during embryonic development but they can also be highly active in any growing tissues. The role of the oncogene in cancer has been a long controversy over whether the neoplastic process involves an overexpression of a normal proto-oncogene at an inappropriate time or if it is an expression of a mutated oncogene. Most common in the latter argument has been the mutation of the ras oncogene at specific amino acid loci. It now appears that these mutations are not common and there are still uncertainties about how oncogenes function in carcinogenesis. Almost every discovery starting with the overexpression of the oncogene and the mutation theory is quickly followed by a host of papers showing that the story is more complex than we first believed it to be. The recognition that the ras oncogene may express a P21 protein that was a non-functioning GTPase of the G protein variety led many to speculate that it would be involved in the regulation of adnylcyclase. At last, the elevation of cyclic AMP cannot be clearly demonstrated and it appears that the system may be more complex than a loss in G protein control of adenylcyclase.

More recently, it has been shown that the ras oncogene can cause changes in cell motility like ruffling along the surface and this may involve an autocrine motility factor. Cell motility has always been an important facet of the cancer cell and now that the autocrine growth factors have been found there appear also to be autocrine motility factors. It is unknown how these factors induce the cell to undergo rapid changes in the membrane that involves a ruffling like motion. Cell motility is broken up into various types and ruffling is only one form of a variety of cell movements. It is this change in motility that probably accounts for the morphological changes that are seen in cells following their transformation in vitro when the cells appear to lose their contact and pile up on one another.

Several investigators have recently reported that the steroid receptor and glucocorticoid receptor contain an homology in their sequence similar to the erbA oncogene. This very intriguing observation leads one to wonder why normal steroid receptors should carry such an homology unless it helps the receptor to bind to specific nuclear proteins. Indeed, the receptors have been shown to bind to the nuclear matrix, the skeletal scaffolding system of the nucleus, and many of the nuclear oncogene products bind to this same type of structure. The nuclear protein binding of oncogene products such as myc, fos and myb is a very active area of research. The binding of the retrovirus oncogene products to the nuclear matrix is similar to the binding of the transformation protein, large T antigen, that is present in SV40 transformation. This would also be similar to the E-1A protein binding seen in the adenoma transformation. In summary, both the retroviruses, polyoma and adenoma viruses make transformation proteins that bind to the nucleus and this is believed to be one of the early events in immortalizing a cell.

Whatever the final transformation step, this leads to a progression that causes genetic instability. It is the genetic instability in cancer that counts for its progression as it spins off a variety of different cells with different genotypes. This shows up in the anaplasia and variance in structure that occurs with the development of cancer. This variance causes tumor cell heterogeneity and it is the outgrowth of resistant clones that makes resistance such a perplexing clinical problem. It is difficult to cause normal cells to induce a resistant clone to almost any form of cancer chemotherapy. However, cancer cells invariably cause clones to develop with high drug resistance. This is true for practically every form of therapy imposed upon the cancer. For example, it is rare for anyone to develop normal resistance to cancer chemotherapeutic agents so that with subsequent treatment their bone marrow becomes more difficult to suppress. In contrast, all cancers become resistant as a cytotoxic drug is administered. It is believed that this difference in resistance is due to the wide variety of clones existing in the cancer cell that result from genetic instability. As the genetic instability continues, many types of translocations and chromosome markers can be observed and changes in the amount of DNA occur producing anuploidy. This type of anaplasia is always characterized by changes in the structural elements of the nucleus and cell. One of the frontiers in the oncogene study now is directed towards how the products of the oncogene affect nuclear and cytoplasmic structures. It is believed that these structural changes may be at the heart of genetic instability. While the clinician awaits the research scientists efforts to unravel this problem, there has been much attention as to how these observations might be applied in a clinical setting. There have been several reports that increased oncogene expression might denote the more aggressive forms of cancer. These reports have been dampened and it has become apparent that many normal tissues and benign cells can also express increased amounts of these oncogene protein products. It would be fair to say that the initial enthusiasm for oncogenes has waned as we run into the complexities and overlap with normal tissues. There will undoubtedly be more excitement in the future as we try to unravel whether oncogene expression is changed or increased by DNA rearrangement, changes in the state of methylation of DNA, or point mutations. As we gain additional insight into these problems, we may gain insight into new therapeutic approaches. At present that goal is exciting but far from clear.

7. Monoclonal antibodies and urologic oncology: antigenic expression on genitourinary tumors

LAURENCE H. KLOTZ and NEIL H. BANDER

Introduction

The development of a technique for the routine production of monoclonal antibodies (mAbs) of defined specificity [1] opened up a new era in tumor immunology. It has created the tantalizing possibility of resolving such basic issues as the existence of tumor-specific antigens in human cancer, and the nature of patients' humoral immune response to their tumors. In addition, the application of mAbs to the diagnosis and therapy of cancer promises to provide a host of powerful and specific modalities for the management of malignancy. While the clinical applications of mabs are in a preliminary phase, this chapter will review mAbs currently available which are of interest in urologic oncology, and their applications to date.

Studies of antibody specificity in general and their interaction with tumor antigens in particular, were complicated for many years by the polyclonal nature of the immune response. Attempts to establish a pure population of antibody producing cells failed as normal lymphocytes could neither survive in long-term culture nor could they be cloned.

The technique of hybridization of an immortal myeloma cell line with an antibody-producing B cell, first described in a landmark paper by Kohler and Milstein in 1975 [1], provided a technique by which monoclonal antibodies could be produced in virtually unlimited quantities. Their strategy was straight-forward and elegant. Although normal lymphocytes could not survive in culture, mouse B-cell tumors (myelomas) could. Kohler and Milstein took normal B-cells from the spleen of an immunized mouse and using the techniques of somatic cell genetics, fused these cells to the immortalized mouse myeloma cells. The resulting fused cells, so-called 'hybridomas', combined the features of both parent cells. From the myeloma cell parent, they derived the ability to survive in culture indefinitely. From the immunized spleen B-cell, they derived the ability to produce a specific antibody molecule. These hybridomas can be cloned to yield individual, pure (i.e. monoclonal) immortal populations of cells, each derived from a single

Ratliff, T.L. and Catalona, W.J. (eds), Genitourinary Cancer. ISBN 0–89838–830–9
© *1987, Martinus Nijhoff Publishers, Boston. Printed in the Netherlands.*

hybridoma parent and therefore each secreting antibody to an individual antigenic determinant – a monoclonal antibody.

This revolutionary technique, for which Kohler and Milstein were later awarded the Novel Prize, eliminated the problems related to dealing with mixtures of antibodies in conventional antiserum. MAbs may be used as probes to precisely determine the antigenic expression of tumor cells, and to 'dissect' the polyclonal immune response into its component antibody populations.

An antigen (Ag) is a molecule which, when introduced into an animal, can induce a detectable immune response. In general, only restricted portions of these molecules, known as determinants or epitopes, are involved in the actual binding with antibody combining sites. A single antigen may contain many such determinants. These average about 6 amino acids or sugar moeities in size. For each antigenic determinant there may be many slightly different antibody molecules which will bind, each with subtle differences in amino acid sequences. In the interaction between the antigen and this narrow spectrum of antibodies, each combination will have a slightly different affinity. This represents the so-called polyclonal response which is, in turn, compounded for each antigenic determinant on a complex antigen., and for each complex antigen on a cell.

The most important property of mAbs is their precise specificity, i.e., their ability to recognize a single antigenic determinant. Any reactivity observed with a given mAb is due to the presence of that particular antigenic determinant. This is in contrast to conventional (polyclonal) antisera which contains antibodies of unknown or unwanted specificity in addition to the desired antibody. Consequently, the finding of reactivity when using polyclonal sera is difficult to evaluate. It may indicate the presence of the appropriate epitope or an entirely different pair of Ag-Ab reactions. In practical terms, the ability to produce virtually unlimited amounts of antibody capable of unequivacably detecting its defined antigen in a complex mixture represents a significant advantage.

There are disadvantages of mAbs. Firstly, they are unable to immunoprecipitate antigens having only one determinant for the antibody. This is due to the inability to form lattices by cross-linking multiple antigen molecules. Secondly, the precise specificity of the antibody, under certain circumstances, may be a drawback. For example, many mAbs fail to recognize denatured or precursor forms of the antigen. Polyclonal sera would generally have at least a small proportion of antibody reacting with all forms of the antigen. Thirdly, while polyclonal antisera contains a spectrum of antibodies with affinity for antigen ranging from low to high, a mAb demonstrates antigen-antibody interaction of only a single affinity constant. If the affinity of the mAb happens to be low, the binding of mAb to antigen will be weak. Lastly, polyclonal response involves the production of antibodies of a variety of immunoglobulin classes. Different classes of antibody have the capacity to recruit various effector mechanisms such as complement fixation and antibody-dependent cell-mediated cytotoxicity. An mAb belongs only to a single subclass and may not mediate a desired effector response.

Classification of tumor antigens

Tumor specific antigens may be defined as those antigens that are expressed solely on tumor cells and not on any normal cell in the body at any stage of differentiation or development. To date, no antigen fulfilling this definition has been identified in humans [8]. A more realistic definition of tumor specific antigens are those antigens that are expressed on tumors and are recognized as foreign by the immune system of the tumor-bearing host. A basic tenet of tumor immunology is that such antigens exists.

The evidence for the existence of tumor specific antigens originated [2, 3, 4] with the demonstration, initially by Gross in 1943, of strong tumor antigens on chemically induced sarcomas in mice [9]. Gross detected these antigens by transplantation techniques and showed that inbred mice could be immunized against these tumors. However, these experimentally induced tumors may be special cases in that most spontaneous tumors do not appear to carry detectable tumor-specific transplantation antigens [5–7]. The best evidence for tumor-specific antigens on human tumors comes from the observation that some cancer patients produce antibodies that detect cell surface antigens which are restricted to their own tumors [8]. To date, neither mouse nor human mAbs have been produced to these unique tumor antigens.

The hope that antigens restricted to human tumor cells could be detected by producing mAbs from mice immunized with these cells has not been fulfilled. None of the antigens so far detected using mouse mAbs have, upon rigorous examination, been shown to be absolutely restricted to tumor cells. However, the search for tumor-restricted antigens is far from over. There are several possible explanations for the failure to detect them to date: 1) human tumor specific antigens do not exist, 2) human tumor specific antigens exist but mice immunized with these antigens either do not recognize or are not capable of producing antibodies to them, and 3) human tumor-specific antigens exist as extremely minor or only weakly immunogenic components of the cell surface, so that whole tumor cells or crude extracts are not sufficiently immunogenic for the stimulation of antibody-producing clones.

It should be pointed out that many mAbs give the appearance of restricted specificity during the early stages of analysis when only a small panel of cell lines or tissue sections has been investigated. The assertion that a tumor specific antibody has been produced is only as strong as its probed antigen panel is long. Antibodies require screening against a large variety of adult, fetal, and malignant tissue sections by immunofluorescence or immunoperoxidase techniques in order to confirm expression of the antigen in tumor samples and exclude its expression on normal tissues not available for study as cell lines. Many of the mAbs described to date have not yet been evaluated in this exhaustive fashion.

Most restricted antigens thus far detected by mAbs are differentiation antigens which fall into 3 groups. The least restricted are characteristic of cells of common embryologic origin (i.e., all neuroectodermal cells). A second group define cells of particular tissue, and the third distinguish cells at a particular differentiation or maturation stage within cells of a given lineage. All three types of mAbs have been described in urologic tumor systems.

Human and murine mAbs

To date, most monoclonal antibodies developed against human tumor cells have been the product of immunized mouse B-cells fused with mouse myeloma cells. Mouse hybridomas are now generated relatively routinely in the laboratory. The repertoire of antibodies produced represent the way the mouse immune system 'sees' the particular immunogen (a human tumor cell). The mouse recognizes foreign antigenic determinants on human tumor cells which are not recognized, or poorly recognized by the patient. This means that antibodies may be produced to tumors which are not immunogenic in the host. Conversely, the mouse may not recognize antigens detected by the human immune system. Accordingly there is great interest in the development of human hybridomas derived from the fusion of human myeloma cells and lymphocytes from patients with cancer. These would allow the dissection of the human serological immune response into its component B-cell populations and therefore allow study of antigens recognized as foreign by the patient. In addition, the administration of human mAb to patients for diagnostic studies or treatment would decrease the potential problems of host sensitization associated with the administration of heterologous mouse proteins.

Human mMbs, however, are proving much more difficult to produce than their mouse counterparts. This is probably due to several factors including: 1) the inability to hyperimmunize patients 2) the lower fusion rate of currently available human myeloma cells, and 3) the difficulty in obtaining stimulated, antigen-primed B-cells from peripheral blood. Various strategies have been utilized to circumvent these problems. One approach fuses human B-cells with mouse myeloma cell lines. These interspecies hybridomas with some exceptions [21] have proven to be generally less stable due to the progressive loss of human chromosomes and the resultant cessation of immunoglobulin production. Another method has been to directly transform (immortalize) human B-cells using the oncogenic Epstein-Barr virus (EBV). EBV-transformed lymphocytes, however, cannot be cloned, secrete low levels of antibody and do so only for a limited period of time.

Despite the problems, human mAbs have been produced by a few groups [12, 15]. The Human Tumor Secrology Laboratory at Memorial Sloan Kettering Cancer Center has produced human mAbs using B-lymphocytes from patients with renal and breast cancer and melanomas. These are currently undergoing analysis but none appears to recognize tumor specific antigens yet. Furthermore, the spectrum of antigens detected by these patients' immune systems is far different from that detected by the mouse system. For instance, over 90% of the human mAbs generated have been to intra-cellular rather than to cell-surface antigens. Because at the present the mouse mAb technology is much further advanced than the human counterpart, the remainder of this discussion will center around the former.

Production of mAbs

The steps in the production of mouse monoclonal antibodies are briefly described.

a) Immunization: Mice, usually BALB/c strain, are injected with the antigen of interest repeatedly over several weeks or months. This may vary from a whole cell preparation to a highly purified substance. An immune stimulant such as Freund's adjuvant is often used. The mouse is then sacrificed, the spleen removed, and a single cell suspension consisting of about 100 million lymphocytes is prepared.

b) Growth of the myeloma: the established, immortal myeloma lines are drug-marked by growth in 8-azaguanine, thereby selecting out those mutants which are deficient in the enzyme hypoxanthine-guanine phosphoribosyl transferase (HGPRTase). These cell are totally dependent on the 'de novo' biosynthetic pathway for nucleic acid production and are unable to utilize thymidine or hypoxanthine in the alternate 'salvage' pathway.

c) Cell Fusion: The suspension of immune spleen B-cells is mixed with myeloma cells. Polyethylene glycol (PEG), a substance which decreases the surface tension of cell membranes, is added to the mixture for 2–3 minutes (longer exposure is toxic to the cells). This allows neighboring cell membranes to fuse, thereby combining two or more cells into one large cell. The probability of a successful fusion between lymphocyte and myeloma cell is small (about $1/200,000$). After the PEG is washed out of the cell suspension, the cells are seeded in tissue culture wells at a density of about 50,000 cells per well. They are fed with medium containing aminopterin, an anti-metabolite which blocks the de novo synthetic pathway of DNA. Any unfused myeloma cells are killed as both of their DNA synthetic pathways have been blocked. Unfused spleen lymphocytes are inherently unable to survive in tissue culture so they too die. The only cells which can survive are the approximately 500–1000 successful hybridomas which have inherited the normal HGPRTase gene from the genome of the normal B-lymphocyte.

d) Growth of hybrids: After approximately two weeks, groups of cells ('clones') become readily visible in some of the wells. These cells secrete immunoglobulin molecules into the tissue culture medium. This immunoglobulin includes that coded for in the DNA of the immune lymphocyte. Since the immune lymphocyte partner which forms each hybridoma is almost a random representative of all the spleen cells and since the mouse's lymphocytes are responding to many diverse antigens, one has to select only those clones secreting antibody to an antigen of interest. This is done using a variety of serological techniques.

e) Selection of hybrids: In the search for tumor related cell surface antigens, the 'spent' tissue culture medium of each clone is screened against a panel of tissue culture cell lines consisting of a range of cancer and normal cell types. Binding of the antibody to the cell surface may be detected by any of the standard immunologic assays such as radioimmunoassay, immunofluorescence enzyme-linked assay, or anti-immunoglobulin-bound erythrocyte rosette assay. From this test, a preliminary 'specific profile' of each hybridoma's secreted antibody is determined. Most of the antibodies from a fusion are broadly reactive; that is, they detect highly immunogenic antigens which are present on most cell types (e.g., HLA antigens). Some antibodies bind antigens which are of intermediate restriction present on some, but not all, cell types. Only a few antibodies detect highly restricted antigens – for example proteins which perform a highly specialized function of a differentiated cell type.

f) Growth of Hybridomas: The few (if any) clones secreting an antibody of apparent interest are then repeatedly subcloned to insure that each clone derives from a single parent cell and is, therefore, producing identical antibody molecules. The clone is then injected intra-peritoneally into syngeneic mice where it forms an ascites-producing tumor. The antibody concentration in ascites fluid is 100–1000 times that of tissue culture medium. This high-titered fluid is utilized to fully characterize and define the antibody and antigen.

g) Immunoprecipitation of antigen: Once a stable population of antibody producing cells has been achieved, the antigen recognized by an mAb can be immunoprecipitated and characterized. Tumor cells expressing the antigen are incubated with ^{3}H glucosamine or ^{35}S methionine which become incorporated into the cell's sugars and proteins. The cells are lysed to release the radiolabelled molecules. The lysate is then incubated with the mAb, and the resulting immune complexes precipitated. The Ag-Ab complexes are de-complexed by boiling, and the resulting solution contains pure, radiolabeled antigen. The molecular weight is then determined by polyacrilamide gel electrophoresis.

h) Further characterization of the mAb requires extensive analysis of its specificity on normal and malignant cell lines in vitro and by immunofluorescence or immunoperoxidase staining of tissue sections of normal, fetal, and malignant tissues. Specificity in vivo is determined by imaging tumors in immunodeficient nude mice and, subsequently, cancer patients using radionuclide-labelled mAb. Finally, the gene responsible for the production of the antigen may be mapped to its chromosomal location using somatic cell hybrids and cloned using transfection techniques.

The potential applications of mAbs in oncology are extraordinary; the following is a brief, general, and undoubtedly incomplete list.

1. Cancer Biology: MAbs can be used as probes to characterize the distribution, significance, and function of cellular antigens, many of which were

previously unknown. Mapping of the antigens permits their further use as molecular probes to analyze the structure of the human genome in both normal and malignant cells.

2. Immunopathology: Specific identification of the antigenic pattern of tumors using a panel of mAbs allows stratification of tumors into subgroups on the basis of their molecular profile. Lymphomas have been stratified in this fashion, and in this chapter advances in the stratification of renal and bladder tumors are presented. This offers the prospect of more precise understanding of tumor natural history and formulation of treatment plans.

3. Immunodiagnosis: Assay of antigen levels in serum and urine may provide a system to detect and follow the course of malignant disease and to stratify patients with cancer relative to risk of recurrence. For example, mAb OC125 reacts with a glycoprotein associated with ovarian cancer [14]. This antigen is found at increased levels in 82% of patients with ovarian cancer but only 1% of healthy controls. Furthermore, rising or falling levels of the antigen correlated with progression or regression of disease in 93% of patients.

Immunoscintigraphy

The use of radionuclide-labelled mAbs for radioimmunodetection and radioimmunotherapy has great potential. Pioneer work performed by Pressman and Bale [17–19] showed that semipurified I-131 labelled rabbit antibodies against poorly defined tumor associated antigens can localize to epithelial tumors in vivo. The concept of paired labelling (specific antibodies labelled with I-131 and control IgG labelled with I-125 injected simultaneously followed by substraction imaging), was already defined in 1957. In 1971 the first attempt to localize human choriocarcinoma grafted into hamster cheek pouches with I-131 labelled rabbit anti-human HCG antibodies produced low specific tumor uptake of antibodies and poor scanning images [20]. In 1974, two groups reported localization of heterografted human carcinoma by external scanning with I-131 labeled goat anti-CEA antibodies [21, 22]. The first successful detection of carcinoma in patients using I-131 labelled purified anti-CEA antibodies, external photo scanning and computerized substraction of blood pool radioactivity following injection of Tc-99m labelled albumin was reported in 1978 by Goldenberg [23]. Subsequently the same group reported detecting 35/41 colon carcinoma tumor sites, 21/24 ovarian carcinomas, 12/17 lung carcinomas, 9/14 breast carcinomas and 28/31 uterine carcinomas using I-131 labelled purified goat anti-CEA antibodies [24]. Indium-111 labelled polyclonal anti-CEA antibodies have recently been demonstrated to detect extra-hepatic metastases [28].

The first successful tumor localization with radiolabelled mAbs (anti-CEA) using both external photoscanning and tomoscintigraphy was reported in 1981 by Mach [25]. In 1983, Buchegger et al. [26] used nude mice grafted with human colon carcinoma and clearly demonstrated that fragments from different anti-CEA mAbs gave better tumor to normal tissue ratios than intact antibodies. The highest ratios were obtained with Fab fragments due to improved penetration of the fragments into CEA containing areas. F(ab')2 fragments have subsequently been shown to be optimal for imaging [27].

In 1984, Delaloye using I-123 labelled F(ab')2 fragments of anti-CEA mAbs and tomoscintigraphy, was able to clearly localize the majority of tumor deposits from patients with colon carcinoma within 6 to 24 hours after injection [30].

Immunotherapy

MAbs may be effective alone in producing specific toxicity for the cancer cell by growth regulation, by inducing cell-mediated phenomena, or via activation of the complement system. The targeting of drugs, toxins, or radioisotopes conjugated to mAbs seems to offer great hope for the development of cancer-specific cytotoxic agents. Small numbers of patients with colon cancer, melanoma, leukemia, lymphoma, and renal cancer have been treated with mAbs alone. The Hammersmith Oncology Group [16] reported the successful management of 3 patients with malignant effusion of the peritoneum, pleural, and pericardial spaces. These patients were treated with a tumor-associated mAb labelled with I-131. They observed no toxicity and good clinical response as defined by loss of tumor cells in the effusion and objective tumor shrinkage. Miller [13] described the complete response of a drug-resistant B-cell lymphoma to the systemic administration of an antibody directed against the variable region of the immunoglobulin expressed on the lymphoma cell surface (anti-idiotype antibody).

The specific mAbs produced against urologic tumors and the extent to which they have been utilized experimentally and clinically will be reviewed in the following section.

Monoclonal antibodies to kidney

The host immune response to renal cancer is widely held to affect the natural history of the tumor. The evidence for this is indirect. Spontaneous regression of tumor, although rare, is more common in renal cancer than any other tumor [31]. Additionally, some patients relapse with metastatic renal cancer 20 or more years after nephrectomy; these lesions presumably were present at the time of surgery but were kept in check by a balance between tumor and host.

Renal cancer is an experimentally accessible system for several reasons. 1) It is easily grown in tissue culture; the success rate of establishing continuous cell lines from primary tumors is 13%, and from metastatic lesions 23% [32]. This yield is far higher than any other human tumor except for melanoma. 2) Normal

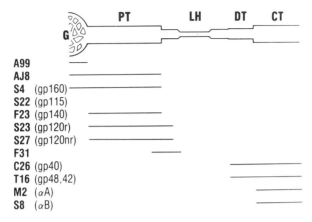

Figure 1. Mapping of the nephron according to antigenic expression of its constituent parts. The nephron is dissected according to its antigenic expression using a panel of mAb's.

renal epithelium can be grown in tissue culture for short periods of time (about 3 months). This means that both the primary tumor and its normal counterpart may be evaluated in vitro, and their antigenic expression and molecular biology compared. This is the only human tumor system where one can compare normal and neoplastic cells from the same (autologous) patient.

MAbs have greatly facilitated the ability to dissect the complex antigenic structure of normal kidney and of renal cell carcinoma (RCC). Much of the work in this area has come from Lloyd Old's group at MSKCC. Their original study [33] described 17 mAbs derived from mice immunized with established cell lines of renal cancer. These mAbs defined 9 cell-surface antigenic systems (Table 1). Immunofluorescence and immunoperoxidase studies demonstrated that these antigens as well as others more recently described [34, 35, 36] were expressed by different cell types comprising the nephron. These mAbs 'map' the domains of the nephron according to the antigenic expression of its parts. Figure 1 shows the immunofluorescence staining of normal kidney by this panel. It is important to point out that with the exception of the blood group antigens and the adenosine deaminase binding protein (ADBP, a proximal tubular antigen previously identified using polyclonal techniques)), none of these antigens had been detected using conventional antisera.

Mab MA99 is derived from a mouse immunized with an ovarian cancer cell line. It detects a glycoprotein complex with subunits of 170,000, 140,000 and 28,000 daltons which is widely distributed on cultured cell lines. In kidney, it stains only glomerular basement membrane. This indicates that an mAb derived from one tissue may be useful in the study of another, unrelated tissue type. MAb S4 was derived from a mouse immunized with a well-differentiated renal cancer cell line (SKRC-7). This mAb immunoprecipitates a glycoprotein of 160,000 daltons (gp160). This antigen is expressed by glomerular and proximal tubular epithelium. Gp160 is also expressed by vessels and interstitial matrix of some tissues including placenta and myometrium, and by a number of sarcomas.

Another group [37] has developed a panel of 7 mAbs which are directed against glomerular antigens. Two of these recognize Fibronectin and type IV collagen respectively, and the other 5 define new carbohydrate or protein determinants which are present on the mesangium or glomerular basement membrane.

MAb AJ8, which precipitates a glycoprotein of 100,000 daltons, also is reactive with glomerular epithelial cells and proximal tubular epithelium. It appears to be identical to the CALLA antigen previously described in leukemia [38] and detected in kidney tissue [39].

MAbs S23, S27 and S6, produced by immunization with a renal cancer cell line, precipitate a glycoprotein of 120,000 daltons which is expressed on proximal tubule brush border and proximal loop of Henle. This antigen has recently been identified as the adenosine deaminase binding protein (ADBP) [40]. The 3 antigens identify distinct epitopes on ADBP. Previous studies with polyvalent antibody to ADBP has shown its presence in kidney, liver, lung, colon, spleen, and placenta, as well as fibroblasts and leukocytes [41, 42, 43]. ADBP also occurs in the body fluids, including serum, saliva and urine. ADBP has been reported to be both present [44] and absent [45] in tumors arising from ADBP + tissues.

Most renal carcinomas arise from proximal tubular cells, and thus, would be expected to share the S4/F23/S23/S27 phenotype of proximal tubular cells. Renal cancers arising in other areas of the nephron would lack expression of these antigens. Distinct subsets of renal cancer can be defined by their antigenic phenotype. Some antigens are expressed by virtually all renal carcinomas, whereas others are expressed by a proportion. In a study of 50 renal cancer specimens typed according to their antigenic expression, 96% expressed at least one proximal tubular antigen. The 4% of tumors which expressed no proximal tubular antigens may be derived from another part of the nephron, and be expected to behave quite differently. Amongst the majority of renal carcinomas of proximal tubular origin, expression of many of the proximal tubular markers are variable and aberrant. For example, although gp100 is expressed by all normal proximal tubular cells, no renal cancers express this antigen. Whether repression of the gene which codes for gp100 is related to the cause of, or the result of, neoplastic transformation is unknown. Conversely, gp115, which cannot be demonstrated on normal proximal tubular cells (or any other normal cells for that matter) is expressed by about 40% of renal cancers. Other proximal tubular antigens may or may not be expressed by a particular tumor. All possible patterns of expression of these antigens have been documented, and the data is consistent with the expression of each of these antigens being independent of one another. Furthermore, there is no clear relationship between degree of differentiation and antigenic expression as is seen in the melanoma and leukemia systems.

Antigenic expression, like other differentiation traits, provides a means to stratify renal tumors into subsets according to their antigenic expression relative

Table 1. Renal MAbs
Reactivity on tissue sections

MAb	Ig class	Ag	Normal tissue	Neoplasms	Group
T138	IgM	gp25	endothelium	epidermal ca.	MSKCC
J143	IgG1	gp 140, 120, 30	G, uroth, esoph, skin thyroid	most carcinomas	MSKCC
AJ8	IgG1	gp100 (CALLA)	G, PT	acute lymphoblastic leukemias	MSKCC
S4	IgG2a	gp160	G, PT	renal cancer, sarcomas	MSKCC
T43	IgG1	gp85	PT, skin	many cancers	MSKCC
F23	IgG2a	gp140	PT, fibroblasts	renal cancers, sarcomas	MSKCC
S23	IgG1	gp120	PT, LH, prost., breast	many carcinomas	MSKCC
S27	IgG1	gp120	PT, LH, prost., breast	many carcinomas	MSKCC
S6	IgG1	gp120	PT, LH, prost., breast	many carcinomas	MSKCC
MK1-1	IgG1	N.D.	PT, panc., breast, lymphocytes	renal cander	ROME
P31	IgM	N.D.	terminal PT, LH, ovary, testis	renal cancer	MSKCC
10.32	IgG1	gp90-Tamm-Horsfall	asc. limb of Henle, DT	N.D.	Cedarlove Labs
C26	IgG21	gp40	DT, CT, uroth	colon cancer	MSKCC
M2	IgM	A-blood group	CT, uroth	many carcinomas	MSKCC
S8	IgM	B-blood group	CT, uroth	many carcinomas	MSKCC
T16	IgG2b	gp48, 42	DT, CT, urothel, prost., uterus, breast, skin, esoph.	bladder & breast	MSKCC
V1	IgG1	N.D.	oveary, adrenal	adrenocortical ca.	MSKCC
S22	IgG1	gp115	none	renal cancer	MSKCC
OKIa1	IgG2	HLA-DR	endoth, mesangium, lymphocytes monocytes/macrophages	melenoma, lymphoma	MSKCC
W6-32	IgG1	HLA, A, B, C,	most cells	leukemia	ORTHO
A6H	IgG1	N.D.	PT	most cancer	COPPEL LABS
D5D	IgG1	N.D.	Bowmn. cap (occ)	R.C., lung, colon ca.	U. MINN
C5H	IgG1	p115	G	R.C.	U. MINN
B1	AgG2a	N.D.	B-cells, fetal ureteral bud	all human cancers	Dana-farber
BA1	IgM	N.D.	B-cells, PMN, Bowm. cap, DT, CT	N.D.	U. MINN

Table 1. Continued

MAb	Ig class	Ag	Normal tissue	Neoplasms	Group
BA2	IgC3	p24	Bowmn. cap, DT, CT	leulemia	U. MINN
SSEA-1	IgM	glycolipid	PT	germ cell ca.	WISTAR
LK-2Y	IgM	N.D.	DT, CT, uroth	chorioca, terato, bladder breast, lung, lymphoma	MSKCC
E6	N.D.	N.D.	none	renal ca.	MAINZ W. GERMANY
B7	N.D.	N.D.	none	renal ca.	MAINZ W. GERMANY
C8	N.D.	N.D.	none	renal ca.	MAINZ W. GERMANY
D8	N.D.	N.D.	none	renal ca.	MAINZ W. GERMANY

Abbreviations: G   Glomerulus
PT   Proximal tubule
DT   Distal tubule
CT   collecting duct
N.D.   not defined

to survival. A correlation between the antigenic profile of renal cancer and the clinical course of the patients can be demonstrated. Cancers that are S4 + /S23 + tend to be well differentiated and slow growing with a 90% 2 year survival rate. Conversely, S4 − /S23 − tumors are rapidly progressive and these patients have only a 10% 2 year survival (34).

MAbs S27 and S23 are of particular interest because the existence of multiple mAbs recognizing different epitopes on the same antigen permits the development of a highly sensitive and specific sandwich assay to detect the presence of this antigen in bodily fluids. An assay for ADBP has been developed using S23 and S27. In the urine, ADBP is a marker for proximal tubular injury [47, 48, 49]. 100% of 37 normal controls and 95% of 40 patients with glomerulonephritis had low levels of urinary ADBP. Conversely, of 79 patients with acute tubular necrosis (ATN), 100% had elevated levels. The marker also appears to differentiate between various forms of urinary tract infection. 6 of 6 patients with acute bacteremic pyelonephritis had high ADBP levels, whereas none of 12 women with acute cystitis had elevated levels. Additional data on transplant patients demonstrated that urinary ADBP is elevated 1 to 7 days prior to the onset of clinical manifestations of rejection, and that sustained elevation following anti-rejection therapy signified a high likelihood of re-rejection following cessation of therapy (Table 2).

ADBP has also been detected in the serum of renal cancer patients by means of this mAb-based assay [50]. It is elevated in 45% of renal cancer patients, compared to 10% of non-renal cancer patients. Patients who have persistent elevation of serum ADBP following nephrectomy appear to be at a high risk for recurrence of disease. These patients had a 17% five year survival rate, compared to 75% for those patients with normal post-operative levels.

Wahlstrom's group has generated a mAb to the endogenous feline retrovirus RB114 p30 antigen. This mAb reacts with an antigen in the tumor cell cytoplasm of 27/27 renal cell adenocarcinomas, and in the lumen of normal tubuli of tumor-bearing kidneys. This antigen was detected in the urine of patients bearing renal cancer, and declined after nephrectomy. Six of 8 patients with persistently elevated p30 antigen post nephrectomy had distant metastases, compared to 2 of

Table 2. Urinary ADAbp and transplant rejection

	Total number of episodes	Urine ADAbp 0.35	Urine ADAbp 0.35
No post-transplant rejection	11 patients	11	0
Urine ADAbp level 1–7 days prior to rejection	29 (19 patients)	0	29
Successful treatment for rejection	18	6	12
Kidney re-rejected post treatment		0/6	10/12 (83%)

7 whose p30 antigen normalized. Urinary p30 antigen may be a marker for residual renal cell carcinoma [53].

Other mAbs stain selectively the loop of Henle (mAb F31), distal and collecting tubules (mAb C26, a product of a colon cancer immunization), and collecting tubules only (mAbs M2 and S8).

Embryologists wishing to study the development of the nephron can study fetal tissue sections or fetal kidney cells in vitro. For example, a 22 week human fetal kidney stained with gp100 demonstrates a progressive increase in staining of tubular structures as one moves from cortex towards medulla, reflecting increased differentiation. Similarly, cultures of normal kidney epithelium have also been evaluated to determine the specific site of origin of the cells which grow in vitro; about 80% of these cells are derived from the proximal tubule [34].

MAbs offer tremendous potential in imaging and treating malignant disease. One group [52] has used 3 mAbs reactive to renal cancer in the radioimmunode-tection and immunoradiotherapy of a human RCC-bearing mouse xenograft model. Renal tumors as small as 40 mg were clearly visualized by radioimmuno-scintigraphy. I-131 labeled mAb was then administered, producing significant inhibitory effects with marked improvement in survival.

Bander et al. at MSCCK [51] have successfully imaged human renal cancer implanted in the thigh of Swiss nude mice with the F(ab′)$_2$ fragment of mAbs S4 and S22. Pilot studies have recently begun at MSKCC to determine the localization and pharmacokinetics of mouse monoclonal antibodies S4, S22, and F23 in patients with advanced renal cancer. Using the same mAbs, therapeutic trials have also been initiated. Preliminary results are encouraging with major responses seen in 2 of 4 patients treated with 10 mg of mAb.

Together, these mAbs represent an invaluable tool for a wide spectrum of investigations including studies of embryogenesis, microanatomy and physiology of the normal kidney, to the analysis of the effects induced by the nephrides and nephrotic syndrome, to the determination of the cellular origins of subsets of renal cancers, and potentially the stratification of renal cancer patients based on the antigenic expression of their tumors.

Monoclonal antibodies to bladder cancer

The heterogeneity of bladder cancer is manifested in the variable natural histology of pathologically similar tumors. Much effort has gone into the analysis of bladder tumors, beyond grade and stage, in an attempt to predict more accurately the subsequent behavior of a given tumor.

Hybridoma technology has been used to create a variety of mAbs directed against antigens expressed on the surface of bladder tumors. To date, all such mAbs have been created by mouse-mouse fusions of murine myeloma cells with spleen cells from mice immunized with established lines of cultured human bladder cancer or lysates of bladder tumors. In this section, the more interesting of these mAbs will be discussed.

Fradet [54] developed 11 mAbs which identify distinct antigens of bladder cancer. These were generated by immunization with bladder cancer cell lines 253-J, 486-P, or T24 or with fresh bladder papillomas. Specificity was determined by direct or absorption tests on a panel of 75 established human cell lines, short-term cultures of fibroblasts and kidney epithelial cells, and immunofluorescence analysis of normal fetal and adult human tissues and tumor specimens.

Table 3 provides data on the patterns of reactivity of these mAbs on cell lines and frozen sections. MAb Om5 identifies an antigen, which is the most restricted of the group. It was expressed by 4 of 18 bladder cancer cell lines, 1 melanoma line and 1 pancreatic line. 4 of 10 fresh bladder tumors expressed the antigen, and all of these had a papillary morphology. None of the poorly differentiated or solid tumors tested expressed this antigen. The antigen has been identified on the cell surface of normal adult urothelium in about 50% of samples tested. This antigen has not been immunochemically characterized.

In contradiction to OM5, 3 other antibodies characterize antigens expressed by more aggressive tumors. T43 immunoprecipitates an 85,000 molecular weight glycoprotein called URO−5. It is an antigen which is widely distributed on most cultured cell types, but not on normal urothelium. Six of 10 bladder tumors were URO−5+, as are normal Kidney proximal tubules and the basal cell layer of skin, cervix and esophagus. MAb T23 was reactive with 3 of 10 bladder tumors and a variety of normal tissues. MAb T138 demonstrated binding to 5 of 10 bladder tumors and a very limited number of other tumors. In spite of their lack of tumor-specificity, these 3 mAbs appear to be expressed preferentially by high grade, invasive tumors. Three other mAbs, J233, JP165, and T101, detected antigens which were not expressed by any normal adult or fetal tissues. J233 was expressed on several cultured bladder and renal cancer cell lines, but not on any frozen sections by immunofluorescence. T101 was expressed on a variety of tumor cell lines, but only on 4/10 bladder tumors, 1 villous adenoma, and 1 breast tumor.

Chopin et al. [55] have developed a pair of mAbs, G4 and E7, which recognize a determinant present on high grade transitional cell carcinoma (TCC) and carcinoma-in-situ (CIS), but not on 16 normal urothelia or a panel of 30 normal or malignant, non-TCC tissues. G4 precipitates an 80 kilodalton (Kd) glycoprotein.

Grossman [56] defined 2 antigens using RT-4 immunized mice. MAb A2 recognizes an antigen present on 2 bladder cell lines, RT4 and 5637 and 1 cervical carcinoma line as determined by extensive absorption analysis.

Koho [57, 58] et al. described 6 mAbs which reacted against bladder tumor cell lines. 3 of these mAbs precipitated the same antigen, a 92 Kd polypeptide. This antigen was expressed by 5 of 7 bladder cancer cell lines but not by normal urothelium. Another mAb reacted with 6 of 7 bladder tumors and a prostatic cancer cell line but not with normal urothelium. Other investigators [59, 60] have described a similar cross-reaction between prostatic and urothelial carcinomas using specific mAbs. Immunofluorescence of fresh tumors and normal tissue was not performed.

The Hellstroms [61] have generated hybridomas to the FANFT-induced mouse bladder tumor. One of these, mAb 2H5, bound to membranes (plated cell extracts) from 5 of 7 transitional cell carcinomas but not to any other of 21 tissue preparations from other origins studied. The antigen was weakly expressed by normal bladder urothelium. Neither IF of fresh tumors, nor evaluation of cell lines was performed. This mAb immunoprecipitated a 140 KD protein.

Masuko et al. [62] have defined 3 antigenic systems using mAbs produced against bladder cancer cell line KU-1. One system, defined by 3 mAbs, is a glycopeptide complex consisting of molecules with molecular weight of 78,000 (major) and 40,000 and 130,000. This antigen is expressed by 5 of 6 bladder cancer cell lines and a portion of human epithelial cell lines. It is not expressed by normal tissues or cells except for one of the 3 epitopes which is expressed by normal epidermis.

Settle et al. [63] developed an mAb which recognizes cytoskeletal keratins of stratified epithelia and bladder carcinomas, but not normal bladder epithelium. This was raised to a mouse bladder tumor using rat immune splenocytes.

MAbs to intermediate filament proteins have been used to study the processes involved in the neoplastic progression of bladder tumors [64]. Normal urothelium expresses cytokeratin 18 in the superficial cell layer only. This pattern is also seen in well-differentiated papillary transitional cell carcinomas. In highly invasive tumors, cytokeratin 18 is expressed throughout the tumor, including the basal cell layer. This is somewhat paradoxical, as normal transitional cells mature into cytokeratin 18-expressing cells at the end stage in their development. One would expect high grade tumor expression to reflect a more primitive phase of cellular maturation.

A, B and H blood group specific monoclonal antibodies have been used in an indirect immunoperoxidase technique to define blood group isoantigen expression by normal transitional epithelium and TCC [65]. Conventional ABH testing using the specific red cell adherence (SRCA) test is technically difficult and subjective. Only 12% of 31 patients who were isoantigen positive by the mAb immunoperoxidase technique progressed to invasive disease compared to 50% of antigen negative patients. A subsequent report refined the method using an avidin-biotin complex technique [65a]. This has resulted in a more reproducible assay as well as consistently strong binding of the H antigen. Nonetheless, the advantages of ABH serotyping over conventional clinical evaluation of bladder tumors by means of grade and stage has yet to be demonstrated conclusively.

Summerhayes et al have generated 9 mAbs from membrane preparations of human bladder cancer which recognise 3 different antigenic systems on the surface of normal human urothelium. These 3 antigenic groups are localized to subpopu-

Table 3. Bladder MAbs
Reactivity on tissue sections

MAb	Ig class	Ag	Normal tissue	Cell line	Neoplasms	Group
OM5	G1	N.P.	none pos		4/10 BT's	MSKCC
T16	G2B	GP 48.000 42.000	distal and collecting duct urothelium, prostate, breast ducts, pluri-stratified epithelia		bladder, breast	MSKCC
T87	G1	GP 60,000	like T16 but neg. on pluristratified epithelia		most human cancers except renal and neuro-ectodermal	MSKCC
J143	G1	140, 120, 30 KD, GP	glomeruli (F & A) thyroid BM, basal cell layer of urothelium, skin, esoph.		all BT's and other epithelial tumours	MSKCC
T43	G1	85 KD GP	(both F&A) prox. tubule kidney basal cell layer of skin, cervix, neg. on normal urothelium		neg. on non-epithelial tumours, pos. 3/8 RCC 6/10 BT	
T23	1gM	N.P.	astrocytes, melanocytes, fibroblasts, smooth muscle		3/10 BT, 2/10 renal, 3/3 lung, 2/2 astrocytoma, 2/2 melanoma, 3/3 sarcoma	MSKCC
T138	1gM	gp 25 KD	endothelial cells		5/10 BT, 2/3 lung, 1/1 sarcoma, 2/2 breast	MSKCC
T110	G1	gp 240KD	fibrillar straining in the extra cellular matrix of all normal and malignant tissues tested			MSKCC
JP165	G1	N.P.	neg. all normal and fetal tissue		2/2 Bt, 2/2 renal	MSKCC
J233	G1	N.P.	neg. on all normal adult/fetal tissue		neg. on tissue pos 4/18 cell lines	MSKCC
T101	G2a	N.P.	neg on all normal adult/fetal tissue		4/10 BT, 1 villous adenoma pos many cell lines	MSKCC
A2	g1	N.K.	not tested		not tested on tissue pos RT4 BT cell lines	U. Michigan
A80	g1					
LBS1, 19 17	NK	N.K.	not tested	pos all epithelial derived cell lines	not tested on tissue pos 2/6 BT lines	Inst. of Urol. London
LBS 2, 8, 15, 17	NK	N.K.	not tested	pos urothelium derived cell lines	not tested tissue	Inst. of Urol. London

Table 3. Continued

MAb	Ig class	Ag	Normal tissue	Cell line	Neoplasms	Group
LBS 10, 20A, 20B, 21, 34	NK	N.K.	neg. on urothelium	pos urothelium derived cell lines	not tested	Inst. of Urol. London
4B5	g1	92 KD	neg. on urothelium	5/7 BT	not tested	Stockholm
7E9	g3	92 KD	neg. on urothelium	similar	not tested	Stockholm
14B11	g1	92 KD	neg. on urothelium	similar	not tested	Stockholm
4E8		polypeptide 190KD 170KD	neg. on urothelium	5/6 BT	not tested	Stockholm
S2CG	g1	polypeptide 50KD	neg. on all crude extracts of normal tissues			
2H5	NK	140KD	normal liver and lung	7/7 BT lines	2/2 crude extracts of BT	Stockholm
1E6	NK	N.P.	(crude extracts)			
A4	IgM	78 40 }KDgp 130	neg. on urothelium	3/5 BT 3/3 colon	3/5 BT no other tumours tested	
MBE3	IgM	same as A4	similar to A4	similar	similar	
HBG9	IgB		similar but pos. on epidermis		similar	
HBE10	IgM		similar to A4	6/6 BT lines 3/3 colon	similar	

Abbreviations: NP   not precipitated
NK   not known
BT   Bladder Tumors

lations of normal urothelium; 1 group is specific for basal and intermediate cells of urothelium, and the others stain superficial and intermediate cell layers. Invasive tumors demonstrated 'one-sided basal staining', characterized by the surface staining of cells at the epithelial-stromal interface. The authors claim this may have predicitive value for invasion [66].

A hemagglutinating IgM mAb, mAb 145 directed against a red blood cell membrane antigen also recognizes an antigen expressed on normal urothelium [67]. In 16 bladder tumors from 12 patients, 7 expressed both ABH and mAb 145 antigens, 7 expressed neither, and 2 were mAb 145 + /ABH − . One patient who progressed to invasive disease had progressive loss of both antigens.

A mAb developed by Lin's group [68] recognizes an antigen expressed by a histologically wide range of bladder tumors. This mAb has been evaluated in the detection of exfoliated tumor cells in bladder washings. The assay appears to be superior to routine cytology in the detection of low grade tumors, although patient numbers were small.

MAb Ca1 recognizes the so-called 'Ca' antigen which is a marker for human epithelial malignant cells [69]. Flow cytometric measurement of Ca antigen visualized by immunofluorescence demonstrated [70] a significant increase in the proportion of fluorescent cells in 11 of 12 aneuploid tumors and 0 of 14 diploid tumors. 7 of 11 tumors with Ca1 + cells were invasive. This pattern is the reciprocal of the expression of blood group antigens which are less likely to be expressed by invasive tumors.

Using urine from bladder cancer patients as the immunogen, McCabe and Lamm developed mAbs to urinary fibrinogen/fibrin degradation products [71]. Using this mAb an enzyme-linked immunosorbent assay (ELISA) was developed to evaluate the level of these products in urine. The assay identified 83% of the specimens from bladder cancer patients with a false positive rate of 5%. The accuracy of the assay was not limited to high grade lesions as well differentiated tumors produced an elevated value as often as did poorly differentiated tumors.

There are numerous potential applications of these antibodies in the management of patients with this disease. The antigenic profile of a tumor, based on immunofluorescence studies with a panel of monoclonals, is easily performed. The ability to type a patient's bladder tumor may provide information about its natural history. For hematopoietic tumors [72] and melanoma [73], diversity in the antigenic expression of tumors is analogous to the diversity in the surface antigens of corresponding normal cells as they differentiate, and for these tumors subsets may be defined on the basis of these antigens. It has been demonstrated by the red cell adherence assay and immunoperoxidase testing that loss of normal blood group antigens on urothelial neoplasms correlates with invasive tumor potential. However, in the bladder antigenic system, data regarding the relationship between antigen expression and the likelihood of invasion and metastasis has not yet been developed.

A second, related application is in the use of flow cytometry in conjunction with monoclonal antibodies. Huffman [74] has described the use of multi-parameter flow cytometry in quantifing the relationship between DNA-RNA content and antigenic expression. Using mAb OM5 [54] which recognizes a differentiation antigen expressed by normal urothelium and well differentiated transitional cell carcinomas, exfoliated epithelial cells in the urine of patients with non-papillary carcinoma-in-situ were examined during and after intravesical therapy with Bacillus-Calmette-Guerin (BCG). 5 of 9 patients with persistence of OM5 positive cells after therapy had recurrent tumor, whereas none of four without detectable antigen-positive cells after therapy had persistent tumor. The analysis of the antigenic characterization of bladder tumors from bladder irrigation specimens may provide a powerful tool to assess clinical status and response to therapy.

Grossman et al. [75] imaged an RT4 bladder tumor growing in a nude mouse with I-125 labelled intact murine mAb A2. Tumor uptake peaked at 24 hours. The uptake of I-125 mAb in the bladder was comparable to levels in other nontarget tissues. High background from blood pool radioactivity remains a problem. Imaging of metastatic bladder cancer with mAbs has not yet been attempted clinically.

A fourth, exciting application is the use of mAbs directed against bladder tumor antigens as intravesical therapy. This is appealing because the potential problems associated with the systemic administration of mouse monoclonals, (sensitization, cross-reactivity with normal tissue bearing the same determinant, etc.) would be diminished. In addition, mAb-toxin conjugates which may be too toxic to be administered systematically may be used intravesically. To date, no experience with the use of intra-vesical mAb has been reported.

MAbs to prostate

In 1964, Shulman et al [77] described an acid phosphatase which was immunologically specific to human prostate. Prostatic acid phosphatase (PAP) has been purified to homogeneity from both the human prostate gland and seminal fluid [78]. PAP is a glycoprotein with a molecular weight of about 100,000. By isoelectric focusing it can be separated into eight or more isoenzymes with isoelectric points between 4.2 and 5.5. [79, 80, 81]. Antiserum raised against purified PAP exhibits, upon appropriate absorption, immunologic reactivity only with purified PAP or prostate tissue extract and not with extracts from other tissues [77, 80].

Recently, Lee et al. described four anti-PAP MAbs of different subclasses (IgG1, IgG2a, IgG3, and IgM) [82]. Initial data indicated that the mAbs of the IgG1 and IgM subclasses were more specific for PAP than were those of the IgG2a and IgG3 subclasses. The binding analysis suggested that the IgG2a and IgG3 mAbs bound to an identical or closely spaced antigenic determinant on PAP. The

Table 4. Prostate MAbs
Tissue sections

MAb	Ig class	Ag	Normal tissue	Neoplasms	Group
aPro 13	NK	40KDgp	endothelium, BPH, 1/7 neg. prostate (ductal epithelium only) 1/1 neg. testicle, 1/1 tonsil	4/16 Ca prostate 1/2 RCC	Duke Med. Centre
aPro 3	NK	175KD gp non reduced		strong absorption from poorly diff. prostate adeno Ca	Duke
aPro 5	NK	54KD gp 34KD gp		well diff. Ca prostate and testis, neg. on 50 normal and malignant tissues. Pos. on prostate, ductal epithelium, and Ca prostate	Roswel Park
F77 129	IgG3	NK	prostate, breast, variable staining in liver and kidney	prostate, breast	Harvard
MHG7	IgM	NK	neg. foreskin, pos. 3/6 BPH otherwise not evaluated	focal (10-35%) pos. staining in 6/10 prostate. Other tumours not evaluated	San Diego
Panel of 8 Mabs	1, 2a, IgM	NK	3 groups: 1) epithelium specific, 2) polyepithelial, 3) stroma specific, other	3 mAbs not tested, 5 mAbs pos. on breast & prostate, no other tumours tested	Stanford
DU83.21	IgM	non reduced: 180 & 110KD reduced: 60 KD chain & 28KD chain	neg. bladder, pos. proximal tubules of normal kidney	1/4 bladder, 11/19 prostate, primaries, 1/6 mets. 0/15 other primary tumours	E. Virginia School of Medicine Norfolk, Va
P6.2	IgM	NK	similar to D83.21	14/19 primary Ca pros., 4/6 mets. Ca prostate, 6/15 other tumours, 3/4 bladder tumours	
KR-P8	NK	NK	3/3 BPH, 5/5 neg. prostate, 0/16 other tissues	15/15 prostate, 1/1 met. lymph node from prostate Ca, 0/5 other tumours	Richmond Va.

Abbreviations: NK, not known

IgM and IgG1 mAbs reacted with two other distinct antigenic determinants, indicating that 3 or more distinct antigenic determinants were detected.

The PAP molecule has been further defined using submaxillary protease digestion to break it into 3 fragments (SP-1, 2 and 3). Anti-PAP mAbs exhibited striking specificity to PAP, particularly to the SP-1 fragment, without binding to other acid phosphatase preparations. By competitive or direct binding assays, three nonidentical and non-overlapping antigenic determinants were recognized to be clustered on the SP-1 fragment. SP-3, the enzyme active site, was an antigenically cross-reactive region, and SP-2 was nonantigenic.

Lillehoj [83] produced 6 mAbs with strict specificity for PAP. Binding to PAP was not inhibited by absorption with lysosomal acid phosphatase, which is similar in its molecular size and kinetic properties.

PAP can be assayed by a number of immunoassays, both serologically and immunohistochemically. MAb assays develop to date have increased specificity, but less sensitivity, than the polyclonal antisera based assays currently in use [84]. Their clinical role has yet to be defined. At least one study [85] has shown no advantage of an mAb-based RIA over conventional polyclonal antibody-based RIA in the evaluation and monitoring of patients with prostate cancer.

In 1980, prostatic antigen (PA) was identified and purified from prostatic tissue by Wang et al. [86]. This has subsequently been identified in seminal plasma, normal, malignant, and hypertrophic prostate, and in the sera of patients with prostate cancer. PA is localized within the cytoplasm of ductal epithelial cells and in secretory material in ductal lumina. It consists of a single polypeptide of MW 34,000. Serologically it is quite distinct from PAP [87].

The specificity of PA has been further defined by mAb F5 [88]. This mAb, defined by competitive binding and immunohistochemical studies, reacted with normal, malignant, and metastatic prostate tissue as well as purified PA. It did not react with other normal or malignant tissues including bladder and kidney. Expression on fetal tissues was not studied. The determinant is resistant to tissue fixation with paraffin. The degree of staining correlated with the degree of cytological differentiation, being most intense in well-differentiated tumors. However, poorly differentiated tumors, whether primary or metastatic, stained well enough to permit differentiation from tumors of non-prostatic origin.

Frankel et al. have generated 3 mAbs (1F3, 2G7, and 1C5) specific for prostatic antigen (PA) [89]. All three mAbs were of the IgG1 subclass. These defined two non-cross-blocking unique determinants on PA, each present as one site per molecule. The antigen has the same tissue distribution as PA. Immunoperoxidase staining of paraffin sections of BPH and prostatic carcinoma revealed strong prostate epithelial reactivity, but no reactivity with prostate membrane preparations. This suggests that PA is an intracellular antigen. The existence of 2 mAbs recognizing different epitopes of the same antigen permitted the detection of serum PA. Six of 6 normal and 4 of 4 non-prostatic cancer patients had PA levels less than 5 ng/ml; 7 of 20 stage D prostate cancer patients had levels of 100 or greater. The sensitivity and specificity of this assay, as well as its relationship to serum PAP levels, has yet to be defined precisely, but it may have a role as a tumor marker for prostatic carcinoma.

Ware et al. [90, 91] described an antigen, p54, defined by mAbs aPro 3 and aPro 5. These mAbs bound preferentially to the surface of the immunizing cell line, PC-3, and reacted less strongly with another human prostatic carcinoma cell line (DU145) and a colon carcinoma line (LoVo). APro 3 also reacted with human breast carcinoma and normal fibroblast cell lines. The mAb competed with serum immunoglobulin from patients with prostatic cancer for binding to p54 antigen. This indicates that the determinant recognized by these patients' serum Ig was identical to that recognized by the aPro 3 mAb. The antigen was detectable in extracts of human normal and malignant non prostatic tissue, as well as in benign prostate tissue. Absorption analysis, however, revealed substantially greater quantities in malignant prostate tissue and testis tumors.

Another mAb (a-Pro 13) developed by the same group [92] defined an antigen (p40) expressed by ductal epithelium of the prostate, renal vascular endothelium, testicle and tonsil. By immunoperoxidase staining, the antigen was expressed by 4 of 16 prostate cancers, 1 of 2 renal cancers, and no other malignant tissue. The antigen was found to be stable on the cell surface of PC-3 cells. The mAb-Ag complex persisted on the cell surface for over 56 hours. This bears on the potential therapeutic role of mAb-toxin conjugates.

Starling et al. [93, 94], using prostatic cancer cell line DU145 as an immunogen, developed a mAB (D83.21) which bound to both prostate and bladder cancer cell lines. It did not bind to a number of other normal or malignant cell lines except for a cytomegalovirus (HCMV) transformed human embryonic lung cell line. Neither normal nor HCMV infected but non-transformed embryonal lung fibroblasts expressed the antigen recognized by D83.21, indicating a shared antigen between urogenital tumors and HCMV-transformed cells [95]. Malignant tissue and liver metastases demonstrated high reactivities, but normal and hypertrophic prostate did not. By immunoperoxidase, 58% of primary prostate carcinomas and 17% of metastatic tumors reacted with D83.21. Subsequent analysis of this antigen [96] indicated that it is a membrane glycoprotein made up of disulfide-bonded subunits. This is a characteristic of a number of membrane molecules which act as receptors, including the transferrin, insulin, and T-cell receptor, and suggests that the D83.21 antigen is involved in the transmission of signals across the membrane.

A second mAb, P6.2 [94] developed by the same group reacted with 68% of primary and metastatic tumors. Marked heterogeneity of Ag expression was identified in most tumors, confirming the well-established concept of multiple subpopulations of prostatic cancer cells constituting a prostatic tumor. Neither antibody reacted with 6 normal or 12 benign prostate specimens, nor any of a variety of other normal human tissues except for the proximal tubules of normal kidney.

Using membrane-enriched fractions of human benign prostatic hyperplasia tissues, Frankel et al. generated eight mAbs reactive with human prostate tissues [97]. These were divided into 3 major groups – epithelium-specific, polyepithelial, and stromal-specific – on the basis of differential binding to the surfaces of various component cells in the prostate and other epithelia. Two of the epithelium-specific mAbs, 35 and 24, defined protein antigens specific for prostate epithelia that did not cross react with PAP or PA. These reacted with normal, BPH and malignant prostatic tissue. MAb 35 reacted only with normal kidney and mAb 24 only with salivary gland; neither reacted with any other normal tissue. MAb 35 reacted with bladder cell line T-24; neither reacted with any other non-prostatic line. Only 5 lines were tested, and the MAbs were not screened against fetal tissue.

Another mAb, KP-P8, prepared against the PC3 cell line, reacted with an Ag expressed on glandular epithelium of all normal, BPH and malignant prostate glands. The antigen was not expressed by a variety of normal tissues nor 4 non-prostatic cancer cell lines [98]. The Ag was not destroyed by paraffin preparation of tissue. It was present in seminal plasma indicating it was a secreted product. The authors conclude that the Ab is prostate 'organ-specific'; however, it is difficult to accept this claim in the absence of more extensive testing against cell lines, fresh non-prostatic tumors, and fetal tissues.

Durkop et al. [99] using prostatic carcinoma line HPC 36 as the immunogen and screening against spent tissue culture medium, generated a mAb directed against an antigen found in the supernatant of HPC 36 cultures. The Ag was also expressed on the surface of tumor cells and by a subpopulation of immature prostatic myoepithelial cells but not by normal mature glandular cells. The mAb precipitated a protein of 65 kD. Whether this Ag is secreted into prostatic fluid preferentially by tumor cells remains to be seen.

Lowe et al. has recently generated a human-mouse hybridoma from the fusion of lymphocytes from a regional lymph node of a patient with prostate carcinoma and murine myeloma cells [100]. This mAb, MHG7, reacted with 3 of 4 prostate carcinoma cell lines and about two thirds of BPH and malignant cells on both frozen and paraffin sections. Certain colon and lung carcinoma cell lines were also MHG7-positive.

Another mAb, F77-129, developed by Carroll et al. [101] to the PC-3 prostate adenocarcinoma cell line, recognized an antigen expressed by prostate and breast cancer. This antigen appears similar to Ware's mAb also raised to PC-3. This system has been used to successfully image a 90 mg tumor in a PC-3 tumor-bearing nude mouse. In addition, the authors have demonstrated that the antibody is internalized in vitro. This is important for the development of therapies involving conjugates between mAbs and drugs, toxins, or radiation-emitting compounds.

Progress in the development of mAbs with specificity to prostate cancer has been slower than in other systems due, in part, to the lack of available prostatic adenocarcinoma cell lines, the slow growth rate of prostate cancer, and perhaps to the inherent nature of the antigenic expression of these cancers. The differential antigenic expression of hormone-responsive and hormone-resistant prostate cancers has yet to be explored. Progress has been made in the analysis of PAP and PA and in the characterization of some prostatic surface antigens, Many of the mAbs described above have great potential usefulness.

MAbs and testicular cancer

The concept that normal antigens may be expressed or shed by solid tumors was recognized early in the course of tumor immunology. The current use of alphafetoprotein (AFP) and beta-human chorionic gonadotropin (BHCG) in clinical practice are prominent examples.

MAb studies of testicular cancers have dealt with cell-surface 'embryonic' antigens. A murine mAb has been developed against murine teratocarcinoma which also binds to murine embryonal carcinoma. The antigen recognized is called stage-specific embryonic antigen 1 (SSEA-1) because it is expressed on the 8-cell embryo [103]. This antigen is also expressed by the ectodermal cells of the early postimplantation embryo, on primordial germ cells, on ejaculated sperm and on kidney and endometrial cells. It is not present on mature ovarian or testicular cells, and is not species specific. It can be detected on yolk sac elements of human germ cell tumors, fetal (but not mature) testicular tubules, and on both fresh embryonal cell carcinoma and established embryonal cell carcinoma cell lines. Another mAb defines an antigen SSEA-3, a developmentally earlier antigen present on mouse fetal testicular cells and human embryonal carcinoma cells, including those of testicular carcinoma in situ, but absent from adult murine testis and teratocarcinoma cells. The antigen is also expressed by other cell types, including vascular and smooth muscle cells, erythrocytes, and myoepithelial cells. These findings suggest that human embryonal carcinoma is a very primitive tumor in terms of its cell of origin, arising from primordial or fetal germ cells rather than mature germ cells [104].

MAbs which recognize distinct epitopes of AFP have been developed [105]. Using these mAbs, the authors have developed a highly specific sandwich assay for AFP which has higher sensitivity and specificity for hepatocellular carcinoma than the conventional polyvalent RIA. Result in a small group of patients with testicular cancer were comparable to conventional RIA.

Another area of great potential clinical value is the use of anticytokeratin mAbs in the detection and diagnosis of epithelial tumors. Keratins are a family of water-insoluble proteins of 40 to 70 KD, and are present in almost all epithelial cells. Keratin filaments are related to, but immunologically distinguishable from, intermediate filaments of other types, such as vimentin of mesenchymal cells, desmin of muscle cells, neurofilaments of neurons, and glial filaments of astrocytes [106].

148

One study reported to date examined cytokeratin staining in germ cell tumors [107]. All seminomas stained negatively for cytokeratin, while all embryonal carcinomas, yolk sac tumors, and choriocarcinomas were at least focally positive. Thus these mAbs will be an adjunct to conventional histology in those cases of diagnostic difficulty, for example between anaplastic seminoma and embryonal carcinoma.

Conclusion

Monoclonal antibody technology offers an unprecedented tool with which to evaluate the molecular expression of tumors, and to utilize these antigens both as a means of detection of occult lesions and a target for tumor toxins. The role of mAbs in diagnosis is well established in a preliminary fashion in specific areas. Their role in the treatment of genitourinary malignancies remains to be elicited.

While much work has been done in defining tumor antigens, it is likely that hundreds or thousands of tumor-associated antigens are expressed by tumors. Monoclonal antibodies will remain a fruitful area for both basic and clinical investigation for the forseeable future.

References

1. Kohler G, Milstein C: Continuous cultures of fused cells secreting antibody of predefined specificity. Nature 256: 495, 1975
2. Gross L: Intradermal immunization of C3H mice against a sarcoma originating in an animal of the same line. Cancer Res 3: 326, 1943
3. Foley EJ: Antigenic properties of methylcholanthrene-induced tumors in mice of the strain of origin. Cancer Res 13: 835, 1953
4. Prehn RT, Main JM: Immunity to methlycholanthrene-induced sarcomas. J Nat Cancer Inst 18: 769, 1957
5. Hewitt HB, Blake ER, Walder AS: A critique of the evidence for active host defense against cancer, based on personal studies of 27 murine tumors of spontaneous origin. Br J Cancer 33: 241, 1976
6. Weiss DM: The questionable immunogenicity of certain neoplasms. Cancer Immunol Immunother 2: 11, 1977
7. Klein G, Klein E: Rejectability of virus-induced tumors and non-rejectability of spontaneous tumors: a lesson in contrasts. Transpln Proc IX, 1977
8. Old LJ: Cancer immunology: the search for specificity. Cancer Res 41: 361, 1981
9. Gross L: Intraderman immunization of C3H mice against a sarcoma that originated in an animal of the same line. Cancer Res 3: 326, 1943
10. Houghton AN, Brooks H, Cote RJ, Taormina MC, Oettgen HF, Old LJ: Detection of cell surface and intracellular antigens by human mabs. Hybrid cell lines derived from lymphocytes of patients with malignant melanoma. J Exp Med: 158: 53, 1983
11. Cote RJH, Morrissey DM, Houghton RN, Beattie EJ, Oettgen HF, Old LJ: Generation of human cell surface and intracellular antigens by mabs. Hybrid cell lines derived from lymphocytes of patients with malignant melanoma. J Exp Med 158: 53, 1983

12. Cote RJH, Morissey DM, Houghton RN, Beattie EF, Oettgen HF, Old LJ: Generation of human monoclonal antibodies reactive with cellular antigens. PNAS 80: 2026, 1983

13. Miller DD, Warnke R: Treatment of B-cell lymphoma with monoclonal anti-idiotype antibody. NEJM 306: 517, 1982

14. Klug TL, Bast RC, Niloff JM, Knapp RC, Zurawski VR: Monoclonal antibody immunoradiometric assay for an antigenic determinant (CA125) associated with human epithelial ovarian carcinomas. Cancer Res 44: 1048, 1984

15. Edwards PAW, Smith CM, Nevill AM, O'Hare MJ: Production of human monoclonal antibodies to tumor antigens. Eur J Immunol 12: 641, 1982

17. Pressman D, Korngold L: Cancer 6: 619–623, 1953

18. Bale WF, Spar IL, Goodland RL, Wolfe DE: Proc Soc Exp Biol Med 89: 564–568, 1955

19. Pressman D, Day ED, Blau M: Cancer Res. 17: 845, 1957

20. Quinones J, Mizejewski G, Beierwaltes WH: Choriocarcinoma scanning using radiolabelled antibody to chorionic gonadotrophin. J. Nucl. Med 12: 69–75, 1971

21. Goldenberg DM, Preston DF, Primus FJ: Photoscan localization of GW-39 tumors in hamsters using radiolabelled anti-carcinoembryonic antigen immunoglobulin G. Cancer Res 34: 1–9, 1974

22. Mach JP, Carrel S, Merenda C: In vivo localization of radiolabelled antibody to carcinoembryonic antigen in human colon cancer grafted into nude mice. Nature 248: 704–706, 1974

23. Goldenberg DM, Deland F, Kim E: Use of radiolabelled antibody to carcinoembryonic antigen for the detection and localization of diverse cancers by external photoscanning. N. Engl J Med 298: 1384–1388, 1976

24. Goldenberg M, Kim EE, Deland FH: Radioimmunodetection of cancer with radioactive antibodies to carcinoembryonic antigen. Cancer Res 40: 2984–2992, 1980

25. Mach JP, Buchegger F, Forn M: Use of radiolabelled monoclonal anti-carcinoembryonic antigen antibodies for the detection of human carcinomas by external photoscanning tomoscinitgraphy. Immunol Today: 239–249, 1981

26. Buchegger F, Haskell CM, Schreyer M: Radiolabelled fragments of monoclonal antibodies against carcinoembryonic antigen for localization of human colon cancer grafted into nude mice. J Exp. Med. 158: 413–427, 1983

27. Wahl RL, Parker CW, Philpott GW: Improved radioimaging and tumor localization with monoclonal F(ab')2. J Nucl Med 24: 316–325, 1983

28. Fairweather DS, Bradwell AR, Dykes PW: Br Med J 287, 167–170, 1983

29. Begent RHJ, Green AJ, Bagshaw KD: Lancet II 739–742, 1983

30. Delaloye B, Bischof-Delaloye A, Grob JP, Buchegger F: Presented at American Congress of Nuclear Medicine, Los Angeles, Cal 1984

31. Everson T, Cole W: Spontaneous regression of cancer. Philadelphia, WB Saunders, CO, 1966

32. Bander NH: Renal cancer: A model system for the study of human neoplasia. In: Genes and antigens in cancer: the monoclonal antibody approach, Reithmuller H, Koprowski von Kleist S (eds). Karges Press, Basel, 1984

33. Ueda R, Ogata SI, Morrissey DM, Finstad CL, Szudlarek J, Whitmore WF, Oettgen HF, Lloyd KO, Old LJ: Cell surface antigens of human renal cancer defined by mouse mAbs: Identification of tissue specific kidney glycoproteins. Proc Natl Acad Sci USA 78 (8): 5122, 1981

34. Bander NH, Cardon-cardo C, Finstad CL, Whitmore WF, Vaughan ED, Melamed M, Oettgen HF, Old LJ: Immunopathology of human renal cancer: Identification of clinically distinct sucsets. In preparation, 1986

35. Cordon-Cardo C, Bander HN, Fradet Y, Finstad CL, Whitmore WF, Lloyd KO, Oettgen HF, Melamed MR, Old LJ: Immunoanatomic dissection of the human urinary tract by mabs. J Histochem Cytochem 32(10): 1035, 1984

36. Bander NH, Cordon-cordo C, Finstad CL, Whitmore WF, Darraccott Vaughan III, Oettgen HF, Melamed M, Old LJ: Immunohistologic Dissection of the human kidney using mabs. J Urol 133(3), 502, 1985

37. Hancock WW, Kraft N, Clarke F, Atkins RC: Production of mAbs to fibronectin, type IV collagen and other antigens of the human glomerulus. Pathology 16: 197, 1984

38. Ritz J, Pesando JM, Noti-McConarty J, Lazarus H, Schlossman SF: A mAb to human acute lymphoblastic leukemia antigen. Nature 283: 583, 1980

39. Metzger R, Borowitz M, Jones N, Dowell B: Distributions of common acute lymphoblastic leukemia antigen in nonhematopoietic tissues. J Exp Med 145: 1249, 1981

40. Andy RJ, Finstad CL, Old LJ, Lloyd KO, Kornfeld R: The antigen identified by a mouse mAb raised against human renal cancer cells sis the adenosine deaminase binding protein. J Biological Chemistry 259 (20): 12844, 1984

41. Finstad CL, Cordon-cardo C, Bander NH, Whitmore WF, Melamed MR, Old LJ: Specificity analysis of mouse mAbs defining cell surface antigens of human renal cancer. PNAS 82: 2955, 1985

42. Schrader WP, Stacy AR: Immunoassay of the adenosine deaminase complexing protein of human tissues and body fluids. J Biol Chem 154: 11958, 1979

43. Trotta PP: Biochemistry 21, 4014, 1982

44. Andy RJ and Kornfeld R: The adenosine deaminase binding protein of human skin fibroblasts is located on the cell surface. J. Biol Chem 257: 7922, 1982

45. ten Kate J, Wijnen JT, van der Goes RGM, Quadt R, Griggioen G, Bosman FT, Khan PM: Quantitative changes in adenosine deaminase isoenzymes in human colorectal cancer. Cancer Res 44: 4688, 1984

46. Bander NH: Comparison of antigen expression of human renal cancers in vivo and in vitro. Cancer 53: 1235, 1984

47. Thompson RE, Piper DJ, Galberg C, Chan TH, Tolkoff-Rubin NE, Rubin RH: Adenosine dimainase hinding protein, a new diagnostic marker for kidney disease. Clin Chem, in press, 1985

48. Tolkoff-Rubin NE, Thompson RE, Piper DJ, Bander NHJ, Finstad CJ, Klotz LH, Old LJ, Hansen WP, Rubin RH: Dignosis of renal proximal tubular injury by urinary immunoassay for a proximal tubular antigen, the andenosine deaminase binding protein. (Presented at the 17th annual meeting of the American Society of Nephrology, Wash DC), 1984

49. Tolkoff-Rubin NE, Cosimi AB, Delmonico FL, Russell PS, Thompson RE, Piper DJ, Hansen WP, Bander NH, Finstad CL, Cordon-Cordo Cordo C, Klotz LH, Old LJ, Rubin RH: Diagnosis of transplant rejection and cyclosporin toxicity by urinary assay for a proximal tubular antigen, the adenosine deaminase binding protein. (Presented at the 17th annual meeting of the American Society of Nephrology, Wash DC), 1984

50. Klotz LH, Bander NH, Thompson RE, Rubin RH, Whitmore WF, Old LJ: Staging and monitoring of renal cancer using a monoclonal based sandwich assay for a proximal tubular serum antigen, the adenosine deaminase binding protein. J. Urol 133:4(2), 165 (abstract), 1985

51. Bander NH, Ramsawak RD, Whitmore WF, Vaughan ED Jr, Oettgen HF, Old LJ: The study of human renal cancer in vitro: 1. Establishment of renal cancer and normal kidney cell lines (in preparation), 1986

52. Chiou RK, Vessella RL, Moon TD, Elson MK, Clayman RV, Gonzalez-Campoy JM, Klicka MJ, Shafer RB, Lange PH: Localization of human renal cell carcinoma xenografts with a tumor-preferential monoclonal antibody. Cancer Res 45: 6140, 1985

53. Wahlstrom T, Suni J, Nieminen P, Narvanen A, Lehtonen T, Vaheri A: Renal cell adenocarcinoma and retrovirus p30-related antigen excreted to urine. Lab Invest 53: 464, 1985

54. Fradet Y, Cordon-Cordo C, Oettgen HF, Old LJ: Cell surface antigens of human bladder cancer defined by mouse monoclonal antibodies. Proc Natl Acad Sci USA 81: 224–228, 1984

55. Chopin D: Monoclonal antibodies against tumor associated antigens on human transitional cell carcinoma. J Urol 133: 4(2), 13, abstract, 1984

56. Grossman HB: Monoclonal antibodies against human bladder cancer. J Urol 130: 610–614, 1983

57. Koho H, Paulie S, Ben-Aissa H, Jondottir I, Hansson Y, Lundblad ML, Perlmann P: Monoclo-

nal antibodies to antigens associated with transitional cell carcinoma of the human urinary bladder. Cancer Immunol Immunother 17: 165, 1984

58. Paulie S, Koho H, Ben-Aissa H, Hansson Y, Lundblad ML, Perlmann P: Monoclonal antibodies to antigens associated with transitonal cell carcinoma of the human urinary bladder II. Cancer Immunol Immunother 17: 173, 1984

59. Moon TD, Vessella RL, Lange PH: MAbs against renal cell carcinoma. 78th AUA abstracts, 169, 1983

60. Starling JJ, Sieg SM, Beckett ML, Schellhammer PF, Ladaga LE, Wright GL: MAbs to human prostate and bladder tumor-associated antigens. Cancer Res 42: 3084, 1982

61. Hellstrom I, Rollins N, Settle S, Chapman P, Chapman W, Hellstrom KE: MAbs to two mouse bladder carcinoma antigens. Int J Cancer 29: 175, 1982

62. Masuko T, Yagita H, Hahimoto Y: MAbs against cell surface antigens present on human urinary bladder cancer cells. JNCI 72: 3, 1984

63. Settle SA, Hellstrom I, Hellstrom KE: A mAb recognizing cytoskletal keratins of stratified epithelia and bladder carcinomas. Experimental Cell Research 157 (2), 1985

64. Ramaekers F, Huysmans A, Meosker O, Schaart G, Herman C, Vooijs P: Cytokeratin expression during neoplastic progression of human transitional cell carcinomas as detected by a mAb and a polyclonal antibody Lab. Invest 53 (1): 31, 1985

65. Finan PJ, Anderson JR, Doyle PT, Lennox ES, Bleehen NM: The prediction of invasive potential in superficial transitional cell carcinoma of the bladder. Dr J Urol 54: 720, 1985

65a. Seal GM, Rowland MG, Thomalla JV, Rudolph RA, Pfaff DS, Kamer M, Eble JN: ABH Antigens in normal urothelium. J Urol 133: 513, 1985

66. Summerhayes IC, McIlhinney RAJ, Ponder AF, Shearer RJ, Pocock RD: Monoclonal antibodies raised against cell membrane components of human bladder tumor tissue recognizing subpopulations in normal urothelium. JNCI 75: 1025, 1985

67. Rearden A, Nachtsheim DA, Frisman DM, Chiu PK, Elmajian DA, Baird SM: Altered cell surface antigen expression on bladder carcinoma detected by a new hemagglutinating monoclonal antibody. J Immunology 131: 6, 3073, 1983

68. Young A, Lin DW, Prout GR: Production and characterization of mouse monoclonal antibodies to human bladder tumor-associated antigens. Cancer Res 45: 4439, 1985

69. Ashall F, Bramwell ME, Harrish: A new marker for human cancer cell: The Ca antigen and the Ca1 antibody. Lancet 2: 1, 1985

70. Czerniak B, Koss LG: Expression of CA antigen of human urinary bladder tumors. Cancer 55: 2380, 1985

71. McCabe RP, Lamm DL, Haspel MV, Pomato N, Smith KO, Thompson E, Hanna Jr MG: A diagnostic-prognostic test for bladder ca using a mAb-based enzyme-linked immunoassay for detection urinary fibrin(ogen) degradation products. Cancer Res 44: 5886, 1984

72. Foon KA, Schroff RW, Gale RP: Surface markers on leukemia and lymphoma cells: recent advances. Blood 60: 1–19, 1982

73. Houghton AN, Eisinger M, Albino AP, Cairncross JC, Old LJ: Surface antigens of melanocytes and melanomas. J Exp Med 156: 1755–1766, 1982

74. Huffman JL, Fradet Y, Cordon-Cardo C, Herr HW, Pinsky CM, Oettgen HF, Old LJ: Effect of intravesical BCG on detection of a urothelial differentiation antigen in exfoliated cells of carcinoma in situ of the human urinary bladder. Cancer Research, in press, 1986

75. Gross MD, Skinner RWS, Grossman HB: Radioimmunodetection of a transplantable human bladder carcinoma in a nude mouse. Invest Radiol 19: 1984

76. Trejdosiewicz LK, Southgate J, Donald JA Masters JRW, Hepburn PJ, Hodges GM: Monoclonal antibodies to human urothelial cell lines and hybrids: Production and characterization. J Urol 133: 533, 1985

77. Shulman S, Mamrod L, Gonder MJ, Soanes WA: The detection of prostatic acid phosphatase by antibody reactions in gel diffusion. J Immunol 93: 474, 1964

78. Chu TM, Wang MC, Merrin C: Isoenzymes of human prostate acid phosphatase. Oncology 35: 198, 1978
79. Chu TM, Wang MC, Lee CL: Prostatic acid phosphatase in human prostate cancer. In: Biochemical Markers for Cancer, Chu TM (ed). Marcel Dekker Inc, New York, 1981
80. Lee CL, Wang MC, Murphy GP, Chy TM: A solid-phase fluorescent immunoassay for human prostatic acid phosphatase. Cancer Res 38: 2871, 1978
81. Lin MF, Lee CL, Wojcieszyn JW: Fundamental biochemical and immunological aspects of prostatic acid phosphatase. Prostate 1: 415, 1980
82. Lee CL, Li YC, Jou YH: Immunochemical characterization of prostatic acid phosphatase with monoclonal antibodies. Ann NY Acad Sci 309: 52, 1982
83. Lillehoj HS, Coe BK, Rose JR: Monoclonal anti-human prostatic acid phosphatase antibodies. Molecular Immun: 19(9): 1199–1202, 1982
84. Shevchuk MM, Romas NA, Ng PY, Tannenbaum M, Olsson CA: Acid phosphatase localization in prostatic carcinoma. Cancer 52: 1642–1646, 1983
85. With MP, de Oliveira JG, Frohmuller HGW: Mab-based RIA compared with conventional enzyme immunoassay in the detection of PAP. Eur Urol 10: 326, 1984
86. Wang MC, Valenzuela LA, Murphy GP, Chu TM: A simplified purification procedure for human prostat-specific antigen. Oncology 39: 1, 1982
87. Papsidero LD, Wand MC, Valenzuela LA: A prostate antigen in sera of prostatic cancer patients. Cancer Res 40: 2428, 1980
88. Papsidero LH, Croghan GA, Wang MC: Monoclonal antibody (F5) to human prostate antigen. Hybridoma 2: 139, 1983
89. Frankel AE, Rouse RV, Wang MC, Chu M, Herzenberg LA: Monoclonal antibodies to a human prostate antigen. Cancer Reserach 42: 3714–3716, 1982
90. Ware JL, Paulson DF, Parks SF, Webb KS: Production of Monoclonal antibody aPro3 recognizing a human prostatic carcinoma antigen. Cancer Res 42: 1215–1222, 1982
91. Webb KS et al: MAbs to different epitopes on a prostate tumor associated antigen. Ca Immunol Immunother, 14: 155, 1983
92. Webb KS, Paulson DF, Parks SF, Tuck FL, Walther PJ, Ware JL: Characterization of prostate-tissue-directed monoclonal antibody, a-Pro 13. Cancer Immunol Immunother 17: 7–17, 1984
93. Starling JJ, Sieg SM, Beckett ML, Schellhammer PF, Ladaga LE, Wright GL: Monoclonal Antibodies to human prostate and bladder tumor-associated antigens. Cancer Res 42: 3084–3089, 1982
94. Wright GL, Beckett ML, Starling JJ, Schellhammmer PF, Sief SM, Ladaga LE, Poleskic S: Immunohistochemical localization of prostate carcinoma-associated antigens. Cancer Res 43: 5509–5516, 1983
95. Cambell AE, Beckett ML, Starling JJ, Sieg SM, Wright Jr GL: Antiprostate carcinoma monoclonal antibody (D83.21) cross reacts with a membrane antigen expressed on cytomegalovirus = transformed human fibroblasts. Prostate 6: 205, 1985
96. Starling JJ, Wright Jr GL: Disulfide bonding of a human prostate tumor-associated membrane antigen recognized by mAb D83.21. Cancer Res 45: 804, 1985
97. Frankel AE, Rouse RV, Herzenberg LA: Human prostate specific and shared differentiation antigens by monoclonal antibodies. Proc Natl Acad Sci USA 79: 903–907, 1982
98. Raynor RH, Hazra TA, Moncure CW, Mohankakumar T: Characterization of a monoclonal antibody, KR = P8, that detects a new prostate = specific marker. JNCI 73 (3): 617–625, 1984
99. Durkop H, Donn F, Loning T, Arndt R: Mabs to secretion products of prostatic carcinoma cells. Presented at European society for urological oncology and endocrinology, 1984
100. Lowe DH, Handley HH, Schmidt J, Royston I, Glassy MC: A human monoclonal antibody reactive with human prostate. Journal of urology 132: 780–785, 1984
101. Carroll AM, Zalutsky M, Schatten S, Bhan A, Perry LL, Sobotka C, Benacerraf B, Greene MI:

MAbs to tissue-specific antigens 1. Characterization of an antibody to a prostate tissue antigen. Clinical Immuno Immunopath 33: 268, 1984

102. Lindgren J, Pak KY, Ernst C, Rovera G, Steplewski Z, Koprowski H: Shared antigens of human prostate cancer cell lines as defined by mAbs. Hybridoma 4 (1), 1985

103. Solter D, Knowles BB: MAb defining a stage-specific mouse embryonic antigen (SSEA-1). Proc Natl Acad Sci USA 75: 5565, 1978

104. Damjanov I, Fox N, Knowles BB, Solter D, Lange PH, Fraley EE: Immunohistochemical localization of murine stage-specific embryomic antigens in human testicular germ cell tumors. AM J Pathol 108: 225, 1982

105. Bellet DH, Wands JR, Isselbacher KJ, Bohuon C: Serum AFP levels in human disease: Perspective from a highly specific monoclonal radioimmunoassay. PNAS 81: 3869, 1984

106. Lazarides E: Intermediate filaments as mechanical integrators of cellular space. Nature 1980: 249, 1980

107. Battifora H, Sheibani K, Tubbs RR, Kopinski MI, Sun TT: Antikeratin antibodies in tumor diagnosis. Cancer 54: 843, 1984

Editorial Comment

THOMAS R. HAKALA

The discovery that animals can immunologicaly recognize tumor transplants from syngeneic animals led to the search for antigens unique to spontaneously arising tumor cells. Production of antibodies to such putative tumor-specific antigens (TSAs) or tumor-associated antigens (TAAs) by conventional immunization, has been largely unsuccessful. However, the requisite specificity and molecular homogeneity of monoclonal antibody preparations has given new life to the search for TAAs.

The properties of enhanced specificity and molecular homogeneity in monoclonal antibody preparations are obviously interrelated. The enhanced specificity represents a quantitative improvement over that found with polyclonal antibodies and is achieved without the need of absorption with control antigen preparations. The molecular homogeneity of monoclonal antibodies is a qualitative distinction from polyclonal antibodies and can be exploited in ways which are impossible with polyclonal antibodies. Most of the efforts to date have focused on the enhanced specificity of monoclonal antibodies to detect TAAs in genito-urinary tumors.

A large number of monoclonal antibodies against spontaneous human tumors have been described. Almost none of them have been shown to be completely unique to a tumor when they have been tested against a wide variety of non-tumor tissue. None the less these antibodies appear likely to be quite useful. The criteria for a useful monoclonal antibody are a function of the use to which the antibody is to be put. If antigen detection in circulating or excreted body fluids is to be the goal, then differences in antigen shedding from tumor and normal cells becomes more important than their relative presence on the cell surface. For the purpose of tumor localization relative cell surface expression is paramount though modest amounts of cross-reactivity with normal tissue may be accepted. If the purpose is to deliver lethal damage to tumor cells, then greater antibody specificity is required of the antibody to prevent the destruction of normal tissue.

In order for an antibody to be useful in detecting or in destroying human tumors, the TAA must be expressed in sufficient quantity to allow a significant amount of binding to occur. It is also desirable to have the TAA expressed on a significant percentage of tumors in order to avoid the necessity for custom antibody production for each individual patient. Of the antibodies thus far described, there appears to be a roughly inverse correlation between the degree of tumor specificity and the percentage of the tumors upon which the antigen is found. That is, those antibodies presented as being the most highly specific to a tumor also appear to be present on the smallest percentage of tumors of a given type. TAA heterogeneity may be overcome with monoclonal antibody mixtures if the pantheon of specificities is manageably small.

The lack of absolute tumor specificity need not be an impediment to the practical application of monoclonal antibodies. Antigen accessibility may be as important as antigenicity. For example the amount of Stage-Specific Embryonic Antigen 1 (SSEA-1) is greater in normal kidney than in some tumors, yet anti-SSEA-1 permits specific localization of these tumors by gamma scintigraphy [1]. Almost no antibody is localized to SSEA-1 containing normal tissue.

The extensive compilation of monoclonal antibodies reported by many investigators and summarized by Drs. Klotz and Bander indirectly points to the need for some system of cataloging the wide variety of antibodies which have been discovered to date. Monoclonal antibody production is straight-forward but the technique itself is expensive and labor intensive. Time and effort required for the detection of TAAs would be reduced if investigators could be spared the characterization of antibodies and antigens reported by others. Uniform criteria of antibody characterization together with practical methods for exchange of antibodies already characterized may be of use in this regard. In some ways the situation is similar to that of the early days of anti-HLA antibody development. Antibody exchange and HLA workshops removed the need for each laboratory to repeat all the efforts of others and helped produce knowledge from data.

Some principles are emerging from the reports of anti-tumor monoclonal antibodies published thus far. In general, those antibodies which are relatively tumor specific have been derived from immunizations using cell lines instead of fresh tissue. Perhaps dividing tissue cultured cells are more likely to display unusual antigens. The reasons for the difference between *in vitro* and *in vivo* antibody specificity are yet to be fully explored.

The search for genito-urinary TAAs is complicated by our meager knowledge about the nature of the antigens we pursue. Classical demonstration of TAAs require tumor transplants and syngeneic populations. Since neither is available to study human tumors most investigators have immunized with complex, uncharacterized mixtures (tumor cell preparations) and sought tumor specificity by reference to antibody binding with normal tissue. An alternate strategy has been to select a defined antigen likely to be associated with oncogenesis. An example of this approach in the development of antibodies against synthetic antigens associated with oncogenes [2]. The intimate relationship between monoclonal antibody and nucleic acid techniques that has been so successful in other areas of biology is amoung the most exciting in the detection and analysis of antigenic expression of genitourinary tumors.

We are at present limited by the immunologic repertoire of a relatively small number of species in the production of monoclonal antibodies. As techniques develop which allow monoclonal antibody production from animals other than mice and rats and improve antibody production from human hybridomas, we may find that the immunological responsiveness of these alternate hosts may change the profile of antigens recognized or at least which antigens are immunodominant. This should expand our resolution of antigenic differences, improve detection of different classes of epitopes and perhaps increase the likelihood of detecting useful antigens which are operationally tumor specific.

The molecular homogenetity of monoclonal antibodies permit manipulations not possible with polyclonal antibodies. Such manipulations include epitope examinations and antibody engineering by biologic selection, chemical modification and DNA modification.

The epitope of a TAA to which a monoclonal antibody binds may not be the most tumor specific even though it may be immunodominant. Isolation of the TAA molecule with the original antibody and immunization with that molecule may produce monoclonal antibodies with greater affinity to the originally detected epitope as well as antibodies to other epitopes on the TAA. Epitope examination has been a useful tool in determining the function of other biologically active molecules and may serve similarly with TAAs.

The immunoglobulin class of a monoclonal antibody of interest may not be suitable for the intended application. Binding of complement, solubility, biologic half-life and other characteristics are largely determined by heavy chain class. Spontaneous and induced immunoglobulin class switching can occur during hybridoma growth. Class switching is infrequent but can be detected by suitable assays. It is thus possible to select and sub-clone hybridomas which produce an antibody with both the binding specificity and heavy chain characteristics most suitable.

Chemical modification of monoclonal antibodies is facilitated by their homogeneity however techniques must be individualized to the antibody class. Coupling to isotopes, chromogens, enzymes and toxins is done with techniques similar to those used with polyclonal antibodies. With monoclonal antibodies however it is possible to produce hybrid molecules with two different binding sites on the same molecule. With DNA transfection the structure of the heavy chain molecule can be altered to incorporate biologically active substituents [3].

Monoclonal antibodies can be used to develop antigens totally free of malignant potential. The work of the Hellstroms [4] in the use of a monoclonal antibody to develop an anti-idiotype antibody illustrate this example. A monoclonal antibody has at its binding surface a rather close approximation of the immunologic surface of the antigen to which it binds. This antibody binding site can serve as a template upon which an 'anti-binding site antibody' (antiidiotype antibody) can be made. The binding site of the antiidiotype antibody can form a positive mold of the immunologic surface of the antigen to which the original antibody was produced. The Hellstoms have shown that animals injected with such antiidiotype antibodies will develop immunity to the antigen to which the first monoclonal antibody was produced.

The applicability of a new technique to an old problem does not necessarily mean that it must be applied in the same way that the previous techniques were used. We are in the early phases of the application of the technique of monoclonal antibody production to the search for tumor-associated antigens. The proliferation of antibodies from independent investigator's laboratories has done much to increase our knowledge. However, if each laboratory is to be spared the waste of reinventing somebody else's wheel, and if the results of this antibody explosion are to provide understanding as well as data, then more effort must be devoted toward developing a unified approach to evaluating new antibodies, toward characterizing correponding antigens and toward developing methods for exchanging and comparing the antibodies developed in separate laboratories.

References

1. Ballou B, Reiland JM, Levine G, Taylor RJ, Shen W, Ryser HJ, Solter D, Hakala Tr: Tumor location and trug targeting using a monoclonal antibody (anti-SSEA-1) and antigen-binding fragments. J Surg Oncology 31: 1, 1986
2. Viola MV, Fromowitz F, Oravez S, Deb S, Schlom J: Ras oncogene p21 expression is increased in premalignant lesions and high grade bladder carcinoma. J Exp Med 161: 1213, 1985
3. Morrison SL: Transfectomas provide novel chimeric antibodies. Science 229: 1202, 1985
4. Lee VK, Harriott TG, Kuchroo VK, Halliday WJ, Hellstrom I, Hellstrom KE: Monoclonal antiidiotypic antibodies related to a oncofetal bladder tumor antigen induce specific cell-mediated tumor immunity. Proc Natl Acad Sci USA 82: 6286, 1985

8. LHRH Agonists and Antiandrogens in Prostate Cancer

FERNAND LABRIE, ANDRÉ DUPONT and ALAIN BÉLANGER

Introduction

Prostate cancer is the second leading cause of death due to cancer in men and the first cause in men aged 60 years or more [1]. With increasing longevity, previously occult cases of prostate cancer have enough time to become clinically important, thus possibly explaining the increasing rate of death from prostate cancer in the West [2]. Due to the presence of bone metastases in the majority of patients at the time of diagnosis, the possibility of treatment of the primary tumor by surgery and/or radiotherapy is limited to a small proportion of cases, while, for all others, hormonal therapy and sometimes chemotherapy are the only alternatives [3–5]. However, the results of chemotherapy have been disappointing [5].

The most promising advance in the treatment of prostatic cancer has clearly been the demonstration of the role of testicular androgens by Huggins and his colleagues in 1941 [6]. These observations opened a new era in the treatment of prostate cancer and were based on the following straightforward rationale: 'In many instances, a malignant prostatic tumor is an overgrowth of adult epithelial cells. All known types of adult prostatic epithelium undergo atrophy when androgenic hormones are greatly reduced in amount or inactivated. Therefore, significant improvement should occur in the clinical condition of patients with far advanced prostate cancer subjected to castration or estrogen administration' [7]. Since these observations of Huggins and his colleagues [6, 7], orchiectomy and treatment with estrogens have been the cornerstone of the management of advanced prostate cancer [8].

These two approaches cause improvement for a limited time interval in 60 to 80% of cases, thus leaving 20 to 40% of the patients without improvement of their disease [5, 9–11]. Moreover, progression of the cancer usually occurs within 6 to 24 months in all those who initially responded [12] with a median survival of only six months [13, 14]. In addition to the uncertain improvement in survival, orchiectomy is often psychologically unacceptable while estrogens cause serious

Ratliff, T.L. and Catalona, W.J. (eds), Genitourinary Cancer. ISBN 0–89838–830–9
© *1987, Martinus Nijhoff Publishers, Boston. Printed in the Netherlands.*

side effects such as gynecomastia, fluid retention, myocardial ischaemia and thromboembolism. These side effects of estrogens by themselves have been reported to cause 15% of deaths during the first year of treatment [15]. The side effects of the two current forms of hormonal therapy and their questionable influence on survival left most physicians undecided about the real benefits of hormonal therapy. There was thus the clear need for more efficient and better tolerated therapies.

The finding that agonists of luteinizing hormone-releasing hormone (LHRH) cause a blockade in testosterone formation in experimental animals [16, 17] accompanied by a loss in prostate weight offered the possibility of replacing orchiectomy and estrogens. In fact, in men, following a transient period of stimulation, serum testicular androgens are reduced to castration levels during chronic treatment with the well-tolerated LHRH agonists [17–22]. However, although LHRH agonists make castration more acceptable and free of important side effects, one cannot expect to improve the prognosis of prostate cancer beyond the results previously achieved with orchiectomy [6] since their effect is limited to the blockade of testicular androgens [17–22].

Before describing the clinical results obtained in advanced prostate cancer using the combination therapy, it appears important to review some data which demonstrate the major importance of adrenal androgens in prostate cancer in men as well as some biological properties of androgen-sensitive normal and cancer tissues as well as the properties of commercially available antiandrogens. Then, a proposal for most appropriate antihormonal therapy will be presented.

Major importance of adrenal androgens in men

Man is unique among species in having a high secretion rate of adrenal steroids which are converted into active androgens in peripheral tissues. Despite its discovery in 1960 [23] and the fact that dehydroepiandrosterone sulfate (DHEA-S) is present in human serum at far higher concentrations than any other steroid, the biological function of this so-called adrenal androgen has so far received little attention.

High intraprostatic concentration of DHT following castration

As illustrated in Figure 1, a high level of the active androgen dihydrotestosterone (DHT) remains in the prostatic cancer tissue following castration, thus clearly demonstrating the importance of androgens of extratesticular origin in the prostate. Although orchiectomy, estrogens, or LHRH agonists (through reduction of gonadotropin secretion) cause a 90 to 95% reduction in serum testosterone (T) levels [17–22, 24–40], a much smaller effect is observed on the really important

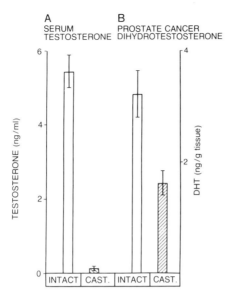

A
SERUM
TESTOSTERONE

B
PROSTATE CANCER
DIHYDROTESTOSTERONE

Figure 1. Effect of surgical castration on the serum levels of T (A) and on the concentration of the active androgen DHT in prostatic cancer tissue (B). Date are from Geller and colleagues [41, 43]. Note the relatively small effect of castration on intraprostatic DHT concentration as compared to the 95% fall in serum T.

parameter of androgenic action in the prostatic tissue, namely the concentration of DHT.

Measurements of serum T and DHT levels have little or no value except as an index of testicular activity since the intraprostatic DHT concentration is the significant parameter indicating the level of active androgen at its site of action. In fact, unexpectedly high concentrations of DHT and 3α-diol (5α-androstane-3α, 17β-diol) have been found in prostatic carcinoma after orchiectomy or DES treatment [41–43]. This is clearly illustrated in Figure 1 where it can be seen that although orchiectomy causes a 90% to 95% fall in serum T level, the intraprostatic concentration of the potent androgen DHT is reduced by only about 50% [41, 43] (Bélanger and Labrie, unpublished data).

Conversion of adrenal androgen precursors

Although, as mentioned earlier, orchiectomy, estrogens, or LHRH agonists decrease by 90% to 95% the circulating androgens with strong intrinsic activity, such as T and DHT [17–22, 24–40, 44, 45], the precursor androgens continue to be secreted at a high rate by the adrenal cortex, thus providing substrates for the intraprostatic formation of the most potent androgenic compound, namely DHT.

The main androgen precursors of adrenal origin are Δ^4-androstenedione

(3 mg/day) and dehydroepiandrosterone (DHEA, 25 mg/day) [46]. The plasma levels of Δ^4-androstenedione are 1.69 ± 0.88 ng/ml, whereas those of T are 4.46 ± 1.57 ng/ml [47]. The serum levels of DHEA and DHEA-sulfate (DHEA-S), on the other hand, are 1.9 ± 0.3 ng/ml and 834 ± 147 ng/ml [29]. These weak adrenal androgens may be converted into strong androgens, not only in the prostatic tissue [48–50] but also at the peripheral level. Skin converts DHEA-S, DHEA and Δ^4-androstenedione into T and DHT [51–54]. Even blood cells can transform androstenedione into T [55, 56] whereas the brain can transform DHEA into T and DHT [57].

Radioactive DHEA-S infused into patients is taken into prostatic tissue and transformed into DHEA, 5α-androstanediol, T, and DHT [49]. Because of such high levels of DHEA-S in the circulation, a small percentage of transformation of this steroid into DHT is sufficient to play a major role in the evolution of prostatic cancer. Androstenedione, another steroid of adrenal origin, may also elicit a stimulatory response in the prostate. Acevedo and Goldziecker have observed that human prostatic tissue can metabolize androstenedione *in vitro* into T, androsterone, and 5α-androstanedione [48]. After *in vivo* infusion, Harper and associates have found an important transformation of this steroid in the prostatic tissue into T, DHT, androsterone, and 5α-androstenedione [49].

5α-androst-5-ene-3β, 17β-diol (Δ^5-diol), a direct secretory product of the adrenals, is another precursor of androgens, especially T [58], and also has intrinsic androgenic activity. Direct production of T and DHT by the adrenals is minimal [59]. Only about 5% of total circulating androgens originate from peripheral conversion from adrenal prehormones, specially androstenedione. The importance of adrenal steroids in prostatic cancer is thus mainly related to the intraprostatic metabolism of DHEA-S, DHEA, androstenedione, and Δ^5-diol.

Based on the above-mentioned data and the intraprostatic levels of DHT measured after castration or estrogen treatment [41, 43] (Bélanger and Labrie, unpublished data), the contribution of the testes and adrenals to the androgenic stimulation of prostatic carcinoma can be estimated to be approximately of equal importance. Such data stress the need to neutralize the activity of the androgens of adrenal origin for an efficient treatment of prostate cancer. The high levels of DHT remaining after surgical castration or treatment with estrogens or LHRH agonists alone are more than likely to have a deleterious effect on the evolution of the cancer. Clearly, a treatment limited to the blockade of androgens of testicular origin only partially relieves the cancer from androgenic stimulation. Moreover, measurements of serum levels of T and DHT, although being excellent parameters of testicular steroidogenic activity, are a poor index of intraprostatic androgenic activity.

Previous clinical evidence for the role of adrenal androgens

That androgen-sensitive cancer cells remain active after surgical castration or high doses of estrogens is clearly illustrated by the finding that 33% to 39% of patients already castrated or treated with estrogens showed a positive response to the pure antiandrogen flutamide [60, 61]. Moreover, after adrenal androgen suppression with aminoglutethimide in patients who had become refractory to orchiectomy and exogenous estrogens, a favorable response was observed in three of seven patients [62]. In a similar study, Robinson and coworkers found palliation in 50% of patients [63].

The first bilateral adrenalectomy in prostatic cancer was performed by Huggins and Scott with appreciable success despite the lack of substitution therapy [64]. Subsequently, bilateral adrenalectomy and hypophysectomy were used in advanced prostatic cancer with a significant rate of remission in previously castrated patients or those already treated with estrogens. In fact, bilateral adrenalectomy has been found to be associated with palliation in 20% to 70% of patients with advanced prostatic carcinoma who had become refractory to castration or estrogen therapy [46, 65–71]. Surgical hypophysectomy has also been found to improve transiently the disease in about 50% of patients [66].

That low levels of circulating androgens can be important in prostatic cancer is further indicated by the close correlation observed between plasma T levels and the evolution of prostatic cancer [72]. Thus, in cases with serum T levels between 0.34 ng/ml and 0.57 ng/ml, partial response was reported in only 37% of cases, whereas when T values were between 0.1 and 0.24 ng/ml, a positive response was seen in 60% of cases. This is further supported by the data of Sciarra and colleagues, who showed that remission after bilateral castration occured in a group in whom serum T decreased to 0.3 ± 0.2 ng/ml, whereas no remission occurred in 10 of 27 patients in whom T levels were 1.4 ± 0.3 ng/ml [73]. That the adrenal androgens were responsible for these high levels of circulating androgens was confirmed by the marked inhibitory effect of dexamethasone on serum androgen levels in these patients. Thus, although serum androgen levels are reduced markedly after surgical or medical castration by estrogens or LHRH agonist treatment remaining basal circulating levels of T are not negligible. Moreover, stress owing to many physical or psychological causes can increase serum androgen levels further.

Biological properties of intact and cancer androgen-sensitive tissues

Characteristics of the biological response to androgens

As illustrated by many examples which will be presented in this section, the biological response to DHT (as well as the response to any biological stimulus)

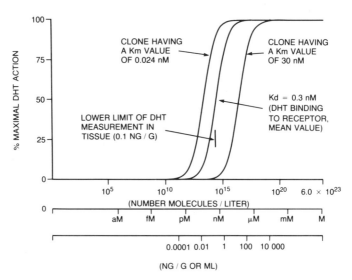

Figure 2. Dose-response curves of 2 clones of androgen-sensitive mouse mammary carcinoma SC–115 cells to increasing DHT concentrations expressed in absolute number of DHT molecules, in molarity and in ng/ml. Comparison is made with the usual mean affinity of binding of DHT to the androgen receptor. Data are from Labrie et al [74] and Simard et al. [89]. The important observation is that levels of DHT below the lower limits of detection of current assays (0.1 ng/ml or g tissue) leave 1.0×10^{14} molecules of DHT per ml, thus offering an extremely large number of DHT molecules with the potential for androgenic stimulation in normal tissues and especially in cancer tissue having hypersensitivity to androgenic stimulation (an example is the clone showing half-maximal growth at 0.008 ng/ml DHT (left curve).

follows a logarithmic instead of a linear rule (Fig. 2). This implies that by decreasing serum DHT levels by 90% causes a much smaller inhibitory effect on the response which is decreased by less than 50% (Figs 2, 3 and 4). This observation is of major consequence since it indicates that by decreasing serum T and DHT levels by approximately 90% by medical or surgical castration leaves more than 50% of the androgenic stimulus on prostate cancer growth.

Another fact of major importance is that our inability to measure a steroid by presently available techniques because of lack of sensitivity should not be interpreted as meaning that the cellular mechanisms are unable to detect and respond to such apparently low levels of hormones. As illustrated in Figure 2, the usual limit of sensitivity of current techniques for DHT measurement in serum or tissue is 0.1 ng/ml or g tissue. It should be realized that approximately 1×10^{14} molecules of DHT per ml or g tissue are left at this concentration of the androgen, thus leaving an extremely large number of DHT molecules for potential stimulation of cancer growth. As illustrated in this Figure, maximal growth of a clone of hypersensitive shionogi mouse mammary cells (SC–115) was obtained at DHT concentrations below the detection limits of presently available assays, the half-maximal stimulation being measured at 0.024 nM or 0.008 ng/ml DHT [74].

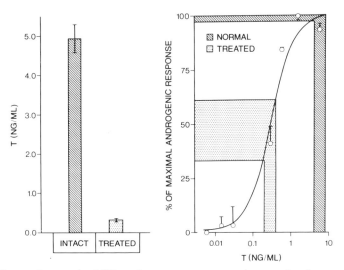

Figure 3. Effect on the growth of Shionogi mouse mammary carcinoma cells of concentrations of testosterone (T) corresponding to the serum values found in intact men (4–8 ng/ml) and the levels achieved after surgical or medical castration (0.2–0.4 ng/ml), respectively (B). Note that a 95% reduction in T concentration causes only a 38 to 64% reduction in cell growth. Panel A shows, as an example, the serum T levels measured before and after 1 month of treatment with an LHRH agonist in adult men suffering from prostate cancer [78].

Importance of low levels of androgens on biological responses

A question which has received little attention is the biological significance of the apparently low levels of serum T and DHT which remain after surgical or medical castration. The particular importance of the subject is suggested by the recent observation that the maintenance of serum T at levels similar to those found in castrated men (0.2–0.4 ng/ml) causes an increase in prostate weight as high as 35–40% of the value found in intact animals [75]. Using the growth of androgen-sensitive Shionogi mammary carcinoma cells as parameter of androgen action [76, 77], the present data show that castration levels of T and DHT can maintain growth of cancer cells in culture at values as high as 38 to 64% of maximal androgen-sensitive growth.

As mentioned earlier, serum T levels in intact adult men usually range between 4 and 8 ng/ml while values of 0.2 to 0.4 ng/ml (5% of control) are observed after surgical or medical castration [24, 25, 78]. As an example, Fig. 3A shows respective values of 4.49 ± 0.35 and 0.31 ± 0.02 ng/ml before and after 1 month of treatment of 12 men suffering from prostate cancer with the LHRH agonist [D-Trp[6]]LHRH ethylamide [79]. As illustrated in Fig. 3B, the important finding is that the apparently low castration levels of serum T at 0.2 to 0.4 ng/ml stimulate growth of the androgen-sensitive mouse mammary carcinoma cells at 38–64% of the maximal growth rate achieved with T levels found in intact men (4 to 8 ng/ml).

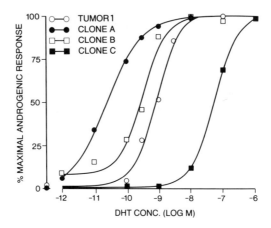

Figure 4. Effect of increasing concentrations of DHT on the maximal androgenic response (DNA content) in the 3 clones obtained from a Shionogi mouse mammary tumor. In order to facilitate visualization of differences in androgen sensitivity, all data are expressed as a percentage of the maximal response to DHT [74].

The same group of patients shown in Fig. 3 had pretreatment and treatment values of serum DHT of 0.55 ± 0.07 and 0.05 ± 0.03 ng/ml, respectively. Again, the impressive finding is that a reduction in serum DHT to 10% of control values decreases androgen-sensitive cell growth only from 74–84% to 27–41% of maximal androgen-sensitive cell growth (data not shown).

Contrary to the widely accepted dogma in the endocrine therapy of prostate cancer [80–82], the present data clearly demonstrate that castration levels of T and DHT exert a significant stimulatory effect on growth in cancer tissue. In fact, the growth of a typical androgen-sensitive carcinoma cell line, namely the Shionogi mouse mammary carcinoma (SC–115) [76, 77] is stimulated at 38 to 64% of maximal growth by castration levels of T or DHT in the incubation medium. These data are in direct contradiction with the belief that the apparently low (5 to 10% of control) serum concentration of serum T and DHT remaining after surgical or medical castration should have little, if any, influence on the growth of prostate cancer [80–82]. This belief was based on the observation of only a 60 to 80% rate of positive response of prostate cancer to castration. However, as will be seen later, further blockade of androgens markedly increases the rate of response to more than 95%.

The present data are in agreement with the elegant study of Barstch et al. [75] who have shown, using Silastic implants of T, that the maintenance in castrated rats of serum T at the concentration found in the serum of castrated men leads to an approximately 10–fold higher concentration of DHT in the prostate tissue, thus causing a stimulation of prostatic weight as high as 30 to 40% of the value found in intact animals. The physiological importance of relatively low levels of

T and DHT has also been demonstrated in rat anterior pituitary cells in culture [78, 84]. Androgens are in fact well known to exert specific inhibitory effects on LHRH-induced LH release in adenohypophysial cells in culture. Using this precise and well-established *in vitro* system, we have observed that reduction of the concentration of T in the incubation medium to the values found in the serum of castrated men reduced the androgenic activity by only 50 to 70%.

The present data, those of Barstch et al. [75], as well as our previous observations [78, 83, 84], clearly demonstrate that low concentrations of androgens are highly active in androgen-sensitive tissues and that variations of these low concentrations of androgens can cause major changes in the responses observed in various androgen-sensitive systems, namely cancer cell growth (these data), growth of the normal rat prostate [75] as well as LHRH-induced LH release in normal rat gonadotrophs in culture [78, 84]. In these three different systems, one common finding is that low castration levels of T at approximately 5% of control can maintain an important level of biological activity at 30 to 60% of the level found under maximal stimulatory conditions. Concentrations of androgens below the physiological range thus have major biological activity. Such data are in agreement with the finding that the prepubertal prostate accumulates DHT in children [85].

Based on the observation that 20 to 40% of patients with advanced prostate cancer do not respond to surgical or chemical castration [9, 10], it was generally believed that 20 to 40% of prostatic carcinomas were already androgen-insensitive at the start of treatment [9, 80–82, 86, 87]. As a more likely explanation, the present data suggest that the circulating levels of T and DHT remaining after castration are responsible for most of the uninterrupted growth of prostatic cancer following standard hormonal therapy limited to the removal of testicular androgens. This is well supported by our recent observation to be summarized later that less than 5% of patients with advanced prostate cancer show progression of their disease when more complete androgen blockade is achieved with the pure antiandrogen Flutamide administered in association with surgical or medical castration at start of treatment in order to neutralize the castration level of androgens [78, 79].

The low levels of serum T and DHT present in the circulation of prostate cancer patients after medical or surgical castration can be directly secreted by the adrenals and/or released into the circulation following transformation in the prostate and other peripheral metabolizing sites from the adrenal precursors DHEA-S, DHEA, Δ^5-diol and Δ^4-dione [48–52]. Direct secretion of T by the adrenals is supported by measurements of T in adrenal vein blood [46]. It is most likely that a significant proportion of T and DHT is released into the circulation from the prostate and other peripheral tissues, especially the skin, which possess the required enzymatic systems [48–52].

The importance of adrenal androgens is particularly well demonstrated by the finding of intraprostatic levels of DHT as high as 1 ng/g tissue (3 nM) following castration or treatment with estrogens [41, 43] (Bélanger and Labrie, unpublished data). Since the K_D value of DHT interaction with the androgen receptor is less than 1 nM [88, 89], it is clear that a concentration of 1 ng/ml or 3 nM DHT in the prostate cancer tissue is more than sufficient to exert a major stimulatory effect on cancer growth.

Wide range of sensitivities of tumor cells to androgens

Clinical evidence in prostate cancer clearly indicates heterogeneity of the sensitivity to androgens and the development of resistance to hormonal therapy. These data pertain to the failure of hormonal therapy in a proportion of previuosly untreated patients and, especially, the low rate of success of hormonal therapy in patients who had previous endocrine manipulations [5, 9–12, 14, 78]. It thus becomes of great interest to study in detail the phenomena of heterogeneity and development of true or apparent androgen resistance in originally androgen-sensitive cells. An excellent model for such studies is the androgen-dependent Shionogi mouse mammary carcinoma 115 (SC–115), a tumor showing rapid growth both *in vivo* and in tissue culture [76, 77].

We have used this model to investigate the heterogeneity of androgen sensitivity following cloning of a tumor and the changes of androgen sensitivity which occur during long-term culture of cloned cells. The present data clearly show that a wide range of hormone sensitivities are found in the clones derived from the original tumor and develop during tissue culture of cloned cells. Such findings have major implications for the efficient treatment of prostate cancer where a population of hypersensitive cells can continue to grow in the presence of the low androgens of adrenal origin left after castration (medical or surgical).

As illustrated in Figure 4, the 3 clones obtained from a Shionogi mouse mammary tumor show marked heterogeneity of sensitivity of DHT action. While the original tumor shows a Km value of DHT action at 0.9 nM, the Km values of DHT action in clones A, B and C were calculated at 0.024, 0.15 and 30 nM, respectively. There is thus a 1250–fold difference in sensitivity to DHT between clones A and C.

After 13 months in monolayer culture in the presence of 10 nM DHT, the original clone B was recloned in soft agar and the growth sensitivity to DHT was again determined. As illustrated in Figure 5, a marked heterogeneity of basal growth (in the absence of androgens), maximal response to DHT and sensitivity to DHT (Km values) was observed among the 10 clones obtained from individual cells. The growth in the absence of androgen varied by as much as 16–fold between clones 6 and 7 while the Km values range from 0.05 to 10 nM between clones 7 and 9 (200–fold range).

The present data indicate that the Shionogi mouse mammary carcinoma tumor can contain cell populations having a marked heterogeneity in terms of sponta-

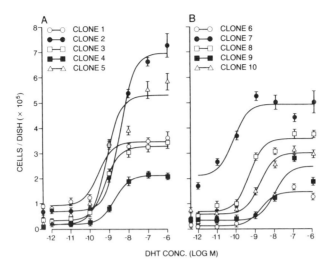

Figure 5. Effect of increasing concentrations of DHT on cell growth of 10 clones obtained after 13 months of culture of cloned cells B (Fig. 4) in medium containing 10 nM DHT [74].

neous growth in the absence of androgens as well as in terms of responsiveness to androgens. Moreover, they illustrate that such heterogeneity can develop under controlled conditions in culture in clones derived from an individual cell. Not only the growth of the various clones shows heterogeneity in the absence of androgens but the maximal response to DHT also shows marked variations. However, the most significant observation is probably the heterogeneity of the sensitivity of cell growth to DHT. In fact, in clones obtained from the original tumor, there was a 1250–fold range of Km values of DHT action while a 200–fold range was obtained in the clones obtained from a single original cell kept in culture for 13 months in the presence of DHT.

Although the origin of tumors is believed to be monoclonal [90], it is clear that most, if not all, advanced tumors are composed of mixed populations of cells having a wide range of phenotypes. That heterogeneity of androgen sensitivity analogous to the one described in this report exists in human prostate cancer is unequivocally demonstrated by the clinical data showing a 30 to 50% response to adrenalectomy, hypophysectomy, Flutamide or aminoglutethimide in patients who relapse after orchiectomy or treatment with estrogens [46, 60–66, 78, 91]. Such a response to further androgen blockage in patients already castrated can only be explained by the presence in these patients of prostatic tumors which were still growing in the 'low' androgenic environment provided by the adrenal androgens following medical or surgical castration.

The situation in human prostate cancer appears to be analogous to the data presented in this study where a proportion of clones show supersensitivity to DHT with half-maximal growth at a concentration of DHT as low as 0.008 ng/ml

(0.024 nM) (Fig. 4). Since the castration levels of serum DHT range from 0.04 to 0.08 ng/ml [78], it is clear that such hypersensitive tumors can continue to grow at a maximal rate following castration. In addition to the second response observed in 30 to 50% of castrated patients following blockage of adrenal androgens, additional proof for the presence of androgen-supersensitive prostatic carcinoma is provided by the recent findings that combined treatment of advanced prostate cancer with an LHRH agonist (or orchiectomy) in association with the pure antiandrogen Flutamide causes a positive response in more than 95% of patients [29–31, 78, 79, 91]. Since only 60 to 80% of patients were responding to castration (medical or surgical) [9–12, 92], the increase in responders from 60–80 to 95% following the combination therapy [29–31, 78, 79, 91, 93, 94] indicates the presence of androgen-hypersensitive tumors in at least 15 to 35% of patients with advanced prostate cancer. These patients were previously thought to be androgen-resistant at start of treatment while, on the contrary, they are androgen-hypersensitive.

The approximately 5% of prostatic tumors which do not respond to combination therapy [78, 93, 94] might be truly androgen-resistant or, alternatively, these tumors could be even more androgen-sensitive and able to grow with the small fraction of free androgens remaining in the prostatic tumors in the presence of therapeutic doses of the antiandrogen. Further blockade of adrenal androgen secretion and/or action will be needed to differentiate between these two possibilities.

Although tumors are monoclonal in origin, they acquire a marked heterogeneity which has to be taken into account for the development of an effective therapeutical strategy. The present data indicate that a marked heterogeneity of sensitivity to androgens exists in the original Shionogi mouse mammary carcinoma in analogy with the clinical evidence in human prostate cancer [46, 60–66, 78, 79, 91, 93]. Moreover, starting with a single cloned cell, the development of similar heterogeneity can be reproduced under controlled conditions *in vitro*. Such data indicate that the Shionogi carcinoma cell line offers an excellent model to investigate in detail the factors controlling the changes in androgen sensitivity and the development of phenotypes having different requirements for androgens.

Antiandrogens

Clinical studies with antiandrogens

As an alternative to bilateral adrenalectomy, antiandrogens have been found to be effective in treating prostatic adenocarcinoma and to cause atrophy of the accessory sex organs in experimental animals and man [60, 61, 95–101]. When the 111 documented cases of patients treated with Flutamide alone at doses ranging from 0.75 to 1.5 g/day are evaluated, an approximately 50% objective response was observed [60, 61, 97, 98, 102–104]. In a typical study in previously untreated stage D carcinoma of the prostate, Airhart and associates have reported that about 50% of patients improve when treated with either flutamide or DES [97].

As mentioned earlier, Flutamide therapy in patients refractory to conventional therapy showed a favorable response of short duration in 23% of cases [60] whereas a 39% response was observed by Stoliar and Albert [61]. Similarly, Airhart and co-workers [97] have observed some improvement by Flutamide in patients already treated with estrogens. Flutamide, a pure antiandrogen, exerts its androgenic activity through inhibition of androgen uptake and competition at the level of the androgen receptor for endogenous steroids [89, 99, 101, 105]. In patients previously untreated, a reduction in size of the local tumor was found in 68% of patients treated with the steroidal compound cyproterone acetate [106–110].

Previous limitations of pure antiandrogens

Pure antiandrogens can neutralize androgens of all sources and thus theoretically represent the ideal form of therapy. However, a secondary increase in gonadotropin and androgen secretion can result from such treatment [95, 96, 98] and progressively higher doses of the drug are needed to neutralize the effect of rising androgen levels [95, 96, 99, 101].

As an example of the neutralizing effect of Flutamide on the inhibitory feedback action of androgens on gonadotropin secretion, plasma T rose from 249 to 484 ng/dl during treatment with Flutamide [104]. Such an elevation of plasma T leads to a progressive reversal of the antiandrogenic action of Flutamide in peripheral tissues. The re-establishment of a new steady-state of gonadotropin and androgen secretion at higher levels needs increasing doses of the antiandrogen, and a point is rapidly reached where the dose of the antiandrogen needed is too high and exceeds the limits of tolerance.

A limitation to the use of pure antiandrogens in prostate cancer was thus the progressive increase in gonadotropin and androgen secretion caused by neutralization of the inhibitory feedback action of androgens at the hypothalamo-adenohypophysial level. This limitation has now been overcome by the combination therapy using orchiectomy or treatment with an LHRH agonist, which blocks gonadotropin secretion [16, 17, 111, 112] and prevents any secondary increase in T secretion [16, 17, 28–40]. This approach was originally suggested by our animal studies, which showed that combined treatment with an LHRH agonist and a pure antiandrogen is highly effective in inhibiting androgenic influence on secondary sex-organ weight during both short-term [95] and long-term [96] treatment in rats.

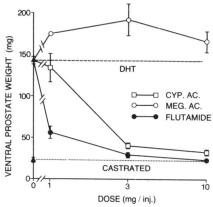

Figure 6. Effect of increasing doses of Flutamide, cyproterone acetate or megestrol acetate on ventral prostate weight in castrated rats receiving dihydrotestosterone (125 µg twice daily) for 14 days starting one day after castration [114].

Importance of using a pure antiandrogen: There is antiandrogen and 'antiandrogen'

An antiandrogen must be strictly defined as a compund which inhibits androgen action at the target tissue level [113]. In agreement with this definition, we should exclusively use pure antiandrogens or compounds devoid of any androgenic, glucocorticoid, progestatin or any other hormonal or antihormonal activity. We have recently compared the properties of three 'antiandrogens' commercially available for the treatment of prostate cancer, namely Flutamide (Eulexin), cyproterone acetate (Androcur) and megestrol acetate (Megace) [114].

It can be seen in Figure 6 that at the dose of 1 mg (twice daily), Flutamide causes a 75% inhibition (p <0.01) of the DHT-induced increase in prostate weight while cyproterone acetate has no significant inhibitory effect and megestrol acetate causes a 28% increase (p <0.05) in prostate weight. At the 3 mg dose, Flutamide and cyproterone acetate inhibit the action of DHT by 94 and 85%, respectively, while megestrol acetate is still stimulatory. At the maximal dose (10 mg), Flutamide causes a complete reversal of the effect of DHT while prostate weight remains at 40% above control (p <0.01) in the group of animals who received cyproterone acetate.

In order to provide a direct measure of the androgenic activity of the 3 compounds used, they were administered alone in castrated animals. While Flutamide shows no effect on ventral prostate weight, cyproterone acetate and megestrol acetate increase prostate weight by 60 and 100%, respectively (p <0.01) [114]. As further proof of the androgenic activity of cyproterone acetate and megestrol acetate, it can be seen in Figure 7 that the simultaneous administration of the pure antiandrogen Flutamide completely prevents the stimulatory action of the two other compounds on prostate weight.

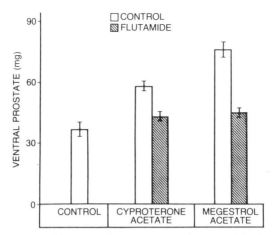

Figure 7. Effect of treatment with megestrol acetate or cyproterone acetate alone or in combination with Flutamide on ventral prostate weight in castrated rats. The compounds were administered subcutaneously twice daily at the dose of 5 mg for 21 days starting one day after orchiectomy [94].

As mentioned earlier, antiandrogens must be strictly defined as compounds which inhibit androgen action at the target tissue level and do not act through inhibition of gonadotropin secretion [113]. An androgenic activity of cyproterone acetate on ventral prostate and seminal vesicle weight in the rat has been previously reported [115, 116]. Moreover, when cyproterone acetate was administered to pregnant rats, all female fetuses showed signs of virilization of the genital tract [117].

The present data show that megestrol acetate has, on a weight basis, an androgenic activity somewhat higher than that of cyproterone acetate. Tisell and Salander [118] have reported that megestrol acetate stimulated the weight of the seminial vesicles as well as that of the coagulating glands in castrated rats while there was no significant effect on the ventral prostate. However, the androgenic effect of megestrol acetate was also illustrated by the histologic appearance of the seminal vesicles and coagulating glands as well as that of the ventral and dorsolateral prostate.

Megestrol acetate (Megace) has been suggested for the treatment of prostate cancer on the basis of its antigonadotropic and antiandrogenic activities [119–121]. The present data show that the antiandrogenic activity of this compound is zero. In order to potentiate its weak antigonadotropic activity and incomplete blockage of testicular androgen secretion, megestrol acetate has recently been administered in combination with estrogens [120, 121]. However, as clearly shown in the present study, megestrol acetate it not an antiandrogen and is thus unable to neutralize the action of the adrenal androgens in the prostatic cancer tissue. On the contrary, megestrol acetate, in common with cyproterone acetate, has some androgenic activity, an action completely opposite to the aim of prostate cancer therapy.

The glucocorticoid activity of cyproterone acetate has been previously described in experimental animals and man [115, 122]. It is reasonable to assume that the use of compounds having intrinsic glucocorticoid activity, such as cyproterone acetate and megestrol acetate, can have a negative influence on the immune defenses against prostate cancer. As mentioned earlier, the ideal or pure antiandrogen should be devoid of any intrinsic hormonal activity. Of the compounds commercially available for the treatment of prostate cancer, the only one which meets these criteria is the nonsteroidal antiandrogen Flutamide. Cyproterone acetate and megestrol acetate have important glucocorticoid and progestational activity [115, 118, 123] (Table 1). In addition, an even more serious limitation of these 2 compounds is their significant androgenic activity.

Of major importance, it should also be added that Flutamide is approximately 2 times more potent than cyproterone acetate [94, 114, 124–126]. Since the usual dose of Flutamide is 250 mg every 8 hours while that of cyproterone acetate is 50 mg, it follows that patients receiving Flutamide probably have 10 times more antiandrogen protection than those receiving cyproterone acetate. It thus seems logical to conclude that among the compounds commercially available, Flutamide is the only one having the properties of a pure antiandrogen, has the best tolerance and is thus the most likely to have optimal benefits for the treatment of prostate cancer.

Table 1. Profile of the antiandrogenic and hormonal activities of Flutamide, cyproterone acetate and megestrol acetate

Activity	Compound		
	Flutamide	Cyproterone acetate	Megestrol acetate
Antiandrogenic	+ (4, 8)	+ (2, 8)	− (8)
Androgenic	− (4, 8)	+ (1, 3, 5, 6, 8)	+ (7, 8)
Progestational	− (4)	+ (1, 2)	+ (7)
Glucocorticoid	− (4)	+ (1, 2)	+ (7)

1) Neri et al., 1967 [115]
2) Neumann et al., 1970 [123]
3) Elger, 1966 [125]
4) Neri et al., 1972 [124]
5) Sufrin and Coffey, 1973 [116]
6) Graf et al., 1974 [117]
7) Tisell and Salander, 1975 [118]
8) Poyet and Labrie, 1985 [114]

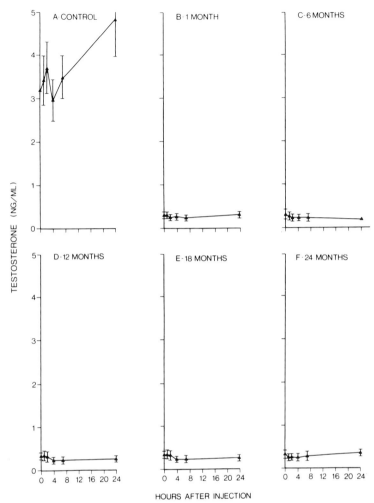

Figure 8. Response of serum radioimmunoassayable testosterone to the administration of the LHRH agonist [D-Trp^6, des-Gly-NH$_2$^{10}]LHRH ethylamide or [D-Ser (TBU)^6, des-Gly-NH$_2$^{10}]LHRH ethylamide on the first day of treatment and after 1, 6, 12, 18 and 24 months of daily treatment (500 µg daily for one month followed by 250 µg daily). The basal levels of testosterone were 3.18 ± 0.49 ng/ml (1 nmole/L = 0.30 ng/ml) [22].

LHRH Agonists

Our finding that agonists of luteinizing hormone-releasing hormone (LHRH) cause a blockade in testosterone secretion accompanied by a loss in prostate weight in experimental animals [16, 17] offered the possibility of an advantageous replacement for orchiectomy and estrogens for the treatment of prostate cancer. In men, following an initial but transient period of stimulation, it is now well established that testicular serum androgens are reduced to castration levels during chronic treatment with these peptides [17, 22, 28–40].

Long-term castration with LHRH agonists

Since our first observations in 1980 [17], during the last 5 years, chronic treatment with potent LHRH agonists has been shown by many groups [17, 22, 28–40, 92, 127] to inhibit serum testicular androgens to castration levels without side effects other than those related to hypoandrogenicity, namely hot flashes and a decrease or loss of libido. It is however most important to make sure that the inhibitory effect of these well-tolerated peptides is maintained during long-term treatment.

As illustrated in Figure 8a, serum T increases slowly during the first 24h following the first administration of the LHRH agonist to reach 50% above control at 24h (p < 0.05). Serum T then decreases to 10% of control at 1 month and remains at this low level thereafter (p < 0.01) (Fig. 8b to 8f). The most important finding is however that no increase in either serum LH or T is observed after the subcutaneous injection of 500 μg of any of the two LHRH agonists used in our study, namely [D-Trp^6]LHRH ethylamide or [D-Ser (TBU)^6]LHRH ethylamide, thus indicating that no escape occurs during chronic treatment with an appropriate dose of these peptides administered by the subcutaneous route.

Loss of biological activity of LH

Despite the decrease in serum testosterone to castrated levels in patients receiving LHRH agonists, serum LH measured by radioimmunoassay (RIA) is only slightly reduced or even sometimes remains normal. Since we had already observed a discrepancy between bioactive and radioimmunoassayable LH in monkeys treated with an LHRH agonist [128], we have measured the bioactivity of LH in the serum of patients with advanced prostatic cancer receiving the combination therapy using an LHRH agonist and the antiandrogen Flutamide in order to determine if the inhibition of serum androgen levels could be due to a loss of the biological activity of circulating LH. Testosterone secretion by a suspension of mouse interstitial cells was used as parameter of LH biological activity.

Figure 9a illustrates the time course of the changes in serum immunoreactive and bioactive LH concentrations in 14 patients with prostatic cancer during the first 90 days of combined treatment with an LHRH agonist and an antiandrogen. After a transient stimulatory period, serum LH levels determined by RIA return to pretreatment values by day 15 and show a 50% reduction at 90 days of treatment (1.1±0.1 on day 90 as compared to 2.2±0.3 ng/ml on day −2). Biologically active serum LH exhibits the same stimulatory pattern at the beginning of the treatment. However, bioactive LH levels, although parallel to radioimmunoassayable LH during the first 2 weeks of treatment, then show a drastic inhibition to 7% of pretreatment values after 30 days of combined antihormonal therapy (0.43±0.04 and 0.030±0.007 ng/ml on days −2 and 30, respectively) and remain low thereafter.

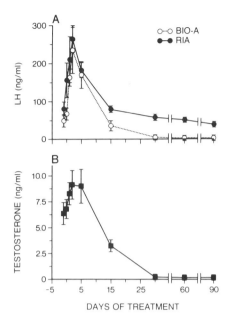

Figure 9. Comparison of the time course of changes in serum levels of bioactive LH, radioimmunoactive LH and testosterone in patients receiving the combined antihormonal therapy with an LHRH agonist and a pure antiandrogen. Blood samples were obtained at 0800h on days −2, 0, 2, 5, 15, 30, 60 and 90 of treatment. Panel A: serum LH assayed by RIA and by the mouse interstitial cell bioassay. Panel B: testosterone measured by double-antibody RIA after purification on LH–20 columns [129].

The changes in serum LH bioactivity thus remain parallel to those of serum testosterone concentrations during the whole course of treatment. As observed for serum bioactive and immunoreactive LH, testosterone levels are stimulated during the first days of treatment, this stimulation being followed by a significant decrease to 50% of control on day 15 (Fig. 9b). Castration levels of the androgen are then reached at later time intervals.

The present data show an almost complete loss of biological activity of LH during treatment of adult men with an LHRH agonist and an antiandrogen while LH measured by RIA was only 50% reduced. Such results illustrate the limitations of RIA measurements for proper evaluation of gonadotropin secretion under at least some experimental conditions in the human. Even though the precise change(s) of the LH molecule remain(s) to be characterized, the close parallelism observed between serum testosterone and bioactive LH levels suggests that the loss of potency of the gonadotropin is mainly, if not exclusively, responsible for the complete inhibition of testicular testosterone secretion observed during chronic treatment with LHRH agonists. Such treatment with LHRH agonists causes a specific and reversible hypophysectomy limited to gonadotrophs or 'gonadotrophectomy'.

Tumor flare with LHRH agonists used alone

Transient increase in testicular androgen secretion

As observed in the first patient with prostate cancer treated with an LHRH agonist [17], the first 5 to 10 days of treatment with these peptides are accompanied by an increase in the serum levels of T and DHT. This transient period of hypersecretion of testicular androgens is observed with any LHRH agonist given by any route of administration at any pharmacologically active dose. This period of increased androgen secretion is due to the stimulated release of pituitary LH induced by the superactive LHRH agonist during the first days of treatment with a secondary hyperstimulation of steroid secretion by the Leydig cells. However, after 5 to 10 days of treatment, desensitization takes place in pituitary gonadotrophs, thus causing a loss of the biological activity of LH and a progressive decrease of androgen biosynthesis in the Leydig cells which are deprived of their obligatory stimulus for steroidogenesis [78, 91, 129].

Tumor flare

It is now well recognized that the transient rise in the serum levels of T and DHT seen during the first days of treatment with LHRH agonists alone carries the serious risk of disease flare or of exacerbation of the signs and symptoms of prostate cancer. The most recent and perturbing report is that of Waxman et al. [130] who have found that 17 of 32 patients (53%) with bone pain at presentation had increased symptoms. Of all the 46 men in the study, 19 of them (41%) had increased symptoms. The 17 patients with increased bone pain experienced additional problems, namely lymphoedema, urinary obstruction, increased serum creatinine and/or signs of cord compression. In two patients, renal and neurological functions were severely compromised. It must be considered that in patients who have no bone pain and are asymptomatic at presentation, an increase in tumor growth is not expected to cause clinical symptoms or signs although such an androgen-induced stimulation, in addition to causing local growth of prostate cancer, is likely to induce the seeding of additional metastases. This recent report on LHRH agonist-induced tumor flare follows a series of previous observations [92, 130].

LHRH Agonists should not be used alone

With this knowledge, one wonders how LHRH agonists can still be used alone for the treatment of prostate cancer. The adverse effects of an increase in serum androgens on the evolution of prostate cancer could easily be predicted from previously knowledge: As early as 1941, Huggins and Hodges [6] have shown hat serum acid phosphatase, a well-known objective parameter of prostate cancer activity, was sharply increased by injecting androgens. There is no reason to believe that an increased secretion of testicular androgens induced by LHRH agonists would not lead to a similar stimulatory effect on serum prostatic acid phosphatase (PAP) and cancer growth. Such a stimulation of serum PAP levels was observed in the report of the Leuprolide Study Group [92] as well as in a study using another LHRH agonist, named Buserelin [37].

It is also of interest that in the early study of Huggins and Hodges [6], there was a decline of serum acid phosphatase to preinjection levels following cessation of testosterone treatment in two patients while, in one patient, this decrease was succeeded by an abrupt spontaneous secondary rise in acid phosphatase. It is of interest that the authors suggested that the subsequent rise could be explained by postulating 'that the cancer cells had been functionally expanded by androgen and therefore responded in an augmented way to hormones...' With the recognized role of androgens in prostate cancer growth, there is no doubt that the interpretation of Huggins and Hodges was correct and that an increase in androgen activity (exogenous or endogenous) is a stimulus for cancer growth and is unacceptable in any regimen of prostate cancer therapy.

Although further proof of the stimulatory action of androgens on prostate cancer growth appears quite unnecessary and even dangerous for the patients, the effect of testosterone administration to 52 patients with metastatic prostatic carcinoma has recently been reported [131]. Signs and/or symptoms of cancer progression were observed in 45 of 52 patients. It should be added that these unforable reaponses were seen extremely early with a median duration of testosterone treatment of only 9 days. It should also be mentioned that 14 or 27% of patients were in remission at the time of androgen administration, thus decreasing the probability of a subjective and/or objective progression being detectable during a short period of treatment with testosterone. In fact, only 7 patients did not experience a progression of their disease during androgen administration. Of these, 6 were in remission at the time of androgen administration and 1 was previously untreated. In all these 7 cases, subclinical disease progression probably took place despite the lack of noticeable sign or symptom. In fact, in all evaluable patients, progression was later seen.

The increase in pain was sudden in onset and severity. Four patients died 2 to 15 days after the start of T administration, presumably as a result of treatment. That the exacerbation of the disease was due to androgen administration itself is supported by the finding of a prompt regression of the unfavorable response in all except 2 of 33 evaluable patients upon cessation of treatment. In the 2 patients who did not experience regression, the complications were in fact similar to those found in patients having tumor exacerbation due to treatment with LHRH agonists alone, namely irreversible paraplegia and pulmonary metastases.

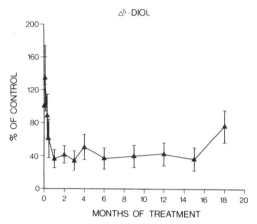

Figure 10. Changes in serum Δ^5-diol in previously untreated patients having clinical stage D2 prostate cancer receiving the combined therapy with a pure antiandrogen in association with orchiectomy or an LHRH agonists. The pretreatment values of serum Δ^5-diol were 0.59 ± 0.07 ng/ml (15 patients) [79].

The most significant and provocative finding is thus the study of Fowler and Whitmore [132] who have observed that 33 of 34 patients (97%) in relapse under endocrine therapy experienced progression of their disease upon administration of androgens. The conclusion of these findings is that even in relapsing patients, 97% possess androgen-sensitive tumors able to respond quickly to androgens even at a late stage of the disease at the time of relapse. The conclusion of these authors is thus most appropriate: 'The occasional catastrophic sequel and the possibility that testosterone may cause significant subclinical prostatic tumor growth dictate caution in further explorations of potential clinical uses of testosterone in patients with prostatic cancer'.

Combination therapy using a pure antiandrogen and an LHRH agonist (or orchiectomy) in previously untreated patients

From March 1982 to September 1985, 131 patients with histology-proven prostatic adenocarcinoma and bone metastases visualized by bone scintigraphy (stage D2) took part in this multicentre study after written informed consent. The criteria for inclusion and exclusion were those of the US NPCP [14]. Of the 131 previously untreated stage D2 patients who had combination therapy, 118 received the combination treatment with the LHRH agonist [D-Trp^6, $_{des}$-Gly-NH$_2$^{10}]LHRH ethylamide or [D-Ser(TBU)^6, des-Gly-NH$_2$^{10}]LHRH ethylamide (Buserelin) in association with the pure antiandrogen 2-methyl-N-[4-nitro-3-(trifluoromethyl)phenyl]propanamide (Flutamide, Eulexin, Euflex) while 13 had orchiectomy (instead of LHRH agonists) in association with the antiandrogen. No difference in the clinical response was observed between chemical or surgical castration. Twenty-three patients were originally started randomly with the Flutamide analog, 5,5-dimethyl-3[4-nitro-3-(trifluoromethyl)phenyl]-2,4-imidazolidione (RU23908). However, the occurrence of visual side effects in 70% of the patients receiving this compound has led to an early change to Flutamide and to the exclusive use of Flutamide in our clinic since June 1983.

The LHRH agonists were injected subcutaneously at the daily dose of 500 µg at 0800h for 1 month followed by a 250 µg daily dose while Flutamide was given three times daily at 0700, 1500 and 2300h at the dose of 250 µg orally. The antiandrogen was started one day before the first administration of the LHRH agonist or orchiectomy.

Complete clinical, urological, biochemical and radiological evaluation of the patients was performed before starting treatment as described [29]. The initial evaluation included history, physical examination, bone scan, transrectal and transabdominal ultrasonography of the prostate, ultrasonography of the abdomen, chest roentgenogram and skeletal survey and sometimes computerized axial tomography (CAT) of the abdomen and pelvis as well as excretory urogram (IVP). Performance status and pain were evaluated on a scale of 0 to 4. The follow-up was as described [29]. The criteria of the US National Prostatic Cancer Project were used for assessment of objective response to treatment [14]. Statistical significance was measured according to the multiple-range test of Duncan-Kramer [129] and the Fisher's exact test [133], when appropriate. The probability of continuing response and survival was calculated according to Kaplan and Meier [134].

In addition to the rapid fall in serum T and DHT mentioned earlier. it is of great interest to see the rapid decrease in the serum concentration of the four adrenal steroids which act as precursors for the biosynthesis of testosterone and 5α-dihydro-testosterone in the prostate cancer tissue. From basal values of 915 ± 75 ng/ml, the serum concentration of DHEA-S is already decreased to 73% of control ($p < 0.05$) between days 1 and 4 of treatment and reaches 61% at one month ($p < 0.01$). Thereafter, the mean concentration of circulating DHEA-S remains at 60% of control or lower ($p < 0.01$).

The serum levels of DHEA follow a pattern almost superimposable to that of DHEA-S. In fact, from basal values of 2.18 ± 0.17 ng/ml, the concentration of serum DHEA decreases progressively to reach 63% of control after one month of treatment ($p < 0.01$). Thereafter, the concentration of DHEA remains approximately constant at mean values ranging between 46 and 67% of control ($p < 0.01$).

An even more striking inhibitory effect is observed on the serum concentration of androst-5-ene, 3β, 17β-diol (Δ^5-diol) (Fig. 10). from basal values of 0.59 ± 0.07 ng/ml, the serum concentration of this adrenal steroid decreases to 44% of control at one month ($p < 0.01$). Thereafter, the mean serum concentration of Δ^5-diol remains at values ranging between 36 and 50% of control

($p < 0.01$) during most of the treatment period. The serum levels of androsten-edione (Δ^4-dione) follow a similar pattern (data not shown). It is of great interest to see that the serum concentration of cortisol remains constant during the whole period of combined antihormonal treatment, the pretreatment value being 184 ± 6.65 ng/ml. During the whole course of treatment, the mean values range between 170 ± 7.10 and 215 ± 11.9 ng/ml.

Starting in March 1982, 131 previously untreated patients with histology-proven prostatic carcinoma and bone metastases identified by bone scan and X-Ray received the combined treatment for more than 3 months as first therapy for an average period of 545 days of treatment and could thus be evaluated (Table 2). Pain was originally present in 66% of patients and it subsided completely in more than 90% of cases during the first month of treatment.

The serum levels of PAP were initially elevated in 87% of the patients, the values ranging between 0.2 and 896 ng/ml, the normal being < 2.0 ng/ml. In all cases, the start of treatment was followed by an extremely rapid fall in serum PAP, a decrease to 21% of control being already reached on days 5 to 10 ($p < 0.01$) after the start of treatment. Serum PAP values returned to normal in all except 8 patients before 6 months of treatment.

Bone scintigraphy performed 3 to 6 months after the start of treatment was an absolute requirement for inclusion of the patients in one of the categories of objective responses. An example of the changes in bone scintigraphy in a patient who showed a complete response at 6 months of treatment is illustrated in Figure 11.

As can be seen in Table 2, a positive objective response assessed according to the criteria of the US National Prostatic Cancer Project [14] has been observed in 95.4% of the patients. Of 131 previously untreated patients with clinical stage D2 prostate cancer, only 6 patients did not show a positive objective response at start of treatment with the combination therapy. Of the positive responses, 30 were complete (23%) while 50 were partial (38%) and 45 were stable (34%). As illustrated in Figure 12 and Table 3, such a high level of complete objective responses is far superior to all previous studies where the treatment was limited

Table 2. Objective response to combined antiandrogen treatment in previously untreated stage D$_2$ prostate cancer patients

Number of patients	Age mean (limits)	Days of treatment mean (limits)	Best objective response				Relapse	Death from prostate cancer	Death from other causes	Arrest of treatment
			Comp.	Partial	Stable	Prog.				
131	67	491	30	50	45	6	31	12	8	10
	(45–86)	(102–1208)	(23%)	(38%)	(34%)	(5%)	(24%)	(9.2%)	(6.1%)	(7.6%)

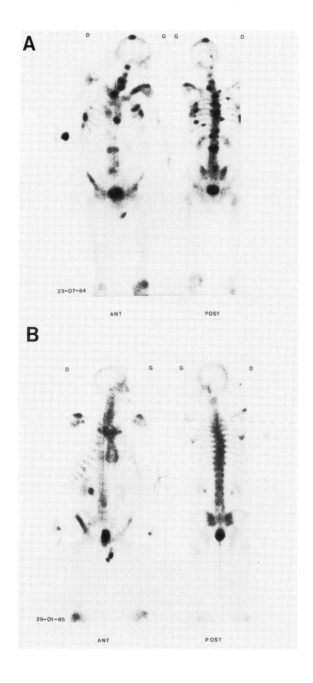

Figure 11. Bone scans with ⁹⁹mTc-labelled methylene diphosphonate of patient treated with the pure antiandrogen Flutamide and the LHRH agonist [D-Trp⁶]des-Gly-NH₂¹⁰]LHRH ethylamide. (A) Before treatment on July 23rd, 1984, showing disseminated bone metastases; (B) January 29th, 1985; 6 months after the start of combined antihormonal therapy. Note the disappearance of all areas of increased uptake [91].

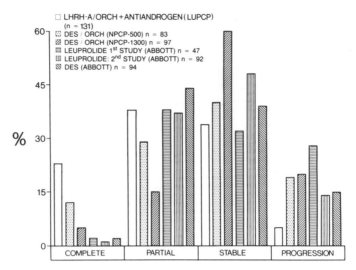

Figure 12. Comparison of the objective response to combination therapy with the results of treatments limited to the blockade of testicular androgens.

to a blockade of testicular androgens. It should be mentioned that the 23% of complete responses observed in the present study includes patients recently entered into the study, a situation which decreases the chances of complete responses which can be achieved at longer time intervals. In fact, for patients who have reached 2 years of combination treatment, 45% of them showed a complete response as best response.

The other striking finding illustrated on Figure 12 is that only 4.6% of patients did show an objective response at the start of combination therapy. In all these cases, however, regression of uptake on the bone scan could be seen in some lesions while disease continued to progress in one or more areas. Such data clearly indicate various levels of androgen sensitivity of different tumors in the same patient. However, subjectively, all patients who had symptomatic disease at start showed a positive response. Thus, while a positive objective response is seen in 95% of cases, a subjective improvement is seen in more than 99% of patients upon start of combination therapy.

In addition to the finding of a much higher proportion of patients who show a complete response to combination therapy, as compared to monotherapy, it can be seen in Table 3 and Figure 12 that the combination therapy markedly reduces the percentage of patients who continue to progress at start of treatment. From values ranging from 14 to 28% following standard therapy, the percentage decreases to 4.6% in the group of patients who received the combination therapy.

In addition to the improved percentage of positive responses at the start of treatment, another most important aspect of the effect of the combination treatment is the marked increase in the duration of the positive response. While the percentage of patients still in remission at 2 years is 60.5% with the combination therapy, it has already decreased to 0% before reaching 2 years with Leuprolide [92] (Fig. 13). There is thus a remarkable advantage of the combination therapy, not only on the percentage of initial responses, but even more strikingly, upon the duration of the positive response. The most medically significant result is however that observed on survival. In fact, as shown on Figures 14 and 15, the probability of survival following combination therapy is 89.2% at 2 years as compared to 40 to 60% by previous therapies ($p < 0.01$).

Combination therapy in previously treated patients

An important question which remains unanswered is the relative benefits of the combination therapy administered as first treatment as compared to the same therapy applied as a second step at the time of disease progression in patients previously orchiectomized or treated with estrogens or LHRH agonists alone. Our data show that the death rate calculated at 2 years is increased by as much as 4-fold in the group of patients where the combination therapy with Flutamide was delayed and given as a second treatment at the time of disease progression.

As illustrated in Figure 15, the survival is markedly increased ($p < 0.01$) in the group of stage D2 patients who received the combined treatment with the pure antiandrogen as first treatment as compared to those who had orchiectomy or received estrogens or LHRH agonists alone prior to the administration of Flutamide. In fact, the survival at 2 years is 89% in the group of patients who received the combination therapy at the start treatment as compared to only 48% in those who had partial androgen blockade for various time intervals before receiving the combination therapy. Up to 2 years of treatment, the death rate is thus increased by more than 4-fold by delaying Flutamide administration (from 10.9 to 51.8%,

Table 3. Comparison of the best objective response to combination therapy versus monotherapy in stage D2 previously untreated prostate cancer patients assessed according to NPCP criteria

Response	Combined anti-hormonal (anti-androgen)		DES/ORCH NPCP-500		DES/ORCH NPCP-1300		Leuprolide 1st study Abbott		Leuprolide 2nd study Abbott		DES Abbott	
	%		%		%		%		%		%	
Complete	30	22.9	10	12	5	5	1	2	1	1	2	2
Partial	50	38.2	24	29	15	15	18	38	34	37	41	44
Stable	45	34.3	33	40	58	60	15	32	44	48	37	39
Progression	6	4.6	16	19	19	20	13	28	13	14	14	15
Totals	131		83		97		47		92		94	

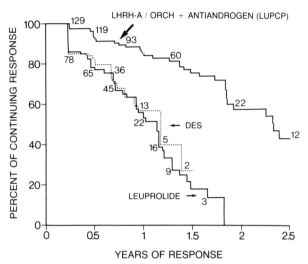

Figure 13. Comparison of the probability of continuing response following combination therapy and the administration of Leuprolide alone [92] or DES [92].

p < 0.01). When only deaths due to prostate cancer are considered, it can be seen in Table 4 that there are 38 deaths in the group of patients who received delayed combination therapy as compared to only 12 deaths from prostate cancer among the patients who had a blockage of both adrenal and testicular androgens at the start of treatment (Table 1).

It can be seen in Table 4 that 24 of 56 (42.9%) of previously treated patients showed a positive objective response to the combined antiandrogen blockade. Patients previously castrated received only Flutamide while those treated with DES or an LHRH agonist alone received [D-Trp⁶]LHRH ethylamide in combination with Flutamide. By contrast, 125 of 131 (95.4%) of previously untreated patients showed a positive objective response at start of treatment (p < 0.01, Fisher's exact test) (Table 1).

In agreement with the present data, 33 to 39% of patients already castrated or treated with estrogens have shown a positive response to Flutamide [60, 61]. Similarly, after adrenal androgen suppression with aminoglutethimide in patients who had become refractory to orchiectomy or estrogens, a positive response was observed in 50% of patients [63]. Bilateral adrenalectomy and hypophysectomy have been associated with palliation in 20 to 60% of cases [78].

As mentioned earlier, there is convincing clinical and laboratory evidence for an important role of adrenal androgens in prostate cancer. The clinical data pertain to the observation in all studies of a 30 to 50% response to adrenalectomy, hypophysectomy, Flutamide or aminoglutethimide in patients who showed relapse after orchiectomy or treatment with estrogens [60, 61, 63, 78, 91]. Such as response can only be explained by the continuing stimulatory action of adrenal androgens on prostate cancer growth following medical or surgical castration.

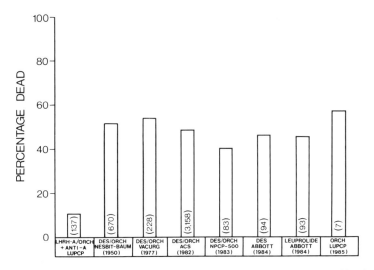

Figure 14. Comparison of the death rate after 2 years of treatment with the combined androgen blockade (Laval University Prostate Cancer Program (LUPCP)) with previous results obtained with no treatment [9] and the standard hormonal therapies (orchiectomy (ORCH) and/or estrogens) in previously untreated stage D patients: Nesbit and Baum's study [9], study of the Veterans' Administration Cooperative Urology Research Group (VACURG) [10]; survey of the American College of Surgeons (ACS) (1982) [92], and study 500 of the USNPCP (1983) [5]; Leuprolide alone (1984) [92]; DES alone [92], and orchietectomy alone (1985) (LUPCP).

As a support to the clinical data obtained following blockade of the secretion or action of adrenal androgens, all the enzymes required for the conversion of the adrenal precursors dehydroepiandrosterone (DHEA), DHEA-sulfate (DHEA-S), androst-5-ene-3β, 17β-diol (Δ^5-diol) and androstenedione (Δ^4-dione) have been described in the prostate cancer tissue [49–52]. Moreover, castrated levels of serum testosterone at 5–10% of control (0.2–0.4 ng/ml) are still effective in androgen target tissues and can maintain androgen-dependent functions at 30 to 50% of control [75, 78]. These findings are in agreement with the observation that the intraprostatic concentration of the most active androgen, namely dihydrotestosterone (DHT), is only reduced by 50% following orchiectomy [43] (Bélanger and Labrie, unpublished observation).

There is thus ample clinical and biochemical evidence for a role of adrenal androgens in prostate cancer. Although it seems logical to remove all androgens as first treatment of androgen-sensitive diseases such as prostate cancer, the relative benefits of early versus late blockage of adrenal androgens had to be determined. The finding of a 95.4% rate of positive objective response at start of treatment following combination therapy in previously untreated patients (Table 1) indicates that prostate cancer, even at the advanced stage of metastases, remains exquisitely sensitive to androgens when continuously exposed to normal levels of androgens. However, when exposed for some time to the low level of

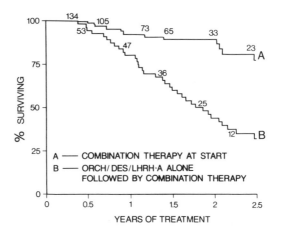

Figure 15. Comparison of the death rate in previously untreated patients having clinical stage D2 prostate cancer who received the combination therapy as first treatment and those who had orchiectomy or received estrogens or LHRH agonsits alone before administration of the combination therapy at the time of progression. Survival was calculated according to Kaplan-Meier from the time of first treatment in the two groups.

adrenal androgens, tumors become autonomous or treatment-insensitive, thus partly loosing their property to respond to the combined antiandrogen blockade in approximately 60% of the cases (Table 4).

It should be mentioned that the development of treatment resistance has been observed in some patients who had received estrogens or had orchiectomy for only 5 to 10 days although the average pretreatment time was 10.9 months. The appearance of autonomous prostate cancer tumors in the human is analogous to the development of androgen resistance in mouse Shionogi mammary carcinoma cells where the phenomenon occurs extremely rapidly and has been found within 2 weeks of exposure to low androgens [135, 136].

The recent finding that the antiandrogen Flutamide can prevent the loss of androgen sensitivity [136] in the presence of low androgen levels may partly explain the favorable results observed in the present study in patients who received the combination therapy at start of treatment. In fact, Flutamide not only blocks the stimulatory action of the adrenal androgens which remain present in prostatic cancer tissue following medical or surgical castration but the drug may well block the spontaneous action of the free androgen receptor [137] and thus prevent or delay the development of androgen-resistant tumors.

The present data confirm that a large proportion of prostatic cancer tumors are autonomous or treatment-resistant at the time of relapse following medical or surgical castration. As a consequence, the delay in administering the combination therapy has a major negative impact on the quality of life and survival, the death rate during the first 2 years being more than 4-fold higher in the group of previously treated patients as compared to those who received the combination therapy as first treatment. Survival, however, was calculated in the two groups from the time of first treatment.

Treatment of patients in relapse following medical or surgical castration

Since the median life expectancy of patients with metastatic disease is of the order of 24 months following standard treatment with castration or treatment with estrogens, the majority of prostate cancer patients seen by the urologist and/or oncologist are those in relapse. In fact, it includes the patients with advanced disease who do not initially respond to standard treatment (20 to 40%) and all those who initially respond but eventually relapse (60 to 80%). All cases of advanced prostate cancer end up in this category of relapse where the therapeutic choices are uncertain and are applied with little uniformity and an absence of defined strategy. Although it is clear that these patients present major therapeutic problems, some points concerning the androgen-sensitivity of their cancer deserve clarification and we will thus attempt to define a strategy for an antihormonal treatment based on the most up-to-date fundamental and clinical information.

Evidence for the androgen-sensitivity of prostate cancer during relapse: need of combination therapy in all patients at all times

The common belief that patients in relapse after castration or treatment with estrogens have exclusively androgen-insensitive tumors should be abandonned. In fact, it is most likely that androgen-sensitive tumors are present at all stages of prostate cancer in all patients and that optimal androgen blockade should be performed in all cases. Instead of being androgen-insensitive, most of the tumors

Table 4. Objective response to combined antiandrogen treatment in previously treated patients in relapse

Number of patients	Months of treat- ment means (limits)	Best objective response				Relapse	Deaths	
		Complete	Partial	Stable	Pro- gression		Pros- tate cancer	Other causes
56	24.3 (6.1– 63.2)	4 (7.1%)	8 (14.3%)	12 (21.4%)	32 (57.1%)	13/23 (54.2%)	38 (63.7%)	2 (3.6%)

which continue to grow after castration are androgen-hypersensitive. These tumors are able to grow in the presence of the 'low' level of androgens of adrenal origin left after castration. Control of these tumors requires further androgen blockade. This affirmation is supported by convincing clinical data as well as by well-established fundamental observation [74, 135].

We will first make a short review of the clinical observations which demonstrate without any doubt that androgen-sensitive tumors remain active after surgical castration or treatment with high doses of estrogens. These pertain to the finding that 33 to 39% of patients already castrated or treated with estrogens showed a positive response to the pure antiandrogen Flutamide [60, 61, 91]. In our own series (Table 4), it can be seen that an objective positive response assessed according to the U.S. NPCP criteria [14], was observed in 42% of patients in relapse. Although the number of complete responses is small (7%), they represent a major achievement in patients who, otherwise, had a life expectance of less than 6 months with a poor quality of life. A decrease of more than 50% in the number of bone metastases was observed in 14% of patients while a stabilization of the disease was seen in 21% of them. Since the antiandrogen Flutamide is extremely well-tolerated and that at least the quality of life is markedly improved in approximately 40% of patients in relapse, it seems logical to recommend addition of Flutamide to any patient showing relapse after medical or surgical castration.

The finding of a 42% positive objective response upon treatment with Flutamide in patients who relapse after castration indicates that a large majority of tumors can be blocked or stabilized at least for some time by the antiandrogen in these patients. In fact, since the average number of bone metastases at the time of relapse is approximately 10, and an arrest or regression of all tumors is seen in approximately 40% of cases. It follows that regression of some tumor(s) must also occur in more than 95% of the other patients who continue to progress globally upon addition of the antiandrogen. In fact, progression does not mean that all tumors progress since a single tumor is sometimes responsible for the progression while all the other tumors are stabilized or even regress. Most of the prostatic tumors, even at the time of relapse, thus have a sensitivity to androgens within the range of action of the antiandrogen. That more than 95% of patients at the time of relapse have androgen-sensitive tumors is clearly demonstrated by the observation of a rapid exacerbation (within 3 days) of the symptoms in 97% of relapsing patients treated with exogenous testosterone [131].

Categories of relapsing patients

Two additional points deserve emphasis: first, patients in relapse following castration and those in relapse following treatment with estrogens or LHRH agonists should not be considered as an homogeneous group of patients. This is an error common to most clinical studies performed in patients in relapse. For those who relapse following orchiectomy, the addition of Flutamide alone is the next logical step. However, in patients treated with estrogens or LHRH agonists alone, measures should be taken to continue to block the testes at the same time as Flutamide is administered. Discontinuation of treatment with estrogens or LHRH agonists implies that testicular androgen secretion will return to normal, thus markedly decreasing the neutralizing ability of Flutamide at the androgen receptor level.

It should be remembered that Flutamide acts by competition with androgens at the receptor level and that maximal efficacy of the drug is necessarily achieved with the lowest level of endogenous androgens [89]. Moreover, a well-known limitation of the use of pure antiandrogens alone is the rise in LH secretion due to neutralization of the inhibitory feedback action of androgens on LHRH and LH secretion, thus resulting in a secondary rise in serum testosterone and a progressive loss of efficacy of the antiandrogen at the receptor level [95, 96]. An absolute requirement for the use of a pure antiandrogen is thus simultaneous blockade of testicular androgen secretion by surgical or medical castration. The androgens left are thus limited to those of adrenal origin and the antiandrogen will have maximal efficacy.

Duration of combination therapy

A second point of major importance which follows the previous one is that one should never stop combined antihormonal therapy at the time of relapse. In fact, it is most likely that some tumors sensitive to androgens are present at all times and that discontinuation of the antihormonal therapy will permit the growth of tumors which could be kept under control by a could well-tolerated therapy. Upon discontinuation of combination therapy, the tumor burden would be increased and tumor growth would then include the growth of tumors unresponsive to the antihormonal treatment as well as those which were kept under control by the antihormonal treatment (but left free to grow upon its cessation).

If one decides to add other therapies such as chemotherapy or local radiotherapy, this should always be done in addition to combined antihormonal therapy, namely antiandrogen and blockade of the testes. This reasoning is even more evident in patients who relapse after monotherapy such as with LHRH agonists alone or DES. Since 97% of patients at the time of relapse have androgen-sensitive tumors [132], it is a major mistake to stop the antihormonal monotherapy before adding other measures such as radiotherapy or chemotherapy. Instead of changing hormonotherapy for these other treatments, the most reasonable approch is first to change to combination therapy and then to possibly add (not change for), those extra measures (if found useful). Local radiotherapy is certainly a most useful treatment for pain due to local mestastases. The benefits of presently available chemotherapy are however questionable [5].

Inhibition of adrenal secretion

Aminoglutethimide, an inhibitor of adrenal steroidogenesis, has been found to induce a positive response in a significant proportion of relapsing patients. Thus, in patients who had become refractory to orchiectomy and exogenous estrogens, a favorable response was observed in three of seven patients [46]. Similarly, Robinson et al. [63] have seen a palliation in 50% of patients. In a recent study, a subjective response of a median duration of 8 months was found in 19 out of 40 (47%) relapsing patients treated with aminoglutethimide while a positive objective response assessed according to NPCP criteria was seen in 6 of 40 cases (15%) [138]. A subjective improvement in a similar group of patients has been reported in 9 of 12 (75%) cases [139]. Complete and partial objective responses (according to US NPCP criteria) have been reported in 7 of 43 patients (15%) [140, 141].

The sum of available clinical data indicates that the administration of amino-glutethimide to relapsing patients offers subjective benefits in approximately 50% of patients. It should be mentioned that in many patients treated with estrogens, the estrogen therapy was stopped and there is every reason to believe that the inhibition of adrenal androgen secretion was more than offset by the return of testicular androgen activity. Better responses could thus be expected if estrogen therapy had been continued or even better replaced by orchiectomy or treatment with LHRH agonists. One should not neglect the testicular androgens when dealing with those of adrenal origin. Since both the testes and the adrenals contribute about equally to the total androgens present in prostate cancer, partial blockade of adrenal androgen secretion with aminoglutethimide in the presence of normal testicular androgen secretion might be even less efficient than the previous treatment with estrogens which blocked 50% of androgens, namely those of testicular origin. As will be described in more detail in the section entitled scale of usefulness of antihormonal therapies, blockade of the testes in association with an antiandrogen is the first step and is an obligatory component of all antihormonal regimens.

Scale of usefulness of antihormonal therapies in prostate cancer

The antihormonal therapy of prostate cancer is based on the principle that prostate cancer development and growth is sensitive to androgens as originally suggested by Huggins and Hodges [6]. The second and recently established principle [28, 78] which is the basis for combined antihormonal therapy, is that two sources, namely the testes and the adrenals, contribute about equally to the total amount of androgens present in the prostate (both normal and tumoral).

If one accepts that androgens stimulate prostate cancer growth, the next logical step in the treatment of this disease is to eliminate, as much as possible, all androgenic influences on prostate cancer with the best available drugs. Since the testes represent approximately 50% of androgens and appropriate means to eliminate this source of androgens are readily available, this should be an essential component of any antihormonal therapy of prostate cancer. The choice is between orchiectomy and the use of LHRH agonists. For the patients who accept surgical castration, this is certainly most valid. However, LHRH agonists are now widely available and there is no doubt that these peptides are a well-tolerated, safe and an efficient way of achieving a complete blockade of testicular androgen secretion [17, 22, 78].

Due to their high rate of serious cardiovascular side effects [15], estrogens, in our opinion, are no longer justified. In addition to a death rate as high as 15% due to estrogens during the first year of treatment, a finding sufficient by itself to prohibit their use, there is also evidence that estrogens can increase the level of prostatic androgen receptors, thus increasing the local activity of androgens [142, 143]. Elimination of approximately 50% of the androgens active in prostate cancer can thus be easily achieved by orchiectomy or treatment with LHRH agonists without any side-effect other than those due to elimination of testicular androgens.

The next easy and also highly efficient step is the oral administration of a pure antiandrogen such as Flutamide. For reasons discussed above, the administration of the antiandrogen should, without exception, start at the same time as orchiectomy or first injection of the LHRH agonists. From our current knowledge on the pharmacokinetics of action of the antiandrogen, the first pill or tablet of Flutamide should be administered 3 hours before injection of the LHRH agonist or orchiectomy. The antiandrogen has a double beneficial action: first, it inhibits by approximately 50% the serum levels of the four adrenal steroids DHEA-S, DHEA, Δ^4-dione and Δ^5-diol, thus decreasing to the same extent the level of androgens from adrenal origin in the prostate cancer [78, 144]; second, it competes with the remaining adrenal androgens for the androgen receptor [89].

While medical or surgical castration causes a decrease of free intraprostatic DHT from approximately 3.0 to 1.5 ng/g tissue (Fig. 1), the addition of Flutamide causes a major additional decrease estimated to leave approximately 0.2 ng free DHT/g tissue. The combination of castration and Flutamide at the dose of 250 mg every 8 hours thus causes an estimated 93% decrease in intraprostatic free DHT. It should be mentioned that this approximately 93% blockade of androgens in prostate cancer tissue is achieved very easily with minimal or no side effects. It should be added that these values of free active DHT are approximate and based on the available affinities of DHT and Flutamide for the androgen receptor and the concentration of the respective substances in the prostate (Bélanger, Dupont and Labrie, unpublished data). Important variations are also expected between patients as well as between individual tumors in each patient.

The next question is the usefulness of further androgen blockade after combination therapy. The response is most likely to be yes if the benefits of the added drug are not compensated by side-effects which affect the quality of life. The approximately 7% of active DHT or 0.20 ng DHT/g tissue left free after combination therapy can well play an important role in prostate cancer growth. The importance of these low levels of DHT is likely to vary with each tumor [141]. In fact, although 0.20 ng DHT/g tissue is at the lower limit of current measurement assays, it might well be in the range of sensitivities of some tumors or clones [74]. As illustrated in Figures 2, 4 and 5, the response of prostate cancer to androgens is logarithmic, thus indicating the importance of low levels of DHT.

In summary, based on our are current endocrinological, urological and biochemical knowledge, the drug that should be used in all cases of advanced prostate cancer is a pure antiandrogen such as Flutamide. It is the single most efficient inhibitor of androgen action in prostate cancer. However, this drug should never be used alone but always in combination with an LHRH agonist or surgical castration. With this combination therapy, excellent results are obtained with minimal side effects limited to hot flashes and a decrease of loss of libido. Although further androgen blockade could be desirable and research efforts should be devoted to this subject, the other available drugs can only achieve a partial blockade of adrenal androgen secretion below the efficiency of Flutamide, a drug that blocks both adrenal secretion and action [78, 144]. If one elects to use further blockade of adrenal secretion, these other drugs or measures should always be in addition to the combination therapy which should be continued for life.

Clinical trials on the benefits of combination therapy versus combination therapy plus aminoglutethimide and low dose hydrocortisone should be undertaken. It is also possible that the addition of ketoconazole during the first two weeks of treatment with LHRH agonists in order to block the transient rise in serum androgens could be advantageous. This drug, however, should never be used alone but always in combination with Flutamide and an LHRH agonist (or orchiectomy) since its inhibitory effect on adrenal steroid secretion is much too weak.

None of the above-mentioned drugs should be used alone, combination therapy with an LHRH agonist (or orchiectomy) in association with Flutamide being the minimal antihormonal regimen for all patients suffering from advanced prostate cancer. Why leave tumors grow when well-tolerated drugs are available. The time for partial blockade of androgens in prostate cancer is something of the past and unacceptable according to the most up-to-date endocrine and biochemical scientific data. The goal of all of us treating advanced prostatic cancer should be the best possible response and not simply a response.

Since the combined antiandrogen blockade provides a much higher rate of positive response at the start of treatment (95.4 vs 60–80%), and provides additional years of excellent quality of life with no side effects other than those related to the blockade of androgens (hot flashes and a decrease or loss of libido) [78, 79, 93, 94], it seems logical to propose that the combination therapy should be given as first treatment with no exception to all patients having advanced prostate cancer and should be continued without interruption for life. For all those who have received previous hormonal therapy, the combination treatment remains the best alternative and can permit a positive response in a large proportion of patients with a good quality of life and most likely prolongs survival. In order to avoid the development of resistance to treatment, compliance is an essential requirement: the combination therapy with an antiandrogen + LHRH agonist (in non castrated patients) should be taken for life without any interruption.

References

1. Silverberg E, Lubera JA: A review of American Cancer Society estimates of cancer cases and deaths. CA 33: 2–25, 1983
2. Tulinius H: Epidemiology of prostate cancer. Recent Results Cancer Res 60: 3–13, 1977
3. Labrie F: A new approach in the hormonal treatment of prostate cancer: complete instead of partial blockade of androgens. Int J Androl 7: 1–4, 1984
4. Williams G, Blooms SR: Treatment of advanced carcinoma of the prostate. Brit Med J ii: 571–572, 1984
5. Murphy GP, Beckley S, Brady MF, Chu M, Dekernion JB, Dhabuwala C, Gaeta JF, Gibbons RP, Loening SA, McKiel CF, McLeod DG, Pontes JE, Prout GR, Scardino PT, Schlegel JU, Schmidt JD, Scott WW, Slack NH, Soloway M: Treatment of newly diagnosed metastatic prostate cancer patients with chemotherapy agents in combination with hormones versus hormones alone. Cancer 51: 1264–1272, 1983
6. Huggins C, Hodges CV: Studies of prostatic cancer. I. Effect of castration, estrogen and androgen injections on serum phosphatases in metastatic carcinoma of the prostate. Cancer Res 1: 293–297, 1941
7. Huggins C: Antiandrogenic treatment of prostatic carcinoma in man, approaches to tumor chemotherapy. Am Ass Adv Sci 379–383, 1947
8. Paulson DF: The role of endocrine therapy in the management of prostate cancer. In: Genitourinary, Cancer (Skinner DG, De Kernion JB, eds), Philadelphia, WB Saunders Co, 1978
9. Nesbit RM, Baum W: Endocrine control of prostatic carcinoma: clinical and statistical survey of 1818 cases. JAMA 143: 1317–1320, 1950
10. Jordan Jr WP, Blackard CE, Byar DP: Reconsideration or orchiectomy in the treatment of advanced prostatic carcinoma. South Med J 70: 1411–1413, 1977
11. Mettlin C, Natarajan N, Murphy GP: Recent patterns of care of prostatic cancer patients in the united States: results from the surveys of the American College of Surgeons Commission on Cancer. Int Adv Surg Oncol 5: 277, 1982
12. Resnick MI, Grayhack JT: Treatment of stage IV carcinoma of the prostate. Urol Clin North Amer 2: 141–161, 1975
13. Johnson DE, Scott WW, GIbbons RP, Prout GR, Schmidt JD, Chu TM, Gaeta J, Saroff J, Murphy GP: National randomized study of chemotherapeutic agents in advanced prostatic carcinoma: progress report. Cancer Treat Rep 61:•317, 1977
14. Slack NH, Murphy GD, NPCP Participants: Criteria for evaluating patient responses to treatment modalities for prostatic cancer. Urol Clin North Amer 11: 337–342, 1984
15. Glashan RW, Robinson MRG: Cardiovascular complications in the treatment of prostatic carcinoma. Brit J Urol 53: 624–626, 1981
16. Labrie F, Auclair C, Cusan L, Kelly PA, Pelletier G, Ferland L: Inhibitory effects of LHRH

and its agonists on testicular gonadotropin receptors and spermatogenesis in the rat. In: Endocrine Approach to Male Contraception, Hansson V (ed). Int J Androl (suppl 2): 303–308, 1978

17. Labrie F, Bélanger A, Cusan L, Séguin C, Pelletier G, Kelly PA, Lefebvre FA, Lemay A, Raynaud JP: Antifertility effects of LHRH agonists in the male. J Androl 1: 209–228, 1980

18. Faure N, Labrie F, Lemay A, Bélanger A, Gourdeau Y, Laroche B, Robert G: Inhibition of serum androgen levels by chronic intranasal and subcutaneous administration of a potent luteinizing hormone-releasing hormone (GNRH) agonist in adult men. Fertil Steril 37: 416–424, 1982

19. Tolis G, Ackman D, Stellos A, Mehta A, labrie F, Fazekas ATA, Comaru-Schally AM, Schally AV: Tumor growth inhibition in patients with prostatic carcinoma treated with LHRH agonists. Proc Natl Acad Sci USA 79: 1658–1662, 1982

20. Warner B, Worgul TJ, Drago J, Demers L, Dufau M, Max D, Santen RJ, Abbott Study Group: Effect of very high dose of D-Leucine[6]-gonadotropin-releasing hormone proethylamide on the hypothalamic-pituitary testicular axis in patients with prostatic cancer. J Clin Invest 71: 1842–1855, 1973

21. Waxman JH, Was JAH, Hendry WF, Whitfield HN, Besser GM, Malpas JS, OLiver RTD: Treatment with gonadotropin-releasing hormone analogue in advanced prostatic cancer. Brit Med J 286: 1309–1312, 1983

22. Labrie F, Dupont A, Bélanger A, Lachance R, Giguère M: Long-term treatment with luteinizing hormone-releasing hormone agonsts and maintenance of serum testosterone to castration concentrations. Br Med J 291: 369–370, 1985

23. Baulieu EE: Esters sulfates de stéroïdes hormonaux. Isolement de l'ester sulfate de 5-androstene-3β-1-17-one dehydroepiandrosterone (dans une tumeur cortico-surrénalienne. CR Acad Sci, Paris, 251: 1421–1425, 1960

24. Shearer RJ, Hendry WF, Sommerville IF, Fergusson JD: Plasma testosterone. An accurate monitor of hormone treatment in prostatic cancer. Br J Urol 45: 668–673, 1973

25. Robinson MRG, Thomas BS: Effect of hormone therapy on plasma testosterone levels in prostatic cancer. Br Med J 4: 391–394, 1971

26. Kent JR, Bischoff AJ, Ardvino LJ, Hellinger GT, Byar DP, Hill M, Kozbur X: Estrogen dosage and suppression of testosterone levels in patients with prostatic carcinoma. J Urol 109: 858–860, 1973

27. Bélanger A, Labrie F, Lemay A, Caron S, Raynaud JP: Inhibitory effects of a single intranasal administration of [D-Ser(TBU)[6], des-Gly-NH$_2$[10]]LHRH agonists, on serum steroid levels in normal adult men. J Steroid Biochem 13: 123–126, 1980

28. Labrie F, Dupont A, Bélanger, A, Cusan L, Lacourcière Y, Monfette G, Laberge JG, Emond JP, Fazekas ATA, Raynaud JP, Husson JM: New hormonal therapy in prostatic carcinoma: combined treatment with an antiandrogen. Clin Invest Med 5: 267–275, 1982

29. Labrie F, Dupont A, Bélanger A, Lacourcière Y, J, Monfette G, Girard JG, Emond J, Houle JG: New approach in the treatment of prostate cancer. Complete instead of only partial withdrawal of androgens. Prostate 4: 579–594, 1983

30. Labrie F, Dupont A, Bélanger A, Lefebvre FA, Cusan L, Raynaud JP, Husson JM, Fazekas ATA: New hormonal therapy in prostate cancer. Combined use of a pure antiandrogen and an LHRH agonists. Horm Res 18:–27, 1983

31. Labrie F, Dupont A, Bélanger A, Lefebvre FA, Cusan L, Monfette G, Laberge JG, Emond JP, Raynaud JP, Husson JM, Fazekas ATA: New hormonal treatment in cancer of the prostate: combined administration of an LHRH agonist and an antiandrogen. J Steroid Biochem 19: 999–1007, 1983

32. Labrie F, Bélanger A, Carmichael R, Séguin C, Lefebvre FA, Faure N, Dupont A: Inhibition of the testicular steroidogenic pathway in experimental animals and men. In: Recent Advances

in Male Reproduction: Molecular Basis and Clinical Implications, D'Agata R, Lipsett MB, Polosa HJ, Van der Molen HJ (eds). Raven Press, New York, 239–248, 1983

33. Labrie F, Dupont A, Bélanger A, Labrie C, Lacourcière Y, Raynaud JP, HUsson JM, Emond J, Houle JG, Girard JG, Monfette G, Paquet JP, Vallières A, Bossé C, Delisle R: Combined antihormonal treatment in prostate cancer: a new approach using an LHRH agonist or castration and an antiandrogen. In: Hormones and Cancer, vol 31, Bresciani F, King RJB, Lippman ME, Raynaud JP (eds). Raven Press, New York, 533–547, 1984

34. Labrie F, Dupont A, Bélanger A, Labrie C, Lacourcière Y, Emond J, Monfette G, Houle JG, Girard JG, Vallières A, Bossé C, Delisle R: Dramatic response of prostate cancer to complete antihormonal treatment. In: Advances in Urological Oncology and Endocrinology, Bracci U, Siverio FD (eds). Acta Medica, Edizione E Congressi, Rome, 233–248, 1984

35. Labrie F, Dupont A, Bélanger A, Emond J, Monfette G: Simultaneous administration of pure antiandrogens, a combination necessary for the use of luteinizing hormone-releasing hormone agonists in the treatment of prostate cancer. Proc Natl Acad Sci USA 81: 3861–3863, 1984

36. Santen RJ, Warner B, Demers LM, Dufau M, Smith J: Use of GnRH hormone agonists analogs. In: LHRH and its Analogues — a new class of contraceptive and therapeutic agents, Vickery B, Nestor Jr JJ, Hafez ESE (eds). MTP Press, Boston, 1984

37. Wenderoth UK, Jacobi GH: Three years of experience with the GnRH analogue Buserelin in 100 patients with advanced prostatic cancer. In: LHRH and its Analogues: Basic and Clinical Aspects, Labrie F, Bélanger A, Dupont A (eds). Excerpta Medica, 349–357, 1984

38. Labrie F, Dupont A, Bélanger A, Members of Laval University Prostate Cancer Program Spectacular response to combined antihormonal treatment in advanced prostate cancer. Labrie F, Proulx L. (eds). Excerpta Medica ICS 652, 450–456, 1984

39. Wenderoth UK, Jacobi GH: Gonadotropin-releasing hormone analogues for palliation of carcinoma of the prostate. World J Urol 1: 40–48, 1983

40. Robinson MRG, Denis L, Mahler C, Walker K, Stich R, Lunglmayr V: An LHRH analogue (Zoladex) in the management of carcinoma of the prostate: a preliminary repost comparing daily subcutaneous injections with monthly depot injcctions. Eur J Surg Oncol 11: 159–165, 1985

41. Albert J, Geller J, Geller S, Lopez D: A method for tissue extraction and determination of prostate concentrations of endogenous androgens by radioimmunoassay. J Ummunol Med 12: 303–321, 1976

42. Farnsworth WE, Brown JR: Androgen of the human prostate. Endocr Res Commun 3: 105–117, 1976

43. Geller J, Albert JD, Nachtsheom DA, Loza DC: Comparison of prostatic cancer tissue dihydrotestosterone levels at the time of relapse following orchiectomy or estrogen therapy. J Urol 132: 693–696, 1984

44. Vermeulen A, Stoice T, Verdonck L: The apparent free testosterone concentration, an index of androgenecity. J Clin Endocrinol 33: 759–767, 1971

45. Sciarra F, Piro C, Toscano V, Petrangeli E, Caiola S, Di Silverio F, Bracci U, Conti C: Plasma testosterone, dihydrotestosterone, androstenedione, 13α- and 3β-androstenediol, free testosterone fraction, and sex hormone binding globulin capacity in prostatic adenocarcinoma. In: Adlercreutz H, Bulbrook RD, VanderMolen HJ, Vermeulen A, Sciarra F (eds). Endocrinological Cancer Ovarian Function and Disease, Séries no. 515, Amsterdam, Elsevier North-Holland, 93–202, 1977

46. Sanford EJ, Paulson DF, Rohner TJ, Drago JR, Santen RJ, Bardin CW: The effects of castration on adrenal testosterone secretion in men with prostatic carcinoma. J Urol 118: 1019–1021, 1977

47. Sciarra F, Sorcini G, Di Silverio F, Gagliardi V: Testosterone and 4-androstenedione concentration in peripheral and spermatic venous blood of patients with prostatic adenocarcinoma. J Steroid Biochem 2: 313–320, 1977

48. Acevedo HF, Goldziecker JW: Further studies on the metabolism of 4-[4-^{14}C]androstane-3,17-

196

dione by normal and pathological human prostatic tissues. Biochim Biophys Acta 97: 564–569, 1965

49. Harper ME, Pike A, Peeling WB, Griffiths K: Steroids of adrenal origin metabolized by human prostatic tissue both in vivo and in vitro. J Endocrinol 60: 117–125, 1974

50. Pike A, Peeling WB, Haerper ME, Pierrepoint CG, Griffiths K: Testosterone metabolism in vivo by human prostatic tissue. Biochem J 120: 443–445, 1970

51. Gallegos AJ, Berliner DL: Transformation and conjugation of dehydroepiandrosterone by human skin. J Clin Endocrinol Metab 27: 1214–1218, 1967

52. Sommerville IF, Flamigni C, Collins WP, Koullapis EN, Dewhurst CJ: Androgen metabolism in human skin. proc R Soc Med 64: 845–847, 1971

53. Sciarra F, Sorcini G, Di Silverio F, Gagliardi V: Plasma testosterone and androstenedione after orchiectomy in prostatic adenocarcinoma. Clin Endocrinol 2: 101–109, 1973

54. Fazekas AG: Metabolism of dehydroepiandrosterone by isolated human hair follicles. Acta Endocrinol Copenh (suppl) 155: 67–119, 1971

55. Blaquier J, Forchielli E, Dorfman RI: In vitro metabolism of androgens in whole human blood. Acta Endocrinol Copeng 55: 697–703, 1967

56. Van der Molen HJ, Groen D: Interconversion of progesterone and of androstenedione and of testosterone in vitro by blood and erythrocytes. Acta Endocrinol Copenh 58: 419–428, 1968

57. Knapstein P, David A, Wu CH, Archer DF, Flickinger GL, Touchstone JC: Metabolism of free and sulfoconjugated DHEA in brain tissue in vivo and in vitro. Steroids 11: 885–896, 1968

58. Kirschner MA, Sinhamahapatra S, Zucker LR: The production, origin and role of dehydroepian-drosterone and delta-5-androstenediol as androgen prehormones in hirsute women. J Endocrinol Metab 37: 183–189, 1973

59. Baird BT, Uno A, Melby JC: Adrenal secretion of androgens and estrogens. J Endocrinol 45: 135–136, 1969

60. Sogani PC, Ray B, Whitmore Jr WF: Advanced prostatic carcinoma: flutamide therapy after conventional endocrine treatment. Urology 6: 164–166, 1975

61. Stoliar B, Albert DJ: SCH 13521 in the treatment of advanced carcinoma of the prostate. J Urol 111: 803–807, 1974

62. Sanford EJ, Paulson DF, Rohner TJ, Drago Jr, Santen RJ, Bardein CW: The effects of castration on adrenal testosterone secretion in men with prostatic carcinoma. J Urol 118: 1019–1021, 1977

63. Robinson RMG, Shearer RJ, Fergusson JD: Adrenal suppression in the treatment of carcinoma of the prostate. Br J Urol 46: 555–559, 1974

64. Huggins C, Scott WW: Bilateral adrenalectomy in prostatic cancer. Ann Surg 122: 1031–1041, 1945

65. Bhanalaph T, Varkarakis MJ, Murphy GP: Current status of bilateral adrenalectomy of advanced prostatic carcinoma. Ann Surg 179: 17–23, 1974

66. Ferguson JD: Limits and indications for adrenalectomy and hypophysectomy in the treatment of prostatic cancer. In: Hormonal Therapy of Prostatic Cancer, Bracci U, Di Silverio F (eds) Cofese Edizioni, Palermo, 201–207, 1975

67. Greene LF, Emmett JL: Further observations on the treatment of carcinoma of the prostate by bilateral orchiectomy. S Clin North Amer 26: 1007–1017, 1946

68. MacFarlane DA, Thomas LP, Harrisson JH: A survey of total adrenalectomy in cancer of the prostate. Am J Surg 99: 562–572, 1960

69. Markland FS, Chiopp RT, Cosgrove MD, Howard EB: Characterization of steroid hormone receptors in the Dunning R-3327 rat prostatic adenocarcinoma. Cancer Res 38: 2812–2826, 1978

70. Menon M, Walsh PC: Hormone therapy for prostatic cancer. In: Prostatic Cancer, Murphy GP (ed), PSG Publishing Co, Littleton, Massachusetts, 175–220, 1979

71. Morales PA, Brendler H, Hotchkiss RS: The role of adrenal cortex in prostatic cancer. J Urol 73: 399–409, 1955

72. Di Silverio F: Histological type of tumor and hormone dependence. In: Hormonal Therapy of Prostatic Vancer, Bracci U, Di Silverio F (eds), Cofese Edizioni, Palermo, 47–58, 1975

73. Sciarra F, Piro, Concolino G, Conti C: Il metabolismo del deidroepiandrosterone as livella cutaneo: Experimenti in vitro. Folia Endocrinol 4: 423–430, 1968

74. Labrie F, Veilleux R: A wide range of sensitivities to androgens develops in cloned Shionogi mouse mammary tumor cells. The Prostate, 8: 293–300, 1986

75. Bartsch W, Knabbe M, Voigt KD: Regulation and compartmentalization of androgens in rat prostate and muscle. J Steroid Biochem 19: 929–937, 1983

76. Matsumoto K, Sato K, Kitamura Y: Roles of androgen and its receptors in mouse mammary tumor. In: BS Leung (ed), Hormonal Regulation of Mammary Tumors, vol 1B Eden Press, Montreal, Canada, 216–244, 1982

77. Stanley ER, Palmer RE, Sohn D: Development of methods for the quantitative in vitro analysis of androgen-dependent and autonomous Shionogi carcinoma 115 cells. Cell 10: 35–44, 1977

78. Labrie F, Dupont A, Bélanger A: Complete androgen blockade for the treatment of prostate cancer. In: Important Advances in Oncology, De Vita VT, Hellman S, Rosenberg SA (eds) Lippincott JB PA, 193–217, 1985

79. Labrie F, Dupont A, Bélanger A, Giguère M, Lacourcière Y, Emond J, Monfette G, Bergeron V: Combination therapy with Flutamide and castration (LHRH agonist or orchiectomy) in advanced prostate cancer: a marked improvement in response and survival. J Steroid Biochem, in press, 1986

80. Scott WW, Menon M, Walsch PC: Hormonal therapy of prostatic cancer. Cancer 45: 1929–1936, 1980

81. Klein LA: Medical Progress: prostatic carcinoma, New Engl J Med 300: 824–827, 1979

82. Elder JS, Catalona WJ: Management of newly diagnosed metastatic carcinoma of the prostate. Urol Clin North Amer 11: 283–295, 1984

83. Marchetti B, Plante M, Poulin R, Labrie F: Dramatic response of prostate weight and ornithine decarboxylase to low levels of testosterone in castrated rats. J Steroid Biochem, 36: 325, 1985

84. Drouin J, Labrie F: Selective effect of androgens on LH and FSH release in anterior pituitary cells in culture. Endocrinology 98: 1528–1534, 1976

85. Hammond GL: Endogenous steroid levels in the human prostate from birth to old age: a comparison of normal and diseased tissue. J Endocrinol 78: 7–19, 1978

86. Barnes RW, Ninan CA: Carcinoma of the prostate: biopsy and conservative therapy. J Urol 108: 897–900, 1972

87. Scott WE, Menon M, Walsh PC: Hormonal therapy of prostatic cancer. Cancer 45: 1929–1936, 1986

88. Asselin J, Mélançon R, Moachon G, Bélanger A: Characteristics of binding to estrogen, androgen, progestin an glucocorticoid receptors in 7, 12-dimethylbenz(a)anthracene-induced mammary tumors and their hormonal control. Cancer Res 40: 1612–1622, 1980

89. Simard J, Luthy I, Guay J, Bélanger A, Labrie F: Characteristics of interaction of the antiandrogen Flutamide with the androgen receptor in various target tissues. Mol Cell Endocrinol 44:261–270, 1986

90. Dexter DL, Calabresi P: Intraneoplastic diversity. Biochim Biophys Acta 694: 97–112, 1982

91. Labrie F, Dupont A, Bélanger A, St-Arnaud R, Giguère M, Lacourcière Y, Emond J, Monfette G: Treatment of prostate cancer with gonadotropin-releasing hormone agonists. Edocrine Reviews, 7: 67–74, 1986

92. The Leuprolide Study Group Leuprolide versus diethylstilbestrol for metastatic prostate cancer. New Engl J Med 311: 1281–1286, 1984

93. Labrie F, Bélanger A, Dupont A, Emond J, Lacourcière Y, Monfette G: Combined treatment with LHRH agonist and a pure antiandrogen in advanced carcinoma of the prostate. The Lancet i: 1090, 1984

94. Labrie F, Dupont A, Bélanger A, Poyet P, Giguère M, Lacourcière Y, Emond J, Monfette G,

Borsanyi JP: Combined treatment with Flutamide and surgical or medical (LHRH agonist) castration in metastatic prostatic cancer. The Lancet p 49, 1986

95. Séguin C, Cusan L, Bélanger A, Kelly PA, Labrie F, Raynaud JP: Additive inhibitory effects of treatment with an LHRH agonist and an antiandrogen on androgen-dependent tissues in the rat. Mol Cell Endocrinol 21: 37–41, 1981

96. Lefebvre FA, Séguin C, Bélanger A, Caron S, Sairam MR, Raynaud JP, Labrie F: Combined long-term treatment with an LHRH agonist and a pure antiandrogen blocks androgenic influence in the rat. The Prostate 3: 569–578, 1982

97. Aihrart RA, Barnett TF, Sullivan JW, Levine RL, Schlegel JU: Flutamide therapy for carcinoma of the prostate. South Med J 71: 798–801, 1978

98. Prout Jr GR, Irwin Jr RJ, Kilman B, Daly JJ, MacLaughlin J, Griffin PP: Prostatic cancer and SCH 13521: II. Histological alterations and the pituitary gonadel axis. J Urol 113: 834–840, 1975

99. Neumann F, Schenck B: New antiandrogens and their mode of action. J Reprod Fertil Fertil (suppl) 24: 129–145, 1976

100. Neumann F, Graf KJ, Hason SH, Schenche B, Steinbeck H: Central actions of antiandrogens. In: Androgens and Antiandrogens, Martini L, Motta L (eds) Raven Press, New York, 163–171, 1977

101. Raynaud JP, Bonne C, Bouton MM, Lagacé L, Labrie F: Action of a non-steroidal antiandrogen, RU23908, in peripheral and central tissues. J Steroid Biochem 11: 93–99, 1979

102. Irwin RJ, Prout Jr GJ: A new antiprostatic agent for treatment of prostatic carcinoma. Surg Forum 24: 536–538, 1973

103. Jacobo E, Schmidt JD, Weinstein SH, Flocks RH: Comparison of Flutamide (SCH-13521) and diethylstilbestrol in untreated advanced prostatic cancer. Urology 8: 231–233, 1976

104. Hellman L, Bradlow HL, Freed S, Levin J, Rosenfeld RS, Whitmore WF, Zumoff B: The effect of flutamide on testosterone metabolism and the plasma levels of androgens and gonadotropins. Clin Endocrinol Metab 45: 1224–1229, 1977

105. Peers E, Henson F, Neri R, Tabackinik I: Effects of non-steroidal antiandrogen SCH14521 on testosterone disposition in rats. Fed Proc 32: 759, 1973

106. Scott WW, Schirmer HKA: A new progestational steroid effective in the treatment of prostatic cancer. Trans Am Assoc Genitourin Surg 58: 54–61, 1966

107. Wein AJ, Murphy JJ: Experience in the treatment of prostatic carcinoma with cyproterone acetate. J Urol 109: 68–70, 1973

108. Tveter KJ, Otnes B, Hannestad R: Treatment of prostatic carcinoma with cyproterone acetate. Scand J Urol Nephrol 12: 115–118, 1978

109. Isurugi K, Kukutani K, Ishida H, Hosoi Y: Endocrine effects of cyproterone acetate in patients with prostatic cancer. J Urol 123: 180–183, 1980

110. Varenhorst E: Metabolic changes during endocrine treatment in carcinoma of the prostate. A prospective study in man with special reference ot cardiovascular complications during treatment with estrogens or cyproterone acetate or after orchiectomy. Linkoping University Med Diss 103, 1978

111. Cusan L, Auclair C, Bélanger A, Ferland L, Kelly PA, Séguin C, Labrie F: Inhibitory effects of long-term treatment with an LHRH agonist on the pituitary-gonadal axis in male and female rats. Endocrinology 104: 1369–1376, 1979

112. Sandow J, Von Rechenberg W, Jerzabek G, Stoll W: Pituitary gonadotropin inhibition by a highly active analog of luteinizing hormone-releasing hormone. Fertil Steril 30: 205–211, 1978

113. Dorfmann RI: Androgens. In: Proc of the Third Int congress on Hormonal Steroids, James V, Martini L (eds) Excerpta Medica, Amsterdam, p 995, 1971

114. Poyet P, Labrie F: Comparison of the antiandrogenic/androgenic activities of Flutamide, cyproterone acetate and megestrol acetate. Mol Cell Endocrinol 42: 283–288, 1985

115. Neri R, Monahan MD, Meyer JG, Alfonso BA, Tabachnick IA: Biological studies on an antiandrogen (SH-714). Eur J Pharmacol 1: 438–444, 1967

116. Sufrin G, Coffey DS: A new model for studying the effects of drugs on prostatic growth. 1. Antiandrogens and DNA synthesis. Inv. Urol 11: 45–54, 1973

117. Graf KJ, Kleinechke Jr RI, Neumann F: The stimulation of male duct derivatives in female guinea pigs with an antiandrogen cyproterone acetate. J Reprod Fertil 39: 311–317, 1974

118. Tisell LE, Salander H: Androgenic properties and adrenal depressent activity of megestrol acetate observed in castrated male rats. Acta Endocrinal 78: 316–324, 1975

119. Johnson DE, Kaesler KE, Ayala AG: Megestrol acetate for treatment of advanced carcinoma of the prostate. J Surg Oncol 7: 9–15, 1975

120. Geller J: Rationale for blockage of adrenal as well as testicular androgens in the treatment of advanced prostate cancer. Semin Oncol 12: 28–38, 1985

121. Geller J, Albert J, Yen SSC, Geller S, Loza D: Medical castration of males with megestrol acetate and small doses of diethylstilbestrol. J Clin Endocrinol Metab 52: 576–580, 1981

122. Girard J, Gaumann JB, Bohler U, Zuppinger V, Haas HG, Staub JJ, Wyss HI: Cyproterone acetate and adrenal functions. J Clin Endocrinol Metab 47: 581–586 1978

123. Neumann F, Elger W, Steinbeck H: Antiandrogens and reproductive development. Philos Trans R Soc London, Ser B Biol Sci 259: 179–184, 1970

124. Neri R, Florance K, Kariol P, Van Cleave S: A biological profile of a non-steroidal antiandrogen, SCH 13521 (4'-nitro-3'-trifluromethylisobutyranilide). Endocrinology 91: 427–437, 1972

125. Elger W: Die rolle der setalen androgen in der sexual disserenzierung des kanichens und ihre. (Partie I and II). Archives d'Anatomie Microscopique et de Morphologie 55: 658–670, 1966

126. Tenniswood M, Abrahams P, Bird C, Clark A: Antiandrogen do not alter androgen-dependent characteristic of acid phosphatase in the rat ventral prostate. Mol Cell Endocrinol 37: 153–158, 1983

127. Allen JM, O'Shea JP, Mashiter K, Williams G, Bloom SR: Advanced carcinoma of the prostate: treatment with a gonadotrophin releasing hormone agonist. Brit Med J 286: 1607, 1983

128. Resko JA, Bélanger A, Labrie F: Effects of chronic treatment with a potent luteinizing hormone-releasing hormone agonist on serum luteinizing hormone and steroid levels in the male Rhesus monkey. Biol Reprod 26: 378, 1982

129. St-Arnaud R, Lachance R, Kelly SJ, Bélanger A, Dupont A, Labrie F: Loss of luteinizing hormone (LH) bioactivity in patients with prostatic cancer treated with an LHRH agonist and a pure antiandrogen. Clin Endocrinol, 24: 21–30, 1986

130. Waxman J, Man A, Hendry WF, Whitfield HN, Besser GM, Tiptaft RC, Paris AMI, Oliver RTD: Importance of early tumour exacerbation in patients treated with long-acting analogues of gonadotropin-releasing hormone for advanced prostatic cancer. Brit Med J 291: 1387–1388, 1985

131. Kahan A, Delrieu F, Amor B, Chiche R, Steg A: Disease flare induced by D-Trp[6]-LHRH analogue in patients with metastatic prostatic cancer. The Lancet i: 871, 1984

132. Fowler Jr JE, Whitmore WF: The response of metastatic adenocarcinoma of the prostate to exogenous testosterone. J Urol 126: 372–375, 1981

133. Armitage T: Statistical methods in medical research. Blackwell Scientific Publications, Oxford, 1971

134. Kaplan EJ, Meier P: Non parametric estimation from incomplete observations. Am Statis Ass J: 53: 457–481, 1958

135. King RJB, Cambray GJ, Jagus-Smith R, Robinson JH, Smith JA. In: Receptors and mechanisms of action of steroid hormones, Pasqualini JR (ed) Marcel Dekker, New York, p 215, 1977

136. Luthy I, Labrie F: Development of androgen resistance in mouse mammary tumor cells can be prevented by the antiandrogen flutamide prostate, in press, 1986

137. Simard J, Labrie F: Unoccupied androgen receptors are biologically active in rat pituitary

gonadotrophs. Proc 7th Int Congr Endocrinology, Excerpta Medica Cong Series 652, Amsterdam, p 973, 1984

138. Ponder BAJ, Shearer RJ, Pocock RD, Miller J, Easton D, Chilvers CED, Dowsett M, Jeffcoate SL: Reponse to aminoglutethimide and cortisone acetate in advanced prostatic cancer. Br J Cancer 50, 757–763, 1984

139. Rostom AY, Folkes A, Lord C, Notley RG, Schweitzer FAW, White WF: Aminoglutethimide therapy for advanced carcinoma of the prostate. Br J Urol 54: 552–55, 1982

140. Worgul TJ, Wanten RJ, Samoj E, Samojlik E, Veldhuis JD, Lipton A, Harvey HA, Drago JR, Rohner TJ: Clinical and biochemical effect of aminoglutethimide in the treatment of advanced prostatic carcinoma. J Urol 129: 51–53, 1983

141. Drago JR, Santen RJ, Kipton A, Worgul TJ, Harvey HA, Boucher A, Manni A, Rohner TJ: Clinical effect of aminoglutethimide, medical adrenalectomy in treatment of 43 patients with advanced prostatic carcinoma. Cancer 53: 1447–1450, 1984

142. Moore RJ, Gazak JM, Wilson JD: Regulation of cytoplasmic dihydrotestosterone binding in dog prostate by 17β-estradiol. J Clin Invest 63: 351–357, 1979

143. Mobbs BG, Johnson IE, Connolly JG, Thompson J: Concentration and cellular distribution of androgen receptor in human prostatic neoplasia: Can estrogen treatment increase androgen receptor content? J Steroid Biochem 19: 1279–1290, 1983

144. Bélanger A, Dupont A, Labrie F: Inhibition of basal and adrenocorticotropin-stimulated plasma levels of adrenal androgens after treatment with an antiandrogen in castrated patients with prostatic cancer. J Clin Endocrinol Metab 59: 422–426, 1984

Editorial Comment

JOSEPH A. SMITH, Jr.

The concept of total androgen suppression in the treatment of patients with metastatic carcinoma of the prostate is not noval. The recognition that prostatic cancer may be stimulated by androgens of adrenal origin has led to previous efforts to ablate adrenal androgen production. Several factors have, however, led to renewed interest in the subject. First, improved biochemical assay methods have allowed identification of what appear to be significant levels of intracellular androgens, even after patients have undergone orchiectomy. Secondly, the development of LHRH analogs and nontoxic anti-androgens has allowed pharmacologic deprivation of both adrenal and testicular androgen from the prostatic cancer cell and decreased the morbidity of treatment. Finally, the enthusiasm and zeal with which Dr. Labrie and colleagues have promoted this subject have generated widespread interest within the lay public.

The role of adrenal anrogens in stimulating the growth of prostatic cancer certainly deserves further study. However, what must be kept in mind is that total androgen suppression is not 'clearly proven beyond any doubt whatsoever' to be superior to traditional methods of hormonal therapy in the treatment of patients with prostatic cancer. Several concepts put forth in the preceding chapter do not offer as irrefutable proof of the superiority of this treatment as is implied and deserve further comment.

Circulating and intracellular androgen levels

Over 90% of circulating levels of serum testosterone are of testicular origin and the adrenal gland contributes only weak androgens to the circulating pool. Therefore, the possibility that adrenal androgens may be of significance in patients with prostatic cancer often has been dismissed. More recent evidence has, however, shown that intracellular dihydrotestosterone levels may be significant even after orchiectomy [1]. The implication is that intracellular conversion of the adrenal steroids androstenedione and dehydroepiandrosterone produces significant amounts of potent androgen dihydrotestosterone. The ability of adrenal androgens to promote secondary sexual characteristics through intracellular conversion to DHT is demonstrated in pathologic conditions such as Cushing's syndrome, idiopathic hirsutism, adrenal hyperplasia or adrenal tumors.

While the demonstrated levels of intracellular DHT after orchiectomy are a possible concern and deserve further study, the contribution of adrenal androgens to the growth of prostatic cancer cells, in either the presence or absence of testicular production of testosterone is uncertain. Dr. Labrie and colleagues estimate that adrenal and testicular androgens contribute equally to intracellular DHT levels and that orchiectomy eliminates only half of the potential androgenic stimulus to prostatic cancer cells. Much of their work regarding cell growth and heterogeneity is based upon the Shionogi mouse mammary carcinoma model. Although their data are interesting and should lead to further study, the unwavering extrapolation that these same phenomena are operative in human prostatic adenocarcinoma is not scientifically sound.

Historical data

The lack of enthusiasm for adrenal androgen blockade among most clinicians treating patients with prostatic cancer is based upon the relatively unfacorable results which have been achieved historically. Certainly, Dr. Labrie and co-workers have derived a much more favorable interpretation of previous results than is commonly held.

Huggins and Scott initially reported adrenalectomy for prostatic cancer patients based upon the belief that adrenal androgen ablation may be beneficial in patients relapsing after primary hormonal therapy [2]. In a literature review, Brendler reported only a six per cent objective response after adrenalectomy [3]. Although 73 per cent of patients reportedly had subjective improvement, most responses were of short duration. Aminoglutethemide produces a medical blockade of adrenal cortical function and has been used as a 'medical adrenalectomy' in prostatic cancer patients. The reported series suggest a favorable response in approximately one third of patients treated with aminoglutethemide after previous hormonal therapy. Most responses are subjective and of short duration and the contribution of concomitantly administered steroids to these results is uncertain.

Pituitary ablation via surgery, cryo destruction, or interstitial irradiation has also been used un patients who fail to respond or relapse after conventional hormonal therapy. Short duration subjective responses of greater than 50 per cent are commonly reported in the literature [4]. However, well documented objective responses are much less common. Indeed, in our series, we observed clear evidence of objective progression in patients with subjective improvement [5]. Hypophysectomy is known to alter levels of endorphins and enkephlins, endogenous opiate peptides which affect subjective pain interpretation and may serve as neuro-transmitters in pain modifying pathways. Since the primary response to hupophysectomy in prostatic cancer patients seems to be subjective improvement in bone pain, the effects of pituitary ablation may be related to alterations in pain perception rather than a favorable impact upon the disease process itself.

Flutamide, as Dr. Labrie correctly points out, is a drug which appears to be relatively unique in that it is a pure anti-androgen. Flutamide has been used in prostatic cancer patients failing alternative endocrine therapy with results somewhat less impressive than implied by Dr. Labrie and colleagues. Sogani and associates reported an objective response of short duration in six of 26 patients with prostatic cancer refractory to conventional hormonal treatment who were treated with flutamide [6]. MacFarlane and Tolley found that 12 of 14 patients failing conventional hormonal treatment had no evidence of a response to 750 mg of flutamide daily [1]. Based upon their own experience, the authors of these papers concluded that flutamide was of little benefit in patients failing standard therapy.

LHRH analogs

The ability of LHRH analogs to suppress serum testosterone levels and maintain them in the castrate region has been well documented and these drugs are now used as an alternative means of endocrine therapy for prostatic cancer patients [8]. However, Dr. Labrie and colleagues wonder how LHRH analogs can be used alone in the treatment of prostatic cancer patients. Their skepticism is based upon analysis of the endocrine response in patients treated with LHRH analogs and seems to ignore the abundant clinical data demonstrating the effectiveness of these agents. While it is true that one should not anticipate a response superior to that achieved with alternative means of hormonal therapy, the equivalent response between patients receiving LHRH analogs and those treated with estrogens and, implicitly, orchiectomy is documented [9].

The issues raised regarding the initial testosterone stimulation in LHRH treated patients and the potential for a 'tumor flare' are important and deserve further comment. Undoubtedly, elevation of serum testosterone in prostatic cancer patients runs contrary to the well established goals of hormonal therapy. As Dr. Labrie points out, administration of exogenous testosterone to prostatic cancer patients relapsing after conventional hormonal therapy is dangerous and has an adverse effect in over 90 per cent of patients. However, in previously untreated patients where circulating levels of serum testosterone may be producing near maximal physiologic stimulation of tumor cells, adverse responses are less common. Nevertheless, there undoubtedly are well substantiated reports of adverse effects observed within the first two weeks of LHRH therapy in prostatic cancer patients. Appropriate patient selection is mandatory and certain patients, including those with impending neurologic compromise, should be excluded from initial LHRH therapy. Using these selection criteria, approximately 10 per cent of our patients have had a modest increase in bone pain during the first week of therapy with an LHRH analog but we have seen no serious adverse response in over 80 patients treated. Also, there seems no clinical justification for the belief that the transient increase in serum testosterone adversely effects survival or duration of response in patients treated with an LHRH analog. Dr. Labrie states that there is a zero per cent response rate at two years in patients treated with an LHRH analog. This clearly runs contrary to most published reports and there seems good evidence that the duration of response is similar to that achieved with orchiectomy or estrogens [9].

A final comment regarding objective response to LHRH analogs is pertinent. Dr. Labrie states that combination therapy with an LHRH analog and an anti-androgen improves the objective response by nearly 40 per cent compared to an LHRH analog alone. Using the same criteria which he espouses, i.e. those of the National Prostatic Cancer Project, patients treated initially with an LHRH analog alone were found to have an 86 per cent objective response [9]. Therefore, the potential for improvement is strikingly more modest than implied in the previous chapter.

Clinical results of treatment with an LHRH analog and flutamide

Initially, enthusiastic reports of LHRH plus anti-androgen treatment were published before large clinical series were available. Reportedly, 95 percent of patients have had an objective response based upon N.P.C.P. criteria although careful review indicates that many patients do not have parameters which would allow accurate definition of response using these criteria. Also, the reported 95 percent response may not be dissimilar to the previously published 86 percent objective response using these same criteria seen in patients treated with an LHRH analog alone. The improvement, if any, with combination therapy may be much less remarkable than is implied.

After patients have failed alternative hormonal therapy, the authors claim a 42 percent objective response in patients treated with flutamide. This response exceeds that reported by other groups using the identical drug. Also, it should be noted that a 48% response of short duration has been reported in patients treated with an LHRH analog after failing estrogen therapy [11]. Since the majority of responses in flutamide or LHRH treated patients are stabilization, one wonders whether this is a true response or simply an observation of the natural history of the disease. Also, it should be questioned whether all of the patients treated by Dr. Labrie and colleagues were true failures on alternative hormonal therapy. Some patients were started on flutamide within five or ten days of orchiectomy or the initiation of estrogen therapy. How could progressive disease be documented within that time? Finally, the advice that hormonal therapy be continued in relapsing patients who are to be treated with palliative irradiation or chemotherapy seems well founded. There is good evidence that some cells maintain their androgen responsiveness in this setting and may increase in size if serum testosterone is allowed to rise. Whether or not flutamide should be instituted after patients have failed orchiectomy is, however, far less certain.

Summary

The concept of total androgen suppression by ablation of both testicular and adrenal androgen production is worthy of study. However, the dogmatic fervor with which this treatment is espoused in the preceding chapter seems unsubstantiated. Neither historical data nor the known hormonal responsiveness of prostatic cancer would imply that this is likely to be a 'remarkable advance'. Fortunately, unlike so many other areas of medicine, this does not seem to be an argument which will persist indefinitely. A large, multi-center study comparing the results of an LHRH analog plus flutamide versus an LHRH analog plus placebo in previously untreated metastatic prostatic cancer patients has recently completed accrual [12]. The results of this study should be forthcoming within the next few years. Dr. Labrie has accepted the results of this study as a foregone conclusion and has suggested another study adding aminoglutethemide or ketoconozale as a third treatment. However, since most clinicians are less convinced of the value of combination therapy with an LHRH analog and flutamide, the results of this initial study will be of great interest. Dr. Labrie deserves credit for increasing the interest in the possibility of adrenal androgenic stimulation of prostatic cancer but the answer as to whether or not such combination therapy improves the results which have historically been obtained with testicular androgen deprivation remains to be determined.

References

1. Geller J, Albert J, Loza D, et al: DHT concentrations in human prostatic cancer tissue. J Clin Endocrine and Metab 46: 440–444, 1978
2. Huggins C, Scott WW: Bilateral adrenalectomy in prostatic cancer. Clinical features and urinary excretion of 17-ketosteroids and estrogens. Ann Surg 122: 1031–1041, 1945
3. Brendler H: Adrenalectomy and hypophysectomy for prostatic cancer. Urology 2: 99–101, 1973
4. Fergusson JD, Hendry WF: Pituitary irradiation in advanced carcinoma of the prostate. Br J Urol 43: 514, 1971
5. Smith Jr JA, Eyre HJ, Roberts TS, Middleton RG: Transphenoidal hypophysectomy in the management of carcinoma of the prostate. Cancer 53: 2385, 1984
6. Sogani PC, Ray B, Whitmore Jr WF: Advanced prostatic carcinoma: flutamide therapy after conventional endocrine treatment. Urology 6: 164–66, 1975
7. MacFarlane JR, Tolley DA: Flutamide therapy for advanced prostatic cancer: A phase II study. Br J Urol 57: 172–174, 1985
8. Smith Jr JA: Androgen suppression by a gonadotropin releasing hormone analog in patients with metastatic carcinoma of the prostate. J Urol 131: 1110, 1984
9. Garnick MB, Glode LM, Smith Jr JA, et al: Leuprolide versus diethylstilbestrol for metastatic prostate cancer. New Engl J Med 311: 1281–86, 1984
10. Labrie F, Dupont A, Belanger A, et al: New approach in the treatment of prostate cancer: complete instead of partial withdrawal of androgens. The Prostate 4: 579, 1983
11. Smith Jr JA, for the Leuprolide Study Group: Clinical effects of gonadotropin releasing hormine analogue in metastatic carcinoma of the prostate. Urology 25: 106–114.
12. Leuprolide plus flutamide versus leuprolide plus placebo. Intergroup study of prostatic cancer.

9. BCG immunotherapy for superficial bladder cancer

DONALD L. LAMM *

Introduction

Transitional cell carcinoma of the bladder is an ideal tumor for the evaluation of cancer immunotherapy. Unlike most tumors, patients with transitional cell carcinoma of the bladder typically present with localized superficial disease which can be readily resected. After tumor resection patients are generally immunologically competent and adequately nourished, but have an approximately 70% risk of tumor recurrence. Such recurrences may be due to the implantation of tumor cells released during transurethral resection. Animal models suggest that traumatized urothelium is particularly susceptible to tumor implantation. Alternatively, tumor recurrence may be due to incomplete resection of the primary tumor, growth of microscopic tumors not visible to the endoscopist, or the generation of new tumors. New tumors may result from continued physical, chemical, or biological carcinogen exposure in a susceptible host or, more likely, from the progression of malignantly transformed cells from occult to overt malignancy. Multifocal atypia, loss of blood group antigens in normal appearing urothelium, and multifocal recurrences in patients with transitional cell carcinoma suggest that malignant transformation is widespread. Such microscopic or submicroscopic disease is accessible for topical therapy. It is presumably the combination of an immunocompetent host with an accessible, antigenic, microscopic or submicroscopic malignancy which has resulted in the successful immunotherapy of bladder cancer.

   BCG immunotherapy for recurrent superficial bladder cancer has been highly successful and has been acknowledged to be currently the most successful form of immunotherapy for human malignancy [1]. Current data to be presented in this chapter suggest that BCG immunotherapy is in fact the most effective intravesical treatment of carcinoma in situ as well as the most effective prohylactic agent for the prevention of recurrence of transitional cell carcinoma.

* Supported in part by NCI 5 ROI CA 42327.

Ratliff, T.L. and Catalona, W.J. (eds), Genitourinary Cancer. ISBN 0–89838–830–9
© *1987, Martinus Nijhoff Publishers, Boston. Printed in the Netherlands.*

Historial background

Tuberculosis has been a primary scourge of mankind. Early morbidity and mortality figures are difficult to obtain and are of questionable validity, but it is estimated that more than 90% of the European population were exposed to tuberculosis and the annual death toll exceeded 275 per one hundred thousand population in the mid-19th century [2]. The prevalence of the tuberculosis bacillus and the mortality rate of infection suggest that this organism may have had a significant influence on evolution. Indeed, in the mouse genetic control of resistance to tuberculosis infection has been documented [3]. It is not surprising, therefore, that bacillus Calmette-Guerin is one of the most potent immune stimulants known. The survival of our ancestors was in part dependent on their ability to mount an immune response to *Mycobacterium tuberculosis*.

Koch demonstrated that the tubercle bacillus was the causative agent of tuberculosis in 1882 [4]. Many researchers initiated attempts to prepare a tuberculosis vaccine thereafter, with preliminary success reported as early as 1886 [4]. Auguste Calmette and Claude Guerin are responsible for the most successful tuberculosis vaccine: bacillus Calmette-Guerin. BCG was isolated at the Pasteur Institute of Lille through progressive attenuation of a virulent strain of *Mycobacterium bovis* that had been previously isolated in 1882 by Nocard. Complete attenuation required 13 years and 231 serial passages which were made possible by adding beef bile to the bacterial emulsions [4]. The first clinical trial of the vaccine was given in 1921. An oral BCG preparation was used to protect a newborn child who was to live in household with active tuberculosis infection. The child suffered no ill effects and did not contract tuberculosis [4]. Since that time more than 1.5 billion BCG vaccinations have been performed with negligible mortality and very little morbidity [5].

Nearly 4 decades elapsed between the application of BCG in tuberculosis prophylaxus and its application in the treatment of cancer. During this interval Freund and other immunologists discovered the remarkable stimulatory effect of BCG on the immune response [6]. BCG was found to be a potent stimulant of the reticuloendothelial system [7], and stimulation of the reticulo-endothelial system had been observed to be associated with the prevention of tumor growth [8]. It was this activity which first prompted investigators in 1959 to evaluate BCG in the inhibition of tumor growth in animal models [9]. The remarkable efficacy of BCG immunotherapy in animal tumor models, the highlights of which will be discussed, was not effectively transferred to man as BCG met with multiple failures in clinical trials. BCG immunotherapy was initially reported to be dramatically successful in the treatment of melanoma, squamous cell carcinoma of the head and neck, lung carcinoma, and, when combined with chemotherapy, acute lyphocytic leukemia and acute and chronic myelocytic leukemia [10]. Unfortunately, with the notable exception of carcinoma of the bladder, most well designed prospectively controlled clinical trials failed to demonstrate significant therapeutic benefit from BCG immunotherapy [11]. The dramatic success in the treatment of human bladder cancer when contrasted with the failures observed in the treatment of other malignancies should provide lessons which will permit the extension of effective immunotherapy to many other human malignancies.

Animal studies

As pointed out by Bast in 1974, clinical investigators have not made optimal use of information obtained from work with animal tumors [9]. Experimental results with animal tumor models cannot be translated directly to the clinic, but the experience gained from such experimentation can significantly improve the design of clinical protocols and expedite the delivery of therapeutic improvements. Experience obtained by a number of investigators and reviewed by Bast [9] suggests that growth of a variety of tumors can be prevented in a wide range of animal species if systemic BCG infection was established by subcutaneous or intravenous inoculation. BCG has been much less effective in the treatment of established tumor grafts. Tumor size has constituted a critical limitation of BCG immunotherapy, with as few as 100,000 cells being a limit of efficacy in some mouse models. In general, admixture of BCG with irradiated tumor ot tumor vaccines has improved the efficacy of BCG. BCG has been effective only when given to immunocompetent hosts. Suppression of the immune response with anti-thymocyte serum, steroids, or irradiation, and thymectomy typically results in failure to develop acquired cutaneous hypersensitivity to PPD and inability to prevent tumor growth. While some nonviable BCG subfractions have demonstrated activity in animal models, in general an adequate number of viable BCG organisms is an essential requirement for successful BCG immunotherapy. In general, approximately ten to the seventh organisms are required. Excessive BCG administration, or administration of nonviable preparations can reduce the efficacy. Close association of BCG and tumor cells results generally produces optimal response. In animal models, intralesional injection is typically highly effective, whereas injection of BCG in areas remote from the tumor typically does not inhibit tumor growth. As with any immunotherapy, BCG can be effective only if there are recognizable antigenic determinants on the tumor cell. It is readily apparent from a review of the suggested requirements for optimal immunotherapy in animal studies, i.e., prophylactic BCG administration, minimal tumor size, immune competent host, administration of adequate numbers of viable organisms, close proximity of BCG to tumor cells, and the presence of an antigenic tumor, that transitional cell carcinoma of the bladder represents an ideal application of the principles of BCG immunotherapy tu human cancer.

Animal studies of BCG immunotherapy in transitional cell carcinoma have also contributed to our knowledge of the factors of importance in effective BCG immunotherapy of bladder cancer. In 1977 Lamm and co-workers observed that intralesional administration of BCG cell walls effectively prevented tumor progression in systemically BCG sensitized rats while no affect was observed when BCG cell walls were injected intralesionally in unsensitized rats [12]. In 1978, deKernion and co-workers observed prolongation of survival, despite an absence of effect on tumor growth, when intramuscular BCG was given on the day of transplantation of the transplantable murine bladder tumor MBT2 [13]. Adolphs, et al., in 1979 observed that cyclophosphamide, which is known to inhibit suppressor T-cells, enhanced the efficacy of systemic BCG immunotherapy [14]. They also observed that systemic BCG alone reduced bladder tumor size relative to untreated controls. Surprisingly, intralesional BCG increased mean bladder weights compared with controls. This increase in bladder weight was no doubt in part related to the mass associated with granuloma formation in BCG inoculated animals. Initial studies by Soloway [15] and Morales [16] suggested that systemic intraperitoneal BCG had no anti-tumor effect, but subsequent studies using higher doses of BCG resulted in very significant protection [17]. The efficacy of high dose systemic intraperitoneal BCG, which is of interest in view of the reported clinical efficacy of oral BCG, has been recently confirmed by Drago in the Nb rat bladder cancer model [18].

Comparison of substrains of BCG in the MBT2 model has demonstrated that Tice and Armand-Frapier preparations in doses ranging from 5×10^5 to 1×10^7 colony forming units per animal were highly effective and superior to immunotherapy with agents such as BCG cell wall skeletons, RE glycolipid or Keyhole Limpet Hemocyanin [19]. Glaxo BCG had no beneficial effect when used in maximal doses in the MBT2 model, but was observed by Pimm and Baldwin to decrease growth of human tumor cell line T24 when admixed at the time of transplantation into nude mice [20]. The immunity induced by BCG has been observed to protect from subsequent tumor challenge for as long as eight months without additional BCG treatment and as long as 15 months if additional BCG was given at the time of tumor inoculation [21]. Animal data clearly confirm that appropriate doses of local and/or systemic BCG inhibit the growth of transitional cell carcinoma. Multiple other non-specific immunotherapeutic agents, including Keyhole-Limpet Hemocyanin, Levamisole, *Corynebacterium parvum*, and interferon inducers have been effective, but to date nothing has been demonstrated to be superior to immunotherapy with live BCG.

Mechanism of action

The wide variety of immunological effects of BCG attests to the wisdom of those who have labeled it a non-specific immune stimulant. While the efficacy of BCG cannot be denied, the mechanism of action which is responsible for the beneficial results observed in cancer immunotherapy remain largely undetermined. There is evidence from animal studies that suggests that BCG may share antigenic determinants with a variety of tumors [22]. BCG is a potent immune adjuvant which heightens the response to antigenic stimulation. Administration of BCG stimulates the reticuloendothelial system resulting in hyperplasia and increased phagocytic and cytolytic activity of macrophages and augmentation of delayed cutaneous hypersensitivity. In animals systemic BCG administration results in hyperplasia of the spleen, which is measurable as increased splenic weight. In our patients given BCG immunotherapy small but statistically significant increase in absolute lymphocyte counts were observed. In animal models, BCG administration has been associated with increased resistance to bacterial and viral infection, enhanced humoral immunity, and increased interferon production. In our patient we have observed an increase in antibody titers to PPD, but no non-specific increase in antibody titers or skin test reactivity to common infectious organisms [23]. We have also observed stimulation of interferon levels in patients who favorably respond to BCG immunotherapy [24].

Intravesical BCG administration results in an intense inflammatory cell infiltration of the bladder with lymphocytes, polymorphonuclear leukocytes, plasma cells, histiocytes, and foreign body giant cells. Some have suggested that the inflammation resulting from intravesical BCG administration is the sole mechanism of action. In view of the multiplicity of responses to BCG and the observation that other inflammatory agents such as DNCB promote rather than inhibit bladder tumor growth [12], inflammation is unlikely to be the sole mechanism of action. Moreover, the efficacy of local BCG immunotherapy is correlated with systemic immune response as measured by PPD skin test reactivity [25, 26], and oral BCG in man [27] and high dose systemic (intraperitoneal) BCG immunotherapy in animals [17, 18] is reported to be effective in the prevention of transitional cell carcinoma without causing local inflammatory reactions. Characterization of the response to BCG immunotherapy in terms of alteration of lyphoid subpopulations is currently under investigation. Preliminary results suggest that, in healthy subjects, BCG vaccination results in a reduction in white cell, lymphocyte, and monocyte counts two days after administration followed by an increase back to baseline levels [28]. Increased NK cytotoxicity was observed on days 10 and 14 and antibody dependent cytotoxicity remained increased through day 21 [28]. On the other hand, BCG vaccination in bladder tumor patients has been observed to prevent the depression of lymphocyte cytotoxicity to bladder tumor cell lines which occurs following transurethral bladder tumor fulguration [29]. The array of responses to BCG suggests that BCG affects a range of different cell types including B cells, T cells, macrophages, killer (K) cells, and natural killer (NK) cells [30]. Since BCG is able to exert an effect in the presence of selective immunosuppressants it is unlikely that it acts through a single mechanism [30]. The induction of cytotoxic T cell immunity is clearly an important mechanism of action of BCG. In experiments by Davies and Sabbadini, tumor immunity in BCG-treated mice could be transferred to non-immune mice by cells having characteristics of T cells [31]. The complexity of immune responses to BCG suggests that multiple factors are responsible for the antitumor effect of BCG. Indeed, as new lymphokines and antitumor factors are identified, it is anticipated that many of these factors will be induced by BCG.

Clinical BCG trials

BCG Prophylaxis: The first clinical trial of intravesical BCG therapy was reported in 1976 by Morales [32]. In this initial report 9 patients with Stage T-0(O) or T-1(A) transitional cell carcinomas were treated with six weekly vaccinations of 120 mg Armand-Frappier BCG in 50cc saline intravesically plus 5 mg of BCG percutaneously using the multiple puncture technique. BCG treatment resulted in a 12 fold reduction in the number of tumors per patient month. Based on these encouraging preliminary results the National Cancer Institute funded two prospective randomized clinical trials of intravesical BCG using Morales' technique. Our initial results were presented in 1979 [33]. The significant advantage of BCG immunotherapy observed at that time has become even more impressive with the passage of time. A total of 94 patients have now been enrolled in randomized studies. Only 10 of 54 (18.5%) patients treated with BCG have had recurrent tumor compared with 19 of 40 (47.5%) control patients (P = 0.003, Chi square). The disease free interval has been prolonged from the mean of 31 months in controls to 58 months with BCG treatment (P = 0.0017). As illustrated in the figure, control patients have continued to have tumor recurrence at the expected rate. However, in the BCG group of patients there is an apparent leveling of the time to recurrence curve. Indeed, of the original group of 30 patients randomized to BCG, 6 were reported to have had tumor recurrence in 1982. Since that time, none of the remaining 24 patients has had tumor recurrence.

The recond prospective randomized trial was performed at Memorial Sloan-Kettering Cancer Center [34]. The same treatment schedule was used but the patient population was quite different and represented a group of patients with superficial bladder tumors who were at very high risk for tumor recurrence as evidenced by the 100% recurrence rate by 8 months in the untreated control group. The dramatic reduction in tumor recurrence from 2.37 tumors per patient month in control to 0.7 tumors per patient month in the BCG group has persisted with continued observation [35].

Multiple investigators have confirmed the efficacy of BCG in the prevention of bladder tumor recurrence. In 1980 Martinez-Pineiro [36] noted 21% tumor recurrence in 29 patients followed for 5 to 42 (mean 15.1) months. In 1982 Brosman noted no tumor recurrence in 49 patients treated with maintenance intravesical BCG and followed for over 2 years [37]. In 1983 Adolphs and Bastien [38] observed only 9% tumor recurrence in 90 patients treated with a single injection of cyclophosphamide and a 6 week course of intravesical and percutaneous BCG [38], and Netto and Lemos reported 6% tumor recurrence in 16 patients treated with high-dose oral BCG [27]. Similar protection from tumor recurrence has been reported by Babayan [39], deKernion [40], Haaf [41], Schellhammer [42], and others.

Two studies stand alone in failing to observe protection from tumor recurrence in patients treated with BCG. These studies are important, since a review of the method of BCG immunotherapy utilized may provide information of use in the design of treatment protocols. The first study by Flamm and Grof [43] observed a 59% recurrence rate in patients treated with Connaught BCG given only intravesically. While this dissappointing recurrence rate may reflect the selection of a high risk population, it is noteworthy that the same strain was highly effective when given both intravesically and percutaneously by Adolphs and Bastien [38] and by members of the Southwest Oncology Group. The second negative study by Stober and Peter [44] is a well performed prospective study comparing transurethral surgery alone versus surgery plus percutaneous BCG. No protection was observed when percutaneous BCG alone was given. These studies suggest that the route of administration is important, and may be particularly important when lower vaccine doses or shorter durations of treatment are used. Low doses of BCG given intravesically alone may be ineffective while combined intravesical and percutaneous BCG, or higher doses given intravesically alone are effective.

Treatment of existing tumor

Despite the observation from animal studies that BCG is rarely effective when tumor burden exceeds 100,000 cells, BCG has been used to treat patients with residual bladder cancer. Surprisingly, such treatment has been remarkably effective and compares very favorably with response rates reported for intravesical chemotherapy. A variety of treatment techniques and BCG substrains have been used. As illustrated in Table 1, complete response rates range from 36 to 83 per cent, with a mean complete response rate of 58%.

While this complete response rate is indeed encouraging, based on the animal data and my own experience in treating patients with bulky disease, I personally make every effort to completely resect all tumor prior to initiating BCG immunotherapy. In two instances patients have had such extensive disease that two separate operations were required to safely remove all visible tumor. These patients, like many others, have remained free of tumor recurrence for several years.

BCG therapy for carcinoma in situ

Carcinoma in situ of the bladder should in theory be an ideal tumor for BCG immunotherapy. Carcinoma in situ is a poorly differentiated and presumably antigenic tumor that is only a few cell layers thick, and is commonly widely dispersed in the bladder. Tumor volume with CIS is small. When confined to the bladder, CIS is most accessible to direct contact with BCG. CIS of the ureter, and perhaps the urethra, is less accessible and more difficult to manage. The complete response rate of 82 percent in a combined experience with 177 patients with CIS of the bladder treated with Armand-Frappier, Connaught, and Tice substrains of BCG exceeds that reported with any other intravesical agent. Reported responses range from 68 percent to 100 percent. Those differences are largely attributable to differences in criteria of qualification for complete response. Morales [49], for example, required complete response without relapse for the duration of the study to qualify as a complete response. Another apparent factor in the difference in reported response rates is the continuation of BCG treatment. Brosman [50] increased his complete response rate from 67% at 12 weeks to 89% at 18 weeks and 100% at 24 weeks in 27 patients who were able to tolerate weekly intravesical BCG treatment. These complete responses are not merely of academic interest since 87% of patients achieving complete response remained disease free during the 5.25 year average follow up period. Excellent responses have been observed with Tice, Armand-Frappier, and Connaight substrains of BCG [51].

The excellent complete response rate of CIS to BCG treatment plus the durability of these responses suggests that BCG is the treatment of choice for carcinoma in situ of the bladder. While invasive or metastatic disease can progress despite a complete response to bladder CIS, and caution must be exercised with meticulous follow up and bladder biopsy to rule out occult invasive disease, it is in my opinion not reasonable to recommend cystectomy as the initial treatment of choice for this group of patients. The complete response rate to BCG is excellent and generally durable. The vast majority of patients who do not respond

Table 1. BCG response rates in residual tumor

First author (ref)	Number	Complete response	Percent
Douville (45)	6	4	67
Morales (46)	17	10	59
Lamm (47)	10	6	60
Brosman (37)	12	10	83
deKernion (40)	22	8	36
Kojima (48)	29	16	55
Schellhammer (42)	22	14	64
Totals	118	68	58

Table 1: Reported response rates in 118 patients with intravesical BCG. Patients with CIS only are excluded.

completely will fail with localized disease, which can be detected and effectively treated. Cystectomy itself has significant morbidity and mortality and there is to date no evidence to suggest early cystectomy will increase overall survival or decrease the morbidity.

Ongoing studies suggest that the superior response rate of BCG in patients with CIS from historical series will prove to be true in randomized prospective comparisons of BCG and intravesical chemotherapy. Adriamycin has a reported complete response rate in CIS of 59 per cent in five series totaling 76 patients. In our ongoing multicenter Southwest Oncology Group trial, BCG has been compared with Adriamycin. Patients randomized to BCG have had an 81% complete response rate compared with a 60% complete response rate in patients treated with Adriamycin ($p < 0.01$).

BCG immunotherapy vs. chemotherapy

BCG has an advantage over intravesical chemotherapy in that its mechanism of action, while not completely defined, is clearly different from that of chemotherapy. Most intravesical chemotherapies are alkylating agents, and resistance to one agent increases the likelihood of resistance to the second. Such cross resistance has not been identified with BCG. In our experience with 22 patients who had failed intravesical chemotherapy, 82 per cent responded favorably to BCG [25]. The high response rate to BCG and the low incidence of significant complications suggest that BCG may be the primary treatment of choice for superficial bladder cancer. Patients who fail BCG treatment will also commonly respond to intravesical chemotherapy.

Two published studies have reported BCG to be significantly superior to Thiotepa in the prevention of bladder cancer recurrence. These studies are

Table 2. BCG therapy for carcinoma in situ

First author (ref)	Number	Complete response	Percent
Morales (49)	7	5	71
Lamm [a]	23	22	96
Herr (51)	47	34	72
Brosman (50)	33	31	94
deKernion (40)	19	13	68
Schellhammer (42)	6	6	100
S.W.O.G. [a]	42	34	81
Totals	177	145	82

[a] Current data from the author's ongoing studies.

particularly impressive when one considers the multiple studies that have been unable to demonstrate that the newer chemotherapies are superior to Thiotepa. In Brosman's randomized comparison of intravesical maintenance BCG with Thiotepa, no recurrences were observed in 27 randomized or 12 nonrandomized patients treated with BCG. In patients treated with Thiotepa 9 of 19 patients (40 per cent) had tumor recurrence [37]. Very similar results were reported by Netto and Lemos with a markedly different BCG treatment protocol [27]. Using Moreau BCG in oral doses of 200 to 800 mg. three times a week, only 1 of 16 patients (6%) had tumor recurrence compared with a 43 per cent incidence of tumor recurrence in patients treated with Thiotepa.

The Southwest Oncology Group has an ongoing multicenter trial comparing intravesical and percutaneous Connaught BCG with Adriamycin. Early results in this study suggested a marked advantage for the BCG group [52]. Currently 139 patients enrolled in this study are evaluable, 85 (61%) with carcinoma in situ and 54 (39%) with superficial transitional cell carcinoma without CIS. Overall, 56 of 70 patients (80%) randomized to receive BCG are disease free compared with 36 of 69 patients (52%) randomized to receive Adriamycin. In patients with CIS 34 of 42 patients (81%) treated with BCG had complete response compared with 26 of 43 patients (60%) treated with Adriamycin. In patients without CIS only 6 of 28 (21%) in the BCG group developed recurrent tumor compared with 16 of 26 (62%) in the Adriamycin group. The observed difference could not be explained on the basis of decreased response to Adriamycin due to previous chemotherapy treatment. Surprisingly, the advantage of BCG was even greater in those who had not received prior chemotherapy. Thirty-one (86%) of 36 BCG treated patients who had received no prior chemotherapy were disease free, compared with only 22 (61%) of 36 patients treated with Adriamycin.

Influence of BCG on tumor progression and survival

BCG and intravesical chemotherapy with Thiotepa, Epodyl, Adriamycin, and Mitomycin C reduce tumor recurrence at least in the short term. The benefit of intravesical immunotherapy or chemotherapy in reducing tumor recurrence beyond 5 years, in reducing tumor progression, or in improving patient survival has not been established. Suggestive but far from conclusive data have been presented to suggest that Thiotepa and Mitomycin C decrease the incidence of tumor progression when compared to untreated controls [53, 54]. Our experience with 90 patients with stage O (Ta) or A (T1) transitional cell carcinoma enrolled in BCG protocols similarly suggests that BCG treatment will reduce tumor progression [55]. Twenty six patients served as controls and initially did not receive chemotherapy or BCG. Sixty four patients were enrolled in randomized BCG protocols. Both groups have been followed for a median of 27 months. The BCG group actually comprised a higher risk population, since only 23% of the control group had lamina propria invasion compared with 69% of the BCG group. In the control group 65% had tumor recurrence, 23% progressed to stage A or greater, and 8% progressed to stage B or greater. In the BCG group 16% had tumor recurrence (p < 0.001), 6% progressed to stage A or greater (p < 0.05), and 3% progressed to stage B or greater (not statistically significant). Progression from stage A to stage B occured in 17% of our controls, 30% of controls in the Group A study [56], and only 4% of our patients treated with BCG. These data must be considered preliminary and must be confirmed by other investigators. If these results are typical, or if other treatment can be developed to reduce the incidence of tumor progression to as low as 6% in patients with stage A disease, marked improvement in survival will result. Since only about 40% of patients who develop muscle invasion can be cured, prevention of progression of noninvasive disease would save over 2000 lives each year in the United States.

BCG in muscle invasive disease

Nonspecific immunotherapy with BCG or any other agent is thought not likely to be effective in the face of significant tumor burden or invasive or metastatic disease. Surprisingly, some documented responses have occured with BCG treatment in patients with residual invasive disease within the detrusor muscle. Only patients who refused cystectomy or had medical contraindications to radical surgery have been offered the alternative of BCG treatment in our studies. We currently have 37 patients with transitional cell carcinoma extending into or beyond the detrusor muscle. These patients have an average age of 75 and have been followed for a median of 41 months. Thirty two per cent of these patients have had no further recurrence of tumor and 43% are alive. While these data compare favoraby with the mean five year survival of 42% in patients with muscle invasive disease treated with cystectomy (with or without preoperative radiation therapy) reported in Whitmore's review [57] one cannot recommend BCG as an alternative to accepted treatment of this lethal disease until prospective long term studies are completed.

BCG immunotherapy technique

When one weighs the known risks, morbidity, and expense of BCG versus the benefits of this treatment, most patients with superficial bladder cancer are cancidates for treatment. An exception would be the patient who presents with a solitary grade I, stage 0 (TA), blood group antigen-positive tumor. These patients will rarely have tumor progression and therefore often require no further therapy. Patients who are at intermediate risk for tumor recurrence, for example those with grade I-II tumors or those who present with more than one tumor, are likely to benefit from an initial 6 week course of BCG but can probably be spared prolonged maintenance protocols. Ideal candidates are those with documented tumor recurrence, carcinoma in situ, high grade tumor, or tumor invading the lamina propria. Patients with resectable muscle invasive disease who are not candidates for cystectomy have also benefitted from BCG in my experience, but one cannot recommend this treatment alternative until the percentage of patients surviving long term is known. Non-invasive carcinoma of the prostatic urethra has not been a contra-indication to BCG immunotherapy. Complete and long term resolution of CIS of the prostatic urethra has been documented in my experience and that of other investigators [42, 50].

Although the optimal protocol for BCG immunotherapy remains undefined, the experience of multiple investigators has provided extensive information from which reasonable though tentative conclusions may be derived. The first question to be answered by the clincian wishing to use BCG is, 'Which substrain is best?' In the United States Glaxo BCG, the most readily available preparation, is marketed in a form which is excellent for tuberculosis prophylaxis but inadequate for the treatment of superficial bladder cancer. This preparation contains only 8 to 26×10^6 colony forming units per ampule, or only about 1% of the commonly used dose. While documented responses using high dose Glaxo BCG have occured [58], our animal data suggest that this preparation does not provide antitumor responses equal to that of Tice or Armand-Frappier substrains [19]. In addition, we have observed that Glaxo BCG is less effective than Tice and Armand Frappier preparations in stimulating human natural cell-mediated cytotoxicity in vitro [59]. Substrains which have been demonstrated by clinical trials to be effective in doses of 40 to 120 mg intravesically include Armand-Frappier, Connaught, Pasteur, Japanese, and Tice. Optimal doses of vaccine have not been established since treatments have been given empirically. Commonly used and effective intravesical doses of these vaccines are 120 mg for Armand-Frappier, Connaught, and Pasteur preparations, 50 mg for Tice, and 40 mg for Japanese BCG.

Most investigators have initiated therapy within 2 weeks of tumor resection in an attempt to provide optimal juxtaposition of BCG and any residual tumor as well as stimulate a strong immune response. In reviewing my own experience, I have not been able to document that patients who have treatment begun within 2 weeks of tumor resection do any better than patients who are tumor free and have an intact urothelium. Since many of my patients travel considerable distances, I have often initiated treatment within 24 to 48 hours after tumor resection. Although febrile responses are more commonly seen in these patients, early treatment can be safely given to patients who have not had extensive tumor resections once gross hematuria has cleared.

Empirically, patients have been treated weekly for six weeks, and it has not been established that longer courses are better or that shorter courses are equally effective. The necessity of maintenance BCG immunotherapy also remains debatable. In theory since it is known that the immune stimulation induced by BCG wanes with time and the proclivity of the urothelium to tumor formation persists, periodic retreatment with BCG should improve long term results. Long term protection from a single course of BCG would suggest the correction of an immune deficit or the induction of specific antitumor immunity. In my experience the initiation of maintenance BCG immunotherapy in patients followed for at least one year of until tumor recurrence reduced the rate of tumor recurrence four-fold, from 1.9 to 0.49 tumors per 100 patient months [25], Preliminary results of Catalona's prospective randomized comparison of maintenance and no maintenance BCG immunotherapy have to date not revealed an advantage for maintenance therapy [25]. One would, of course, not expect to see any advantage of maintenance therapy until the protective effect of primary treatment has waned. Preliminary observations in such an investigation may therefore be misleading. A multicenter evaluation of the role of maintenance BCG immuno-therapy has been recently initiated by the Southwest Oncology Group.

Equally undecided is the advantage of concurrent percutaneous BCG adminis-tration. Clearly excellent results can be obtained with high-dose intravesical BCG alone, as documented by Brosman [37] and others. Flamm and Grof, on the other hand, observed no significant reduction in tumor recurrence with 6 to 12 weekly Connaught BCG treatments given by the intravesical route alone [43]. My ex-perience with Armand-Frappier BCG given only intravesically was equally dis-appointing, with 40 per cent of patients developing tumor recurrence [25]. How-ever, both Catalona and Herr have observed reduction in tumor recurrence with Armand-Frappier BCG given intravesically alone [25]. Antitumor responses to BCG appear to be related at least in part to systemic immunity as measured by PPD skin test conversion. Our experience and that of Kelley and co-workers [60] suggests the PPD skin test conversion correlates with response to BCG treatment. We observed tumor recurrence in only 1 of 22 patients (4.5 per cent) who converted to PPD skin test positive compared with a 32% incidence of tumor recurrence in 38 patients who were skin test positive before BCG or remained negative after treatment ($p = 0.017$ [25]. One should *not* conclude that patients who are PPD skin test positive are not candidates for BCG immunotherapy since these patients, as well as those who fail to convert to skin test positive with BCG, have recurrence rates which are still significantly lower than those who are not treated with BCG. Many patients who remain skin test negative after intravesical BCG, or have tumor recurrence, will respond to continued treatments with both skin test conversion and freedom from tumor recurrence. However, only prospec-tive randomized studies will be able to answer these questions, since Herr has observed prolonged protection from tumor recurrence with a single course of intravesical BCG despite the absence of PPD skin test conversion [25].

Until controlled studies further define optimal BCG treatment protocols, clinical treatments can be individualized to each patient. Since concurrent percu-taneous BCG administration may be more effective and does not increase the expense or morbidity of treatment, I have elected to continue its use. It is clearly less toxic and less expensive than monthly intravesical treatments. Effective systemic immunization can be accomplished with the multiple puncture technique. One simply applies 0.5cc of the suspension to be instilled in the bladder on the cleansed inner thigh and punctures the dermis four times with a 25–28 guage needle. Caution must be exercised to never inject BCG intradermally, subcutaneously, or intramuscularly. Superficial injections will cause ulceration and necrosis, and intramuscular injection has resulted in severe local pain and symptoms of systemic BCG infection. Continued inflammation of percutaneous inoculation sites suggests ongoing immune response or infection. Therefore patients who develop annoying skin reactions can discontinue percutaneous inoculation without concern. No apparent increase in bladder or skin toxicity has been apparent in my experience in patients who are PPD skin test positive.

The decision to give maintenance BCG treatments might logically be based on patient risk factors, since it is unlikely that all patients will require continued BCG treatment. It would appear that PPD skin test negativity will be a useful risk factor. It is important to note that some patients will require more than a single 6 week course of treatment to prevent tumor recurrence [53] or to completely eradicate carcinoma in situ [37]. These studies suggest that one should not consider a patient to be a BCG treatment failure therefore unless he has had at least two 6 week courses of BCG or developed increasing disease while on treatment. This recommendation must be balanced by the admonition that high risk patients should not continue on ineffective intravesical therapy while the disease progresses beyond the limit of surgical excision.

Complications of BCG treatment of bladder cancer

Intravesical BCG produces cystitis with frequency and dysuria in over 90% of patients. Symptoms usually begin after the second or third instillation and persist for about 2 days. Mild gross hematuria is common and about one fourth of patients will have constitutional symptoms consisting of low grade fever, malaise, or nausea. Major complications have been recently reviewed [61]. The most frequent complication observed was fever of over 103 degrees which occured in 3.9% of patients. Granulomatous prostatitis, which is occuring with increasing frequency, occured in 1.3%. While generally asymptomatic, the induration produced by granulomatous prostatitis can be confused with carcinoma of the prostate. Systemic BCG infection with pneumonitis or clinically significant hepatitis occured in 0.9%. BCG typically retains sensitivity to isoniazid, but life threatening acute infection with septic or anaplylactic shock can occur. Such patients require a combination of antituberculous antibiotics including cycloserine, since other antibiotics require several days for response. Arthritis or arthralgia occured in 0.5%, hematuria requiring catherization or transfusion in 0.5%, and skin rash or skin abscess from percutaneous inoculation in 0.4% each. Ureteral obstruction secondary to cystitis or ureteritis occured in 0.3%. Ureteral obstruction occured more commonly in patients with carcinoma in situ of the bladder or ureter. Patients with vesicoureteral reflux have not been excluded from BCG treatment protocols. In the face of ureteral carcinoma in situ, reflux may in fact be advantageous. We have not noted any increase in complications in patients with reflux, with the exception of one patient who developed renal granulomas secondary to intravesical BCG. Bladder contracture has occured in 2 patients (0.2%), epididymoorchitis in 0.2%, and hypotension and cytopenia each in 0.1%. As more patients receive BCG the list of complications will undoubtedly increase, but increased experience will also improve our ability to prevent such complications. Since most patients have increasingly severe cystitis and systemic symptoms prior to the onset of severe BCG complications, the more liberal use of isoniazid in such patients may significantly reduce the toxicity of BCG treatment. Our experience and that of Brosman support this proposition.

Conclusions

BCG immunotherapy represents a major advance in the treatment of superficial transitional cell carcinoma of the bladder. Controlled studies have demonstrated that it significantly reduces the incidence of tumor recurrence when compared to no treatment or chemotherapy with Thiotepa or Adriamycin. Responses in the treatment of carcinoma in situ of the bladder average 82%, and a multicenter study has found BCG to be superior to intravesical chemotherapy with Adriamycin. Fifty-eight per cent of patients with unresectable or residual tumors within the bladder respond with complete resolution of disease. Early experience suggests that disease progression to muscle invasion or metastasis is reduced five fold with BCG treatment. If confirmed, such reduction in progression would result in major improvement in the survival of patients presenting with superficial bladder cancer. While not yet approved by the Food and Drug Administration, continuing experience suggests that BCG is both highly effective and safe in the management of transitional cell carcinoma.

References

1. Kelly DR, Catalona WJ: BCG therapy for superficial bladder cancer. Urol Oncol, Ratliff TL, Catalona WJ (eds). Baton Rouge House Publishers, p 169, 1984
2. Gregg ERN: The archana of tuberculosis with a brief epidemiological history of the disease in the USA. Parts I and II. Am Rev Tuberculosis 78: 151, 1958
3. Gros P, Skamene M, Forget A: Cellular mechanisms of genetically controlled host resistance to *mycobacterium bovis* (BCG). J Immunol 131: 1966, 1983
4. Crispen RG: BCG vaccine in perspective. Sem oncol 1: 311, 1974

5. Lotte A, Wafz-Hockert O, Poisson N, Jimmy-Dumitoescu N, Verron M and Couvet E: BCG complication: estimated risks among vaccinated subjects and statisticam analysis of the main characteristics. Adv Tuberc Res 21: 107, 1984

6. Freund J: The mode of action of immunologic adjuvants. Adv Tuberc Res 7: 130, 1956

7. Biozzi G, Benacerraf B, Grumback F, et al: Etude de activité: Granulopexique du système réticulo-endothélial au cours de l'infection tuberculeuse expérimentale de la souris. Ann instit pasteur 87: 291, 1954

8. Bradner WT, Clarke DA, Stock CC: Stimulation of host mice defense against experimental cancer. I. Zymosan and sarcoman 180 in mice. Canc Res 18: 347, 1958

9. Bast Jr RC, Zbar D, Borsos T, Rapp HJ: BCG and cancer. NEJM 290: 1413, 1974

10. Bast Jr RC, Zbar B, Borsos T, Rapp HJ: BCG and cancer. NEJM 290: 1458, 1974

11. Terry WD, Rosenberg FA: Immunotherapy of human cancer. Excerpta Medica New York Proufaca, Elsevier North-Holland Inc, New York, 1982

12. Lamm DL, Harris SC, Gittes RF: Bacillus Calmette-Guerin and dinitrochlorobenzene immunotherapy of chmically induced bladder tumors. Invest Urol 14: 369, 1977

13. deKernion JB, Rammin KP, Fraser K: A bladder tumor model: response to immunotherapy. Nat Canc Inst Monograph 49: 333, 1978

14. Adolphs HD, Fiele J, Kiel H: Effective intralesional and systemic BCG application of a combined cyclophosphamide BCG treatment on experimental bladder cancer. Urol Res 7: 71, 1979

15. Soloway MS: Effectiveness of Long Term Chemotherapy and/or BCG on murine bladder cancer. Nat Canc Inst Monograph 49: 327, 1978

16. Morales A, Djeu J, Herberman RB: Immunization by irradiated whole cells or cell extracts against experimental bladder tumor. Invest Urol 17: 310, 1980

17. Pang AS, Morales A: Immunoprophylaxis of a murine bladder cancer with high dose BCG immunization. J Urol 127: 1006, 1982

18. Drago JR, Sipio J: Characterization of Nb Rat Bladder Cancer Model. Surg Forum 36: 654, 1985

19. Lamm DL, Reichert DF, Harris SC, Lucio RM: Immunotherapy of murine transitional cell carcinoma. J Urol 128: 1104, 1982

20. Pimm MV, Baldwin RW: Tumor models for screening immunomodulators: Suppression of tumor growth by delayed hypersensitivity reactions. Behring Inst Mitt 74: 214, 1984

21. Reichert DF, Lamm DL: Long term protection in bladder cancer following intralesional immunotherapy. J Urol 132: 570, 1984

22. Minder P: Shared antigens between animal and human tumors and micro-organisms. In BCG in cancer immunotherapy: Jamoureux G, Turcotte R, Portelance V (eds). New York: Grune and Stratton, 73–81, 1976

23. Winters WD, Lamm DL: Antibody responses to bacillus Calmette-Guerin immunotherapy in bladder cancer patients. Canc Res 41: 2672, 1981

24. Winters WD, Lamm DL: BCG-induced circulating interferon, antibody, and immune complexes in bladder cancer patients during immunotherapy. 13th Int Cancer Congress 13: 313 (1775), 1982

25. Lamm DL: BCG immunotherapy in bladder cancer. J Urol 134: 40, 1985

26. Kelley DR, Lage J, Bauer WC, Catalona WJ, Ratliff TL: Prognostic value of PPD skin test and granuloma formation in patients treated with intravesical BCG. J Urol (In press)

27. Netto Jr NR, Lemos CG: A comparison of treatment methods for prophylaxus of recurrent superficial bladder tumors. J Urol 129: 33, 1983

28. Thatcher N, Crowther D: Changes in non-specific lymphoid (NK, K, T cell) cytotoxicity following BCG immunizations of healthy subjets. Canc Immunol Immunother 5: 105, 1978

29. Antonaci S, Ticcinno A, Lucivero G, Miglietta A, Ticcininno A, Bonoma L: The effect of BCG immunotherapy on cell media and cytotoxicity in bladder cancer patients following surgical treatment. Tumori 67: 177, 1981

30. Davies M: Bacillus Calmette-Guerin as an antitumor agent. The interaction with cells of the mammalian immune system. Biochem Biophys Acta 651: 143, 1982

31. Davies M, Sabbadini E: Mechanisms of BCG Action. Cancer Immunol Immunother 14: 46, 1982

32. Morales A, Eidinger D, Bruce AW: Intracavitary bacillus Calmette-Guerin in the treatment of superficial bladder tumors. J Urol 116: 180, 1976

33. Lamm DL, Thor DE, Harris SC, Reyna JA, Stogdill VD, Radwin HM: Bacillus Calmette-Guerin immunotherapy of superficial bladder cancer. J Urol 124: 38, 1980

34. Camacho F, Pinsky CM, Kerr D, Braun Jr DW, Whitmore Jr WF, and Oettgen HF: Treatment of superficial bladder cancer with intravesical BCG in immunotherapy of human cancer. Terry WT, Rosenber SA. (eds). Elsevier, North Holland, New York, p 309, 1982

35. Herr HW, Pinsky CM, Whitmore Jr WF, Oettgen HF, Melamed MR: Intravesical bacillus Calmette-Guerin (BCG) therapy of superficial bladder tumors. Abstract 307, Am Urol Assoc 78: 1983

36. Martinez-Peneiro JA: BCG Vaccine in the treatment of non-infiltrating papillary tumors of the bladder. In: Bladder Tumors and Other Topics in Urologic Oncology, Pavone-Macabew M, Smith PH, Edsmyr F (eds). Plenum Press, New York, p 173, 1980

37. Brosman SA: Experience with bacillus Calmette-Guerin in patients with superficial bladder cancer. J Urol 128: 27, 1982

38. Adolphs HD, Bastian HP: Chemoimmune prophylaxis of superficial bladder tumors. J Urol 129: 29, 1983

39. Babayan RK, Krane RS: Intravesical BCG for superficial bladder cancer. Abstract 393. Am Urol Assoc, 80th Ann Mthn., Atlanta, Ga, May 1985

40. deKernion JB, Huang MY, Lindner A, Smith RB, Kaufman JJ: The Management of superficial bladder tumors and carcinoma in situ with intravesical bacillus Calmette-Guerin. J Urol 133: 598, 1985

41. Haaff EO, Kelley DR, Dresner SM, Ratliff TL, Catalona WJ: Results of retreatment with intravesical BCG therapy for patients failing the initial BCG course. Abstract 289. Am Urik Assoc 80th Ann Mtng, Atlanta, Ga, May 1985

42. Schellhammer PF, Ladaga LE: Bacillus Calmette-Guerin for therapy of superficial transitional cell carcinoma of the bladder. J Urol 135: 261, 1986

43. Flamm J, Grof F: Adjuvant local immunotherapy with bacillus Calmette-Guerin (BCG) in treatment of urothelial carcinoma of the urinary bladder. Wien Med Wochenschr 131: 501, 1981

44. Stober U, Peters HH: BCG-immunotherapie zur rezidiuphylaxe bein harnblasenkarzinom. Therapiewoche 30: 6067, 1980

45. Douville Y, Pelouze G, Roy R, Charrois R, Kibrite A, Martin M, Dionne L, Coulonval L, Robinson J: Recurrent bladder papillomata treated with bacillus Calmette-Guerin: a preliminary report (Phase I Trial). Cancer Treat Rep 62: 551, 1978

46. Morales A, Ottenhof P, Emerson L: Treatment of residual, non-infiltrating bladder cancer with bacillus Calmette-Guerin. J Urol 125: 649, 1981

47. Lamm DL, Thor DE, Stogdill VD, Radwin HM: Bladder cancer immunotherapy. J Urol 128: 931, 1982

48. Kojima H, Ishida Y, Mori C: Eradication of superficial transitional cell carcinoma of the bladder by intravesical instillation of bacillus Calmette-Guerin (BCG). Am Urol Assoc 80th Ann Mtng, Atlante, Ga, p 212, abstract 295, May 1985

49. Morales A: Treatment of carcinoma in situ of the bladder with BCG. A Phase II Trial. Cancer Immunol Immunother 9: 69, 1980

50. Brosman S: The Use of Bacillus Calmette-Guerin in the therapy of bladder carcinoma in situ. J Urol 134: 36, 1985

51. Herr HW, Pinsky CM, Whitman Jr WF, Oettgen HF, Melamed MR: Effect of intravesical bacillus Calmette-Guerrin (BCG) on Cancinoma in situ of the bladder. Cancer 51: 1323, 1983

52. Lamm DL, Crawford ED: BCG versus adriamycin in bladder cancer: a southwest oncology group study. Proc ASCO 4: 109–(c424), March 1985

53. Green DF, RObindon MRG, Glashan R, Newling D, Dalesio O, Smith PH: Does intravesical chemotherapy prevent invasive bladder cancer? J Urol 131: 33, 1984

54. Huland H, Otto U, Droese M, Kloppel G: Long term mitomycin C instillation after transurethral resection of superficial,bladder carcinoma: influence of recurrence, progression and survival. J Urol 132: 27, 1984

55. Reynolds RH, Stogdill VD, Lamm DL: Disease progression in BCG-treated patients with transitional cell carcinoma of the bladder. AUA Proc 133: 390 (392) April 1985

56. Heney NM, Ahmed S, Flanagan MJ, Frable W, Corder MP, Haferman MD, Hawkins IL: Superficial bladder cancer: progression and recurrence. J Urol 130, 1983

57. Whitmore Jr WF: The management of invasive bladder cancer. Sem Oncol 1: 1983

58. Robinson MR, Richards B, Adib R, Abdas A, Rigby CC, Push RC: Intravesical BCG (Bacillus Calmette-Guerin) in the management of T1NxMx transitional cell tumors of the bladder: a toxicity study. In: Bladder Tumours and Other Topics in Urological Oncology, Pavone-Macaluso M, Smith PH, Edsmyr F (eds). Plenum Press, New York, Vol 1, 528 p, 1980

59. Kierum Jr CA, Reichert DF, Mori K, Lamm DL: Differential stimulation of human natural cell mediated cytotoxicity (NCMC) by Gloxo and Pasteur Bacillus Calmette-Guerin (BCG) in vitro. AUA 86the Ann Mtng, Atlanta, Ga, abstract 840, May 1985

60. Kelley DR, Ratliff TL, Catalona WJ, Shapiro A, Lage JM, Baur WC, Haaff EO, Dresner SM: Intravesical bacillus Calmette-Guerin therapy for superficial bladder cancer: effect of Bacillus Calmette-Guerin viability on treatment results. J Urol 134: 48, 1985

61. Lamm DL, Crispen RG, Stogdill BJ, Stogdill VD: Complications of BCG immunotherapy in 1278 patients with bladder cancer. J Urol 135: 212, 1986

Editorial Comment

ALVARO MORALES

This chapter provides a concise historical perspective and a comprehensive review of the place of BCG in the urological armamentarium. ?r. Lamm has highlighted the importance of basic research and its contribution in establishing the role of non-specific active immunotherapy for the treatment of cancer in humans. He has rightly emplasized that the frequently reported success of immunotherapy in experimental tumor systems has rarely been reproduced in their clinical counterparts. Part of the problem resides in the inherent behavioral differences between species but the disappointing clinical results, in many cases, can be traced to trial design in which the experience of basic investigators were largely ignored. In this context it is worth reiterating that the successful introduction of BCG as an effective anti-neoplastic agent in the particular situation of superficial vesical carcinoma was not fortuitous. It represents the clinical application of experimental studies carried out by a number of investigators not necessarily involved in the specific field of bladder cancer. Perhaps the most relevant, early work was that of Coe and Feldman [1] who elegantly demonstrated that the bladder is an ideal and unique organ for the extracutaneous induction of delayed hypersensitivity reactions. A second, important piece of information resulted from a series of well-constructed experiments aimed at establishing the effectiveness of non-specific active immunotherapy in a well defined animal model (reference 9 in the chapter). These experiments provided the cornerstone for the design of clinical protocols employing immune modulators. With this information available, it was apparent that superficial bladder cancer is an ideal candidate for regional BCG therapy: According to Coe and Feldman the bladder would exhibit a strong cellular-mediated response to antigenic stimuli and the human organ-tumor system would completely fulfill the postulates for successful therapy enunciated by Zbar and his group.

The effectiveness of BCG in the treatment of superficial bladder cancer has now been established. Additional improvements, however, may occur by modifying existing protocols, defining the most effective strains of the vaccine, and minimizing annoying side effects. However, further research is needed to elucidate the mechanisms of action of BCG. It has been recently reported [2] that live BCG administered to humans produces an exopolysaccharide glycocalyx which provides the most intimate contact between the bacterial cell wall and the bladder urothelium. It appears that this exopolysaccharide mediates the antigenic and the inflammatory reactions detrimental to tumor development and growth. If this hypothesis can be confirmed, it would be possible to administer a more accurate immunization and to avoid some of the systemic side effects observed with the live bacteria.

Important contributions to the armamentarium of the urologist could be made by basic investigations as well as improvement of currently available protocols. There is a need for comparative studies to determine the individual merits of immune modifiers (i.e. BCG, interferon) and chemotherapeutic agents (adriamycin, mitomycin-C). The dismal response of metastatic bladder cancer to our present therapies may be improved by combined approaches. To expect immunotherapeutic successes where surgery, chemotherapy and radiation have previously failed is beyond reasonable expectations.

The judicious and well timed combination of these modalities may prove to be a worthwhile and fruitful endeavour.

References

1. Coe JE, Feldman JD: Extracutaneous delayed hypersensitivity, particularly in the guinea pig bladder. *Immunology* 10:127, 1966
2. Nickel JC, Morales A, Heaton JP, Costerton JW: Ultrastructural study of the interaction of BCG with bladder mucosa after intravesical treatment of bladder cancer. J Urol 133: 26A, 1985

10. Expectant management of stage a nonseminomatous testicular tumors

ARTHUR I. SAGALOWSKY

The dramatic improvements in patient survival following treatment for even advanced stages of nonseminomatous germ cell testicular tumors (NSGCTT) with multiagent combination chemotherapy and surgery including primary retroperitoneal lymph node dissection (RPLND) and debulking procedures have given rise to legitimate questions of how much, or more accurately, how little therapy is required for low stages of disease. Recently clinical trials of observation alone following orchiectomy for clinical stage A NSGCTT have been in progress. This article will review the data from those trials and pose a number of questions regarding optimal management of this disease.

A postulated 'natural history' of clinical stage A NSGCTT following radical orchiectomy is depicted in Figure 1. Approximately 73 percent of patients were pathologic stage A and were cured by orchiectomy alone. Clearly this group of patients does not benefit from RPLND but suffer its risks if subjected to surgery. Approximately 7 percent of patients will suffer pulmonary relapse despite negative nodes at the time of RPLND. Hematogenous dissemination is the most likely explanation for this pattern of metastasis. Finally, 20 percent of patients will have retroperitoneal and or pulmonary metastases. If early RPLND is not performed will this group of patients be as curable when relapse is first detected? Would some of these patients have been cured by RPLND or at least moved to the less frequent group who have hematogenous metastases? For patients who were initially pathologic stage B_1 (fewer than 5 nodes positive, microscopically only) is cure by RPLND preferable to cure by combination chemotherapy with or without subsequent surgical debulking? For patients who initially were pathologic stage B_2 (greater than 5 nodes positive, or nodes grossly positive) does early RPLND make subsequent cure by chemotherapy at the time of relapse more likely? Will fewer courses of chemotherapy be required? Will the need for surgical debulking following chemotherapy be reduced?

One of the central issues regarding management of testicular tumors is the reliability of clinical staging. From collected series lymphangiography has an overall specificity of 84 percent in pathologic stage A and overall sensitivity of

Ratliff, T.L. and Catalona, W.J. (eds), Genitourinary Cancer. ISBN 0–89838–830–9
© *1987, Martinus Nijhoff Publishers, Boston. Printed in the Netherlands.*

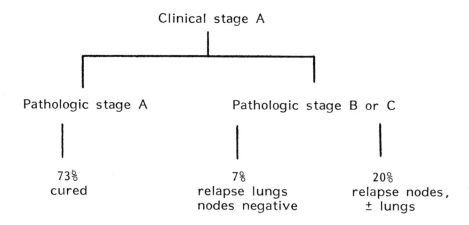

Figure 1. Hypothetical natural history of patients with clinical stage A NSGCTT.

67 percent in pathologic stage B NSGCTT respectively (Table 1) [1]. Abdominal computerized tomography (CT) has an overall specificity of 82 percent and sensitivity of 76 percent in detecting NSGCTT retroperitoneal metastases in pathologic stages A and B respectively (Table 2). The production of tumor markers alphafetoprotein (AFP) and beta subunit human chorionic gonadotropin (beta HCG) by many testis tumors is of great value in initial staging and followup. The overall specificity and sensitivity of these two tumor markers is 93 and 67 percent respectively in pathologic stages A and B NSGCTT (Table 3). The reported incidences of sustained complete remissions following orchiectomy and RPLND for pathologic stages A and B NSGCTT are 89 and 66 percent respectively (Table 4). The higher sustained complete remission rates in the more recent series are attributable to widespread availability of tumor markers and computerized tomography.

Patient survival for clinical stages A, B_1 and B_2 NSGCTT treated by orchiectomy and RPLND is nearly 100 percent [2, 3]. Results of all future treatment modifications must be compared to this standard. Patient survival for advanced NSGCTT (stage B_3 advanced retroperitoneal, stage C pulmonary) treated with platinum based multiagent chemotherapy is 82 percent [3]. The impact of tumor volume on response is shown most clearly in cases with advanced metastases (Table 5) [2]. Einhorn reported 93 and 96 percent of cases with minimal pulmonary or minimal pulmonary and minimal abdominal metastases respectively treated with platinum, vinblastine and bleomycin became tumor free [2]. In contrast only 65 and 66 percent of patients with advanced abdominal or advanced pulmonary disease respectively fully responded. Therein lies the greatest fear in observation protocols following orchiectomy for clinical stage A NSGCTT. There can be little doubt that a patient who initially is pathologic stage B_2 and is observed because of false negative clinical staging is at major risk of relapsing with advanced disease and having a substantially lower cure rate. The following case from the author's personal experience illustrates this point.

G.S. is a 23 year old rodeo bull rider who presented with a 2 month history of a hard mass in the right resticle which he believed was due to trauma. On 8/16/84 he underwent right inguinal orchiectomy for removal of a mixed germ cell tumor that contained embryonal cell carcinoma, teratocarcinoma and chorio-carcinoma. The tumor did not extend through the tunica albuginea or invade the epididymis or spermatic cord. There were numerous areas of vascular invasion (venules and lymphatics) by choriocarcinoma and embryonal carcinoma elements within the testis. Chest x-ray, and chest and abdominal CT were negative. Both serum AFP and beta HCG were elevated prior to orchiectomy (165 ng/ml and 690 mIU/ml respectively) and declined at a rate following orchiectomy consistent with the known serum half-lives for these markers (Fig. 2). Both tumor markers became negative by 18 days following orchiectomy.

This patient was advised of his clinical stage A status and of current observation protocols and results to date. Nevertheless, I recommended he undergo RPLND due to the presence of extensive vascular invasion within the tumor by both choriocarcinoma and embryonal cell carcinoma. A semen specimen was collected for possible cryopreservation but was not of adequate quality to warrant storage. The patient consented to RPLND and at exploration the nodes were grossly normal except for prominent vascularity. Histologic sections revealed embryonal cell carcinoma and teratocarcinoma in 12 of 59 major lymph nodes. There were no metastases of choriocarcinoma. Following a smooth postoperative recovery,

Table 1. Reliability of lymphangiography for detecting nonseminomatous retroperitoneal lymphatic metastases[a]

Series	Pathologic stage A		Pathologic stage B	
	No. Pts	Specificity	No. Pts	Sensitivity
Wallace (1970)	42	98%	25	68%
Maier (1972)	21	86%	48	88%
Hultén (1973)	14	86%	25	84%
Jonsson (1973)	10	90%	12	83%
Kademian (1977)	13	92%	32	88%
Storm (1977)	25 72%	20	50%	
Sago (1978)	18	50%	11	45%
Vugrin (1980)	–	–	60 38%	
Ehrlichman (1981)	4	100%	12	58%
Totals	147	84%	245	67%

[a] Fowler Jr JE: Nonseminomatous germ cell cancer of the testis: current management, future possibilities. Monographs in Urology 3: 162–186, Stamey TA (ed). Princeton NJ, Custom Publishing Services Inc, 1982

228

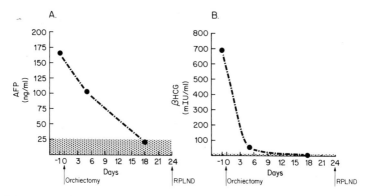

Figure 2. Time course of serum tumor markers in a patient with clinical stage A NSGCTT. Serum AFP and beta HCG were both elevated prior to orchiectomy and normalized before RPLND. The shaded area represents normal values for AFP and beta HCG.

the patient received 2 courses of platinum, vinblastine and bleomycin and has been continuously free of disease for 14 months.

This patient had considerable pathologic stage B_2 disease and inexplicably developed negative tumor markers despite initial marker abnormalities. One may speculate on whether or not he would still have been stage B_2 when relapse was detected if he chose observation, or if he would have had less chance of cure. However, he certainly would have had a greater tumor burden and would have required at least two more courses of first line chemotherapy than he received and possibly surgical debulking following chemotherapy.

Table 2. Reliability of computerized tomography for detecting nonseminomatous retroperitoneal lymphatic metastases[a]

Series	Pathologic stage A		Pathologic stage B	
	No. Pts	Specificity	No. Pts	Sensitivity
Burney (1979)	10	80%	28	82%
Williams (1980)	17	82%	15	93%
Ehrlichman (1981)	2	50%	15	60%
Richie (1981)	10	90%	20	65%
Totals	39	82%	78	76%

[a] Fowler Jr JE: Nonseminomatous germ cell cancer of the testis: current management, future possibilities. Monographs in Urology 3: 162–186, Stamey TA (ed). Princeton NJ, Custom Publishing Services Inc, 1982

With all the preceding information as background I now would like to review the results presented thus far by several authors on surveillance protocols for clinical stage A NSGCTT. Peckham and associates at the Royal Marsden Hospital reported on 53 patients studied from February, 1979 to June, 1981 (Table 6) [4]. Criteria for entry included: 1) normal chest x-ray and CT, excretory urogram, abdominal CT and sonography, lymphangiogram and liver function tests; 2) no tumor at the surgical margin of the spermatic cord; and 3) serum tumor markers negative preoperatively or returned to normal postoperatively. Followup was monthly for the first year, bimonthly for the second year and quarterly for the third year and included serum tumor markers at each visit and CT scans at every other visit for two years! Preorchiectomy serum AFP and/or beta HCG were measured in 32 of 53 patients and one or both were elevated in 75 percent of patients (24/32). There was a slightly higher incidence of marker positivity (78.3 percent, 18/23) when both markers were checked. With a mean followup of 16.7 months (range 6 to 40 months) 17 percent of patients (9/53) had relapsed. Eight relapses occurred at less than 6 months and the remaining relapse occurred by 12 months. Sites of relapse were: marker elevations only, retroperitoneal nodes only, and pulmonary lesions in 1,5, and 3 cases respectively. All 9 patients with relapse became free of disease following chemotherapy. The probability of relapse correlated with the cell type of the primary tumor. Relapse occurred in 42.8 percent (6/14) of cases with embryonal cell carcinoma ('malignant teratoma undifferentiated', British nomenclature) versus 3.4 percent (1/29) of cases with teratocarcinoma ('malignant teratoma intermediate'), p less than 0.05. Pre-orchiectomy tumor markers were available in 4 of 9 patients who

Table 3. Reliability of tumor markers (AFP and HCG) for detecting nonseminomatous retroperitoneal lymphatic metastases[a]

Series	Pathologic stage A		Pathologic stage B	
	No. Pts	Specificity	No. Pts	Sensitivity
Scardino (1977)	22	100%	15	67%
Lange (1977)	13	92%	15	87%
Skinner (1980)	67	85%	44	64%
Javadpour (1980)	53	100%	65	85%
Fowler (1980)	9	100%	11	82%
Vugrin (1980)	–	–	60	45%
Ehrlichman (1981)	3	100%	17	65%
Totals	167	93%	227	67%

[a] Fowler Jr JE: Nonseminomatous germ cell cancer of the testis: current management, future possibilities. Monographs in Urology 3: 162–186, Stamey TA (ed). Princeton NJ, Custom Publishing Services Inc, 1982

relapsed and were normal in two of these cases. These few cases suggest that normal initial tumor markers do not reflect a decreased tendency for the tumor to metastasize. Also patients with initially elevated markers that returned to normal following orchiectomy were not at greater risk for relapse than patients who never had marker elevation. In a later presentation on 120 patients entered into the surveillance protocol, Peckham reported relapse to the retroperitoneum or to the lungs in 10 percent and 9 percent of cases respectively [5].

Johnson and coworkers at the M.D. Anderson Hospital reported on 31 patients with clinical stage A NSGCTT entered into a surveillance protocol since October, 1981 (Table 6) [6]. Staging included chest x-ray, abdominal CT, bipedal lymphangiogram, serum AFP and beta HCG in all cases. Followup included chest and abdominal x-ray and serum tumor markers every 2 months and abdominal CT every 6 months. The mean length of followup was 10 months (range 2 to 18 months). Eighty-four percent of patients (26/31) remained continuously free of disease and 16 percent (5/31) relapsed between 2 and 6 months of followup. In analyzing this series one must acknowledge the unique experience at the reporting institution with skilled interpretation of lymphangiograms. Relapses were identified in the retroperitoneum and/or in the lungs in 1 and 3 cases respectively and by marker elevation only in one case. All five patients with relapse became free of disease following chemotherapy. Patients with embryonal cell carcinoma relapsed more often than did those with teratocarcinoma (30 versus 11 percent) and relapse was more likely to present in sites other than retroperitoneal nodes

Table 4. Sustained complete remissions after orchiectomy and retroperitoneal lymphadenectomy alone in pathologic stages A and B nonseminomatous tumors[a]

Series	Pathologic stage A		Pathologic stage B	
	No. Pts	Sustained CR[b]	No. Pts	Sustained CR[b]
Whitmore (1968)	49	88%	16	56%
Castro (1969)	32	88%	5	20%
Boctor (1969)	13	62%	7	71%
Skinner (1971)	–	–	4	100%
Walsh (1971)	25	96%	4	75%
Staubitz (1973)	36	86%	17	71%
Johnson (1976)	72	90%	–	–
Skinner (1976)	30	90%	–	–
Donohue (1980)	57	93%	24	71%
Totals	314	89%	77	66%

[a]Fowler Jr JE: Nonseminomatous germ cell cancer of the testis: current management, future possibilities. Monographs in Urology 3: 162–186, Stamey TA (ed). Princeton NJ, Custom Publishing Services Inc, 1982
[b]CR, complete remission

(i.e. lung, 25 versus 10 percent). Johnson sites the fact that 10 to 15 percent of patients with positive nodes at RPLND will develop other metastases. From Johnson's findings one might argue that patients with embryonal cell carcinoma are more likely than patients with other tumors ultimately to require chemotherapy for hematogenous metastases and should be spared RPLND. Conversely, one might apply the results from Johnson's and from Peckham's series to suggest that patients with clinical stage A embryonal cell carcinoma should not enter surveillance protocols. In neither case is the percent of patients who had pulmonary metastases without retroperitoneal nodal metastases known. Thus, one could also argue that some of the patients who developed pulmonary metastases may have been cured by early RPLND and never have required chemotherapy.

Johnson and coworkers acknowledge that the morbidity of RPLND is low (7 to 15 percent) and that the mortality risk is extremely low. The major morbidity from RPLND is loss of seminal emission and this has been a key factor for patients seeking an alternative to RPLND. However, concern over fertility in patients with NSGCTT must be kept in perspective. Data on the intrinsic fertility potential of patients who develop testis tumor are few. In one study Bracken and Smith found that only 4 percent (1/25) of patients have semen parameters suitable for cryopreservation at the time the testis tumor is diagnosed [7]. A number of authors report that modifications in the technique of RPLND which preserve the autonomic nerves in the presacral and thoracolumbar regions and the use of sympathomimetic agents postoperatively preserve or allow return of normal ejaculation in up to 50 percent of patients [8–10]. The present author has not seen return of ejaculation in patients who were aspermic after RPLND and were treated with alpha adrenergic agents. However, I have several patients who continue to have normal ejaculation after the surgical modifications of RPLND described above. These modifications of technique pose no real threat to the thoroughness of RPLND in patients who are pathologic stage A or B_1. It must also be remembered that surveillance protocols accept that pathologic stage B_1

Table 5. Response by extent of disease[a]

	Total	NED
A. Minimal pulmonary	30	28 (93%)
B. Advanced pulmonary	38	25 (66%)
C. Minimal pulmonary + minimal abdominal	24	23 (96%)
D. Advanced abdominal	54	35 (65%)
E. Elevated markers only	11	11 (100%)
F. Other	7	6 (86%)
Totals	164	128 (78%)

[a] Einhorn LH: Testicular Cancer as a model for a curable neoplasm: The Richard and Hilda Rosenthal Foundation Award Lecture. Cancer Reserach 4: 3275–3280, 1981

patients will relapse and require chemotherapy which in itself may produce infertility. Fertility should assume less importance than patient survival in treatment plans. No patient should choose surveillance over RPLND based primarily on concerns over fertility without knowing that his baseline semen parameters suggest that he is fertile in the first place. Cryopreservation should be offered to suitable patients before RPLND.

Jewett and associates in Toronto found a relapse rate of 40 percent during a mean followup of 16.6 months (range 3 to 33 months) in 30 patients with clinical stage A NSGCTT treated by orchiectomy alone (Table 6) [11]. Staging included chest x-ray, whole lung tomograms, bipedal lymphangiogram, abdominal CT, and serum tumor markers. Followup included monthly chest x-ray and tumor markers and abdominal CT every three months. Three patients relapsed with markers and CT positive, 6 with markers only positive and 3 with CT only positive. The median time to relapse was 5 months (range 2.5 to 8.5 months). In this series embryonal cell carcinoma and teratocarcinoma had a similar tendency to relapse. At progression all 12 patients received RPLND or chemotherapy and 11 patients became disease free. The remaining patient had partial remission of disease.

Sogani and coworkers at Memorial Sloan-Kettering Cancer Center reported their early findings in 36 clinical stage A NSGCTT patients treated by orchiectomy alone (Table 6) [12]. Staging included chest x-ray, bipedal lymphangiogram, abdominal CT, and serum tumor markers. Followup included monthly chest x-ray and tumor markers and abdominal CT every 3 months. Eighty-one percent (29/36) of patients remained continuously free of disease and 19 percent (7/36) of patients relapsed between 4 to 7 months followup. Recently the same authors presented their longer followup on the original 36 patients plus 9 additional patients in the surveillance protocol [13]. The relapse rate in these 45 patients with a mean followup of 37 months (range 20 to 63 months) was 24.4 percent (11/45) and 75.6 percent of patients (34/45) remained continuously free of disease. Relapse was identified in retroperitoneal nodes, lung, or by tumor marker elevation in 8, 2 and 1 case respectively. Nine of the 11 patients with relapse (81.8 percent) became free of disease for a mean followup of 22 months (range

Table 6. Relapse rates in surveillance protocols for clinical stage A NSGCTT.

Series	(ref.)	n	Followup, mean	months (range)	Percent relapse
Peckham	(4)	53	16.7	(6–40)	17
Johnson	(6)	31	10	(2–18)	16
Jewett	(11)	30	16.6	(3–33)	40
Sogani	(13)	45	37	(20–63)	24.4
Javadpour	(15)	60	26	(24–60)	16.7

15 to 47 months) following further therapy with disease following RPLND and an incomplete response to VAB6 chemotherapy. One patient died of progressive central nervous system involvement by tumor. One might argue that CNS spread of tumor may have been hematogenous in origin and would not have been prevented by early RPLND. Nevertheless the fact remains in this group of patients with NSGCTT who were originally clinical stage A, the one death and the other patient with progressive disease, whose prognosis must be guarded, reveals 4.4 percent of patients (2/45) had a less than optimal result within the early period of followup. Relapse occurred in 57 percent of patients with embryonal cell carcinoma (4/7) and in 25 percent of patients with teratocarcinoma (7/28). Vascular invasion was present in the primary tumor in 57 percent of cases who relapsed versus 18 percent of cases who remained disease free. Based on the experience in these 45 cases the physicians at Memorial Sloan Kettering have made two substantive changes in the surveillance protocol. First, patients with vascular invasion in the tumor no longer are considered candidates for the protocol. Second, patients who are entered into the protocol undergo repeat abdominal CT every 6 weeks instead of every 3 months. I am afraid this degree of followup becomes almost prohibitive from a cost and practicality standpoint.

Javadpour has reported on limited excision of 'primary landing zone lymphatics' and on surveillance following orchiectomy for clinical stage A NSGCTT [14, 15]. Relapse occurred in 10 of 60 patients (16.7 percent) with clinical stage A tumors who were treated by orchiectomy alone and followed for a mean of 26 months (range 24 to 60 months) (Table 6). Embryonal cell carcinoma with or without elements of choriocarcinoma had the highest relapse rate, p less than 0.01. Size of the primary tumor did not correlate with the risk of relapse. However, two histologic features in the primary tumor were very prevalent in patients suffering relapse: vascular or lymphatic invasion and tumor extension into the epididymis (80 percent, p less than 0.001 and 60 percent, p less than 0.01 respectively). Based on this experience Javadpour currently proposes that only patients with clinical stage A NSGCTT and no histologic predictors of a high relapse rate be entered into a post orchiectomy surveillance protocol. Patients who are in the protocol are followed with physical exam, serum tumor markers and chest x-ray every month for 1 year, then every 3 months during the second year and annually thereafter. The need for followup abdominal CT is individualized. The assumption that early relapse will be detected by tumor markers or chest x-ray is a flaw in the protocol in my opinion. Javadpour recommends patients who have one or more of the histologic predictors of relapse (cell type, vascular, lymphatic, or epididymal invasion) undergo surgical staging of the primary lymphatic landing zones of testicular tumors. Nodes from the left renal pedicle, right pericaval, aortocaval and ipsilateral spermatic vessels are carefully inspected and frozen sections are obtained. If frozen sections are positive for tumor a complete RPLND is performed; if specimens are negative all nodal areas are 'meticulously inspected' prior to closing the abdomen. This approach relies heavily on the accuracy of frozen sections which are performed hurriedly and on limited samples. Meticulous visual inspection of the nodes should offer the surgeon little confidence in the microscopic status of the nodes. I had the personal experience of performing a complete bilateral RPLND in a patient with a left sided embryonal cell carcinoma and resecting 119 lymph nodes the majority of which were grossly enlarged and firm. Microscopic evaluation revealed 4 nodes with tiny foci of embryonal cell carcinoma and all of the remaining nodes showed only tremendous inflammatory response with reactive hyperplasia. The assumption that primary landing zones are invariably positive if contralateral sites bear tumor is justified by the extensive experience of Donohue in greater than 270 cases of complete bilateral RPLND [16].

Moriyama and associates retrospectively studied 45 patients with NSGCTT for factors associated with relapse [17]. Metastases developed in 4 of 19 patients (21.1 percent) who had negative nodes at the time of RPLND. Patients with vascular invasion in the primary tumor were far more likely to have metastases than patients without vascular invasion (25 of 29, 86 percent versus 3 of 16, 19 percent). Choriocarcinoma was associated with metastases in 5 of 6 cases and vascular invasion in the testis in all cases. Preorchiectomy levels of AFP and beta HCG did not predict which cases had metastases. The stage of the primary tumor specimen correlated with metastases. High stage lesions (pT2-4, UICC classification) had metastases more often than did low stage (pT1) lesions (17 of 21, 81 percent versus 6 of 24, 25 percent).

In summary, what conclusions may be drawn from the preceding data? I am reminded of the politician who when asked where he stood on a difficult issue replied 'Some of my friends are for it, and some of my friends are against it. As for me, I am for my friends'. All of the referenced series on surveillance protocols following orchiectomy for clinical stage A NSGCTT were performed by highly skilled physicians at major centers with a vast experience in the management of testis tumor patients. Each aspect of the results from the accurate interpretation of initial staging, to the application of multiagent primary and salvage chemotherapy, to surgical debulking when appropriate, must be considered in this context when discussing the good results obtained. Surely a surveillance protocol requires the utmost in patient compliance with followup and sound physician judgment at key intervals. It would be an error to assume that urologists and medical oncologists treating an occasional testis tumor patient with variable followup will obtain the same results as described above.

The experience to date from surveillance protocols allows the following conclusions. The early relapse rate has been approximately 20 percent in all but one series and is in keeping with the accepted false negative rate for current staging modalities. Relapse rates can be expected to become slightly higher with longer followup barring an improvement in staging techniques. The great majority of relapsing patients have become free of disease following combination chemotherapy and/or surgery. At least one patient in a surveillance protocol has died of

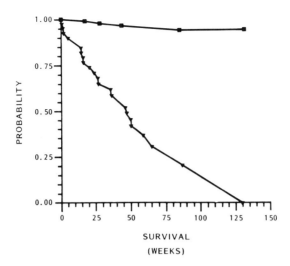

Figure 3. Survival in patients with complete remission or disease-free status after chemotherapy and surgery (squares) compared with that in patients with only partial remission or less (triangles) [18]. 'Reproduced by permission of authors and publisher'.

tumor progression and several other patients continue to have disease after incomplete response to chemotherapy. Previous experience with chemotherapy for testis tumors teaches us that not all patients respond completely to primary or salvage regimens and partial response with persisting active tumor carries a guarded prognosis (Fig. 3) [18]. Therefore, one can predict a finite albeit small number of such patients from surveillance protocols as well. Patients with vascular or epididymal invasion in the primary tumor are at high risk for metastases and should not enter surveillance protocols. Patients with embryonal cell carcinoma are at higher risk for metastases than patients with teratocarcinoma.

Some of the questions posed in the introduction to this article are not answerable at this time. Nevertheless they are vital if we are to devise optimal management for patients with NSGCTT. Surveillance protocols will identify relapse at small tumor volumes in the majority of cases. However, the case cited from my personal experience indicates that some patients believed to be stage A are in fact pathological stage B_2 and will have a considerable tumor burden when relapse is detected even by the most careful followup in a surveillance protocol. Therefore, the majority of patients with relapse will enjoy a high probability of cure but others will not. Following initial enthusiasm for surveillance protocols after orchiectomy in all patients with stage A NSGCTT, investigators clearly are shifting back to additional therapy for patients having any of the histologic predictors in the primary tumor of a significant risk of relapse. Some investigators have suggested two courses of adjuvant chemotherapy in this setting. Patients with pathologic B_1 disease would be cured by RPLND in all but a few percent of cases and never require chemotherapy. Whether or not cure by RPLND is preferable to cure with chemotherapy cannot be answered yet. The risks of RPLND in experienced hands are very low. The acute toxicities of multiagent platinum based chemotherapy are considerable but can be diminished by judicious use of drugs and careful patient preparation. However, chronic toxicities including paresthesias and decreased hearing from high cumulative doses of platinum, and interstitial pulmonary fibrosis from bleomycin are unavoidable currently. The possibility of additional long term consequences of these agents remains. The answers to all of these questions will only be obtained from carefully controlled studies. We must avoid a casual attitude in the management of clinical stage A NSGCTT or the spectacular results achieved to date will surely decrease. We must advise these patients of the options for RPLND or surveillance in a fully informed manner regarding the limits of experience and results to date. The dilema of how best to manage clinical stage A NSGCTT and still maintain near 100 percent patient survival is a happy circumstance that we have yet to enjoy in any other area of urologic oncology.

References

1. Fowler Jr JE: Nonseminomatous germ cell cancer of the testis: current management, future possibilities. Monographs in Urology 3: 162–186.
2. Einhorn LH: Testicular Cancer as a model for a curable neoplasm: The Richard and Hilda Rosenthal Foundation Award Lecture. Cancer Research 4: 3275–3280, 1981
3. Richie JP: Changing concepts in the treatment of nonseminomatous germ cell tumors of the testis. J Urol 131: 1089–1092, 1984
4. Peckham MJ, Husband JE, Barrett A, Hendry WF: Orchidectomy alone in testicular stage I non-seminomatous germ-cell tumors. Lancet 2: 678–680, 1982
5. Peckham MJ: Surveillance in clinical stage I nonseminomatous testicular cancer. Presented to the 5th International Symposium on Urologic Cancer, Sicily, Italy, 1983
6. Johnson DE, Lo RK, von Eschenbach AC, Swanson DA: Surveillance alone for patients with clinical stage I nonseminomatous germ cell tumors of the testis: preliminary results. J Urol 131: 491–493, 1984
7. Bracken RB, Smith KD: Is semen cryopreservation helpful in testicular cancer? Urology 15: 581–583, 1980
8. Nijman JM, Jager S, Boer PW, Kremer J, Oldhoff J, Koops HS: The treatment of ejaculation disorders after retroperitoneal lymph node dissection. Cancer 50: 2967–2971, 1982
9. Lange PH, Narayan P, Vogelzang NJ, Shafer RB, Kennedy BJ, Fraley EE: Return of fertility after treatment for nonseminomatous testicular cancer: changing concepts. J Urol 129: 1131–1135, 1983
10. Proctor KG, Howards SS: The effect of sympathomimetic drugs on postlymphadenectomy aspermia. J Urol 129: 837–838, 1983
11. Jewett MAS, Comisarow RH, Herman JG, Sturgeon JFG, Alison RE, Gospodarowicz MK: Results with orchidectomy only for stage I non-seminomatous testis tumor. Presented at American Urological Association, New Orleans, May 9, 1984
12. Sogani PC, Whitmore JR WF, Herr H, Bosl G, Golbey R, Watson R, DeCosse J: Ochiectomy

alone in treatment of clinical stage I nonseminomatous germ cell tumors of testis (NSGCTT). Proc Amer Soc Clin Oncol, abstract C-547 2: 140, 1983

13. Sogani PC, Whitmore Jr WF, Herr HW, Morse MJ, Bosl G, Fair WR: Long term experience with orchiectomy alone in treatment of clinical stage I nonseminomatous germ cell tumor of testis (NSGCTT) presented at American Urological Association, Atlanta, May 16, 1985
14. Javadpour N, Moley J: Alternative to retroperitoneal lymphadenectomy with preservation of ejaculation and fertility in stage I nonseminomatous testicular cancer: a prospective study. Cancer 55: 1604–1606, 1985
15. Javadpour N: Changing concepts in the management of clinical stage I nonseminomatous testicular cancer: significance of prognostic factors. J Urol 134: 427, 1985
16. Donohue JP, Zachary JM, Maynard BR: Distribution of nodal metastases in nonseminomatous testis cancer. J Urol 128: 315–320, 1982
17. Moriyama N, Daly JJ, Keating MA, Lin W, Prout Jr GR: Vascular invasion and other prognostic factors in nonseminomatous testicular germ cell tumors. Presented at American Urological Association, Atlanta, May 16, 1985
18. Einhorn LH, Williams SD, Troner M, Birch R, Greco FA: The role of maintenance therapy in disseminated testicular cancer. NEJM 305: 727–731, 1981

Editorial Comment

ROBERT R. BAHNSON

The surveillance protocols for patients having clinical stage A nonseminomatous germ cell testicular tumors (NSGCTT) have evolved from observations that retroperitoneal lymphadenectomy (RPLND) has adverse effects on fertility, and combination chemotherapy can salvage the vast majority of patients having metastatic testicular cancer. Dr. Sagalowsky has carefully reviewed the early results of reported surveillance trials and posed meaningful questions suggesting that the preferred management of these patients is still undetermined.

Perhaps the greatest impediment to the acceptance of surveillance protocols is the inability of current staging techniques to detect metastatic disease in 20 to 25% of patients. Microscopic nodal metastases in this group currently are detected only by RPLND. Improvement in staging accuracy should decrease relapse rates in surveillance protocols to approximately 10%, which is the relapse rate observed in patients with *pathologic* stage A disease who have undergone RPLND [1]. However, until new or improved staging modalities are available, a 20% incidence of relapse can be expected after orchiectomy alone for clinical stage A patients. Furthermore, in patients who do not comply with follow-up protocols, relapse may not be detected until advanced disease is present and the prospect for cure is less likely.

Recent data on poor semen quality in patients with NSGCTT and modification of the surgical technique for RPLND in low stage disease diminish the importance of fertility as a major issue in designing treatment plans for clinical stage A patients. Several studies indicate a majority (52 to 77%) of patients with testicular tumors have sperm counts of less than 20 million before or immediately after orchiectomy [2, 3, 4, 5]. Lange et al [6] postulate that expectant management of stage A patients would result in only a 16% increase in potential fertility over patients treated by traditional RPLND and chemotherapy. Pizzocaro et al [7] reported that unilateral RPLND in patients with clinical stage A NSGCTT preserves antegrade ejaculation in more than 80% of patients without compromising survival. By contrast, Narayan et al [8] observed spontaneous return in ejaculation in only 45% of patients treated with an extended bilateral dissection. Limited (staging) lymphadenectomy is appealing because careful mapping studies of the metastatic pathways of NSGCTT performed by Donohue et al [9] have demonstrated the doubtful need for a full contralateral dissection in patients having clinical stage A disease. In these patients, limited node dissection accurately stages the disease while preserving antegrade ejaculation in the majority of cases.

An important observation from the collected series of patients is the identification of factors prognostic of tumor recurrence in low stage NSGCTT. It is apparent that vascular invasion and/or lymphatic invasion in the tumor, extension of the tumor into the epididymus and/or spermatic cord, embryonal histology and possibly size of tumor are important predictors of relapse. It would seem advisable to exclude these patients from surveillance protocols.

Expectant management of clinical stage A NSGCTT is still experimental and the optimal management can be determined only from carefully controlled studies as Dr. Sagalowsky suggests. At present,

I believe the best therapeutic alternative to bilateral complete RPLND for low stage NSGCTT is a staging lymphadenectomy limited to the primary zones of metastatic spread. For right sided tumors this would involve a right paracaval, precaval, interaortocaval, preaortic, right suprahilar, and right iliac dissection. For left sided cases it would involve full dissection in and around the renal vessels on the left extending to the mid-precaval zone while omitting the right paracaval, right iliac, and suprahilar zones. This would eliminate most staging errors, preserve ejaculatory function in many patients, and identify patients who should be treated with a thorough extended bilateral dissection and post operative adjuvant chemotherapy.

References

1. Bredael JJ, Vugrin D, Whitmore Jr WF: Recurrences in surgical stage 1 nonseminomatous germ cell tumors of the testis, J Urol 130, 476–478, 1983
2. Drasga RE, Einhorn LH, Williams SD, Patel DN, Stevens EE: Fertility after chemotherapy for testicular cancer, J Clin Oncol 1: 179–183, 1983
3. Thachil JV, Jewett MAS, Rider WD: The effects of cancer and cancer therapy on male fertility. J Urol 126, 141–145, 1981
4. Fossa SD, Klepp O, Molne K, Aakvaag A: Testicular function after unilateral orchiectomy for cancer and before further treatment, Int J Androl 5: 179–184, 1982
5. Bracken RB, Johnson DE: Sexual function and fecundity after treatment for testicular tumors, Urology 7: 35–38, 1976
6. Lange PH, Narayan P, Fraley EE: Fertility issues following therapy for testicular cancer, Sem Urol 2: 264–274, 1984
7. Pizzocaro G, Salvioni R, Zanoni F: Unilateral lymphadenectomy in intraoperative stage I nonseminomatous germinal testis cancer, J Urol 1343, 485–489, 1985
8. Narayan P, Lange PH, Fraley EE: Ejaculation and fertility after extended retroperitoneal lymph node dissection for testicular cancer, J Urol 172, 685–688, 1982
9. Donohue JP: Metastatic pathways of nonseminomatous germ cell tumors, Sem Urol 2: 217–229, 1984

11. The role of flow cytometry in urologic oncology

KENNETH R. STONE

Introduction

Flow cytometry has evolved as a powerful laboratory tool in both research and clinical settings. The modern flow cytometer is designed to record a variety of simultaneous measurements on individual cells as the cells, aligned by the laminar flow of a surrounding sheath of liquid, pass in single file through a sensing region of the instrument. The flow cytometer, with the aid of a supporting computer, can perform several simultaneous analytical functions on a complex mixture of cells by examining each cell individually at the incredible rate of several hundred to several thousand cells per second. In some instruments, the computer can also utilize the analytical data collected on the individual cells to instruct the flow cytometer to effeciently sort the cells into sub-groups based upon the information collected. A minor component of a complex mixture can therefore be effectively cloned for later examination using alternative techniques. This sorting procedure can be performed aseptically so that cells can be cloned, placed into *in vitro* culture or injected into animals for further propagation.

The historical development and intricate workings of the flow cytometer are beyond the scope fo this article. There are several excellent reviews available which elegantly describe the details of the development [1, 2] and function of this instrument [3–7]. It is sufficient to know that the flow cytometer makes two basic measurements on a cell – scatter of an incident beam of light (usually argon laser or high intensity mercury lamp) and fluorescence emission by appropriate probes attached to or internalized within the cells. The measurement of light scattered by the cell is a rough measurement of the size, as well as to the granularity, of the cell; any fluorescent label which can be excited by the incident beam of light can be used to label the cells or cell compartments. Addition of multiple light sources such as a complementary krypton laser [8–10] or the relatively new dye laser [11–13] greatly extend the capabilities of the flow cytometer since even more simultaneous measurements can be made using multiple fluorescent probes which are excited and which emit at alternative wavelengths.

Ratliff, T.L. and Catalona, W.J. (eds), Genitourinary Cancer. ISBN 0–89838–830–9
© *1987, Martinus Nijhoff Publishers, Boston. Printed in the Netherlands.*

The most important restriction for analysis of a specimen by flow cytometry is that the cells generally must be in the form of a single cell suspension and not be clumped or aggregated. This restriction often creates a major obstacle to the practical application of the flow cytometer to the examination of certain properties of solid tissues, an example of which is a measurement of the expression of cell surface antigens. The procedures necessary to obtain a single cell suspension from a solid tissue usually alters the antigenic properties of the cell surface so that the data obtained do not adequately represent the cells as they existed *in vivo*.

Type of information generated by flow cytometry

The variety of information that a multiparameter flow cytometer could conceivably generate seems almost limitless (reviewed by Shapiro [14]); however, the instrument has only been routinely applied to a limited number of the tasks of which it is potentially capable. The bulk of the clinical and biological information so far generated by flow cytometry falls into two categories – cell cycle kinetic analysis and immunobiology. Cell cycle analysis involves stoiciometric labelling of the cellular DNA with any of several fluorescent probes such that the amount of DNA within the cell can be quantified. The flow cytometer then counts the number of cells, or free nuclei, containing variable amounts of DNA and produces a histogram which depicts the number of cells in each compartment of the cell cycle (Fig. 1). In general, a DNA histogram obtained from a flow cytometric analysis of normal human tissue contains a prominant peak of cells with diploid amounts of DNA, representing cells in the G0/G1-phase of the cell cycle. These cells contain 46 chromosomes (2N) and are representative of the bulk of normal somatic human tissues. A second, smaller peak is normally present at double the channel number of the first peak and represents cells with tetraploid amounts of DNA, corresponding to cells in the G2/M-phases of the cell cycle (4N). Between these two peaks, and overlapping to some extent with them, are found the cells involved in active DNA synthesis corrsponding to the S-phase of the cell cycle. In normal tissues, such as the urinary bladder, the number of cells in the S- and G2/M-phases of the cell cycle are usually small in number, representing less than 10% of the total cells in the tissue. Any of several mathematical models, which make different assumptions about the distribution of cells within the histograms, can be used to quantitate the number of cells in the various cell cycle compartments [15–21].

Many tumor tissues, however, contain cells with abnormal amounts of DNA so that new peaks appear on the histograms corresponding to the appearance of aneuploid clones of cells growing within the tumor (Fig. 2). Increased rates of DNA synthesis are also present in many tumors so that the percentage of cells in the S-phase of the cell cycle is greatly increased. Thus, DNA analysis by flow

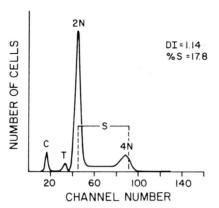

Figure 1. Flow cytometric DNA histogram for the human fibrosarcoma cell line HT 1080 illustrating a near diploid profile. The histogram shows increasing fluorescence on the horizontal axis, as expressed as channel numbers, and the relative number of cells at each flurescence level on the vertical axis. The cell cycle compartments are indicated: 2N = G0/G1-phase, S = S-phase, and 4N = G2/M-phase of the cell cycle. C = chicken erythrocytes. T = trout erythrocytes.

cytometry provides several pieces of information about the proliferative potential of a tumor and about the degree of abnormality within a tumor cell population. Internal markers of known DNA content can be added to the samples in order to define the relative peak positions on the resulting histograms (note Figs 1 and 2). The most commonly used internal markers have been nucleated chicken erythrocytes (CRBC'S), trout erythrocytes (TRBC'S) and human lymphocytes [22, 23]. Chicken erythrocytes have approximately 35%, and trout erythrocytes approximately 80%, of the DNA content of normal human diploid cells [23] and are thus ideal internal standards since they can routinely be added to the clinical sample without interfering with the resulting histogram. Only in cases where a hypodiploid clone is present does the potential exist for these internal standards to interfere with the analysis of the resulting histograms.

Immunological analyses performed on the flow cytometer have usually dealt with the appearance of differentiation and tumor specific antigenic properties of cells. As indicated above, the major constraint encountered in assessing the antigenicity of solid tumors, such as the urologic tumors, is the requirement for the tissue to be reduced to a single cell suspension, prior to analysis in the flow cytometer, using techniques which alter many of the interesting cell surface antigens. Therefore, immunological analysis in the flow cytometer has generally involved examination of lymphoid cells, although internalized antigens of solid tumors can also be analyzed on the instrument [7, 24].

DNA analysis by flow cytometry

A variety of DNA specific fluorescent labels have been used to examine cell cycle

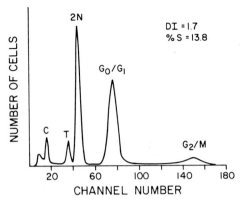

Figure 2. Flow cytometric DNA histogram from a Grade IV transitional cell carcinoma from the urinary bladder with a major aneuploid cell population. The peaks are defined as C = chicken erythrocytes, T = trout erythrocytes, 2N = diploid human cells, G0/G1 = tumor G0/G1 peak, G2/M = tumor G2/M peak. The normal 4N peak corresponding to the diploid 2N cells would be located under the tumor G0/G1 peak on this linear scale. DNA Index (DI) = ratio of modal G0/G1 peak for Tumor Cells to that of normal diploid standards.

characteristics in a variety of tumors (reviewed by Goerttler and Stöhr [25]), one of the most popular of which is acridine orange. This dye is unique in that it binds both to double-stranded DNA to fluoresce at one range of wavelengths (green) and to single-stranded RNA to produce a different range of fluorescence (red). Thus, acridine orange can be used to stain both types of nucleic acid simultaneously [26–28]. Melamed and coworkers [29–36] have used acridine orange to stain bladder tumor cells, utilizing the staining properties of this dye to help identify and gate out of their histograms several contaminating cell types, such as leukocytes and squamous cells.

Other fluorescent dyes which are commonly used to label cellular DNA in urological tissues are ethidium bromide [37], ethidium bromide plus Mithromycin [38], propidium iodide [39], 4'-6-diamidino-2-phenylindole (DAPI) [40], and the Hoescht dyes [41, 42]. The Hoescht dyes are vital dyes and can be used to temporarily label the DNA of living cells, often without irreversibly damaging them. The chemistry of many of these fluorescent dyes has been reviewed by Latt [43] and Darzynkiewicz [44]. Each of these dyes, if utilized as intended, can provide much information about the DNA content of solid tumor cells.

Limitations of DNA analysis by flow cytometry

It is necessary to discuss certain limitations of flow cytometry as it is applied to DNA analysis. The validity of DNA measurements made in the flow cytometer rests upon being able to demonstrate the same type of information by alternative techniques. It has been adequately shown, in several tumor systems, that a major characteristic of malignant cells is the appearance of aberrant chromosomes and chromosome numbers [45–49]. Also, several laboratories, using the technique of absorption cytofluorometry (a microscope-based analysis of the total cellular DNA content), have provided data similar to that obtained from the flow cytometer [50–53]. It is important to realize that flow cytometric analysis provides only a measure of the total DNA content per cell and not of the distribution of this DNA amongst the chromosomal complement of the cells, information which might be obtained from a karyotypic analysis. A chromosomal rearrangement without a substantial net gain, or loss, of DNA would not be detected by flow cytometry. A diploid histogram in a tumor, therefore, does not necessarily mean a normal chromosomal complement. In at least one report by Granberg-Öhman et al. [54] DNA analysis by flow cytometry was compared with the results of a chromosomal analysis on the same cells. They reported that the flow cytometric analysis provided DNA contents 20% higher than the quantity estimated from chromosomal analysis. Barlogie et al. [55], on the other hand, compared the DNA Index (ratio of the modal G0/G1 peak for tumor cells to that of normal diploid standards) with the Karyotype Index (ratio of modal chomosome number to the diploid chromosome number of 46) for several tumors and found that in many cases there was a linear relationship between the two values. There were, however, a number of diploid or near-diploid tumors by chromosome analysis which had aberrent DNA contents by flow cytometry. The discrepencies between laboratories and with different specimens could reflect differences in stainability of the cells as well as procedural differences employed by various laboratories. Thus, the DNA values obtained from the flow cytometer should be regarded as relative values rather than as absolute values.

Some of the fluorescent dyes bind not only DNA but double-stranded RNA as well (e.g., the intercalating dyes propidium iodide and ethidium bromide) so that it is necessary to use ribonuclease (RNAase) in the preparation to destroy this interaction. Other factors such as ionic strength, pH, type of fixation, type of dye and dye concentration are also vitally important in the quality of the staining reaction. In addition, different physical states of DNA can result in differential staining of cells in that the degree of condensation of the DNA or the binding of different proteins could greatly affect the amount of dye bound [56]. This problem is most apparent in flow cytometric analysis of abnormal testicular tissue and sperm [57, 58]. Many of these factors have been addressed by the authors listed above for the use of each of the individual stains.

It is also possible that there could be differences in the way different tissues interact with some of these reagents. We have noted, for instance, that the Krishan reagent (propidium iodide) as used in our laboratory [19, 39, 59] works well for preparation of all epithelial cells and tissues examined so far, including a variety of carcinomas and adenomas. The presence of the non-ionic detergent NP-40 in the reagent adequately releases single nuclei from these cells, even when the cells are badly clumped. Fibroblastic tissues and fibroblasts in short term tissue culture, however, do not behave as well in this staining solution since there is only partial release of the nuclei from the cells and there is a strong tendancy for the released nuclei to form aggregates. Thus, the resulting histograms have much broader peaks than found for the epithelial tissues and there are fewer free nuclei available for analysis per milligram of tissue. Supplementation of the staining solution with additional detergents, mild sonication, or even dounce homogenization, have not resulted in a significant increase in the release of free nuclei from these cells (unpublished observations).

DNA ploidy in urological tumors

It is clear, in several tumor systems, that there is a direct correlation between the appearance of abnormal DNA contents within the tumors and the degree of clinical involvement (reviewed by Barlogie et al. [55]; Frankfurt et al. [40, 60]). Several laboratories have used flow cytometry to examine this relationship in urological tumors. As discussed above, the search for DNA aneuploidy by flow cytometry is not a sufficient criterian, by itself, to identify all urological tumors; diploid, or near-diploid, tumors and those with chromosomal rearrangements which do not have a net loss or gain of DNA content might not be detected by this technique. In addition, sampling errors can also lead to false-negative results since small tumors, or tumors buried deeply within the tissue, can be missed depending upon the procedures used to collect specimens. Still, a large body of information indicates that flow cytometry can be very effective in identifying many of the urological tumors based solely on abnormalities in the resulting DNA histograms.

One of the earliest flow cytometric studies on bladder cancer was reported by Tribukait and Esposti [61] using bladder washings from 288 patients. Their method of preparation consisted of fixation of the cells in 96% ethanol, ribonuclease (RNAase) treatment, release of the cell nuclei by pepsin digestion and subsequent staining of the DNA with ethidium bromide. The results obtained by flow cytometry were correlated with standard cytological and histological analyses. Their preliminary data implied that, in bladder tumors, the presence of aneuploidy was an indication of malignancy. Comparison of the appearance of aneuploidy to tumor grade showed that aneuploidy was present in 7% of the histological grade 0 and grade 1 tumors, in 35% of the grade II tumors and in 79% of the grade III tumors. Thus, there was an apparent direct correlation between the presence of aneuploidy and tumor grade. Further subdivision of the grade II tumors according to the degree of cellular atypia illustrated that tumors with only slight nuclear atypia had a lower incidence of aneuploidy (9%) compared with the more atypical tumors within this group (68% aneuploidy). Also, correlation with cytological grading showed that tumors with benign appearence were aneuploid only 8% of the time while poorly-differentiated tumors expressed

96% aneuploidy. Pedersen et al. [62], in another early study using either propidium iodide or ethidium bromide to stain tumor cells [63], also noted a direct correlation between the degree of anaplasia and the appearence of aneuploid peaks. These early flow cytometric studies therefore illustrated that the flow cytometer was capable of obtaining data similar to that provided by more laborious techniques such as chromosome analysis [45–49] and microscope-based absorption cytophotometry [50–53].

Tribukait et al. [64] later reported on 100 untreated, newly-diagnosed bladder cancer cases where the flow cytometric results were correlated with the TNM system of clinical assessment of tumor involvement [65]. Tumors with tetraploid stemlines were grouped with the aneuploids in this study. A tumor was labeled as having a tetraploid stemline if the number of tetraploid cells (G2/M, 4N) exceeded the average value of the 4N peak of cells from normal bladders by 3 times the standard deviation (in their experience, $4.1 \pm 2.0\%$ for bladder washings and $3.9 \pm 1.3\%$ for biopsies). One third of the T1 tumors showed evidence of aneuploidy while, with only one exception, all of the T2, T3, T4 and TIS tumors had aneuploid stemlines. Examination of the relative positions of the aneuploid peaks of the different members of the T-series indicated that there was a progressive shift from a hypotetraploid position for T1 aneuploid tumors to a hypertriploid position for T3 tumors; therefore, there was an apparent loss of DNA with increasing clinical involvement. There also appears to be a relationship of T-series with the histological grade [66] since grade 3 tumors of the T-series congregated in the hypertriploid region while grade 2 tumors were centered in a more tetraploid region. Frankfurt et al. [40], while examining biopsy material with either propidium iodide or DAPI stains, also noted an interesting correlation between the degree of aneuploidy and the degree of differentiation in bladder tumors. Only in poorly-differentiated tumors did they find DNA Indices (DI) in the range of 1.4 to 2.2. (DI = 1.0 for diploid cells) whereas in well- and moderately-differentiated tumors the DNA Index was usually near diploid. They also noted that there was a progression of aneuploidy with clinical stage in bladder tumors since most T0 and T1 tumors were diploid while most T2 to T4 tumors were aneuploid. They found no correlation between the presence of metastatic lesions and the degree of aneuploidy in the small number of cases they examined. These results indicate that low grade and low stage bladder tumors are generally either diploid or near-tetraploid while more advanced tumors are hypertriploid in DNA content.

Farsund et al. [67, 68] reported observations comparing cell cycle analyses made on multiple aspirations of bladders taken during cystoscopy using a technique developed earlier that allowed selective aspiration of cells from different regions of the bladder [38, 69]. The aspirated cells were fixed with ethanol and stained with ethidium bromide plus Mithramycin. Utilizing this technique, they showed that one could map the DNA distribution of the bladder mucosa and found that, in at least some cases, the distribution of diploid and aneuploid cells varied with location around the tumor. They felt that this technique of selective aspiration was superior to bladder barbotage for sampling tumor cells since, in the latter case, all relationship of cells to their site of origin was lost. Also, there was greater potential for dilution of tumor cells with excessive numbers of normal cells by the bladder barbotage technique which could produce false negative results by flow cytometry. Utilizing the selective sampling technique, they reported that histological grade 2 tumors [66] were 43% aneuploid while 91% of the grade 3 tumors were aneuploid. Examination of the degree of aneuploidy in a number of tumors yielded two main classes of aneuploidy distribution – one with a hypertriploid distribution and one with a hypotetraploid pattern. It was noted that there was more extensive involvement of surrounding bladder mucosa in cases where the aneuploid stemline was hypertriploid than hypotetraploid. This result correlated well with the results of Frankfurt et al. [40] indicating that the more aggressive bladder tumors had DNA contents in the near triploid range.

Melamed and coworkers have examined more than 500 urologic patients by flow cytometry in an extensive study which has been in progress for several years [30–36, 70]. Tumor cells obtained by either bladder irrigation or tumor biopsy were stained with acridine orange so that both DNA and RNA content of the cells could be analyzed simultaneously in the flow cytometer. The combined analysis of RNA and DNA, along with light scatter characteristics of the cells, allowed them to distinguish several contaminating non-tumor cells which were subsequently eliminated by gating from their analysis results.

Collste et al. [30] examined 39 cancer patients by both biopsy and bladder irrigation. Comparison of the results obtained by flow cytometry with those obtained histologically showed that 34 of the 39 bladder tumors were identified in the irrigation samples by flow cytometry as a result of the appearance of either a distinct aneuploid DNA peak or of an increase in the number of hyperdiploid cells above a baseline level (cells with a DNA content above 2N but not showing a distinct aneuploid peak). Four of the five false-negative patients, not detected by flow cytometric analysis of the irrigation fluids, had well-differentiated papillomas and one had a low-grade papillary carcinoma. There were occasional differences between the histograms obtained from the two methods of sample collection. Most often, the specimen with the most variability in the number of DNA stemlines present was that obtained by irrigation, a result which might be expected for a technique which samples a larger portion of the bladder surface than examined by biopsy methods. This data indicated that the irrigation technique might be superior to biopsy procedures for diagnosis of bladder cancer using flow cytometry. Studies involving multiple biopsy sites obtained around a tumor indicated that different stemlines of tumor can be growing at different locations within the bladder, a result supported by the work of Farsund et al. [67, 68] using multiple aspirations of the bladder surface mucosa.

Klein et al [31] extended this study to encompass nearly 400 urologic patients including 100 normal controls. The criteria chosen to identify a positive bladder tumor was that the cells should either: 1) possess a distinct aneuploid peak by flow cytometry, or 2) the percentage of hyperdiploid cells should exceed 15% of the total cells. The overall results showed that the more a tumor progressed the more likely it was to be detected by flow analysis of the DNA content. Thus, flow cytometry was positive for 31% of the papillomas, 86% of the noninvasive carcinomas, 97% of the flat carcinomas *in situ* (CIS) and 92% of the invasive carcinomas. Similar results were noted concerning the appearance of aneuploidy by itself within these tumors. Fifty-five percent of the papillomas were aneuploid compared with 40% of the noninvasive papillary carcinomas, 84% flat CIS, and 67% of the invasive carcinomas. Only two false-positive cases were encountered and both of these involved patients with severe cystitis and bladder calculi associated with benign prostatic hyperplasia, situations which might have induced cellular proliferation within the bladder mucosa. Neither of these cases showed the presence of aneuploidy. More importantly, there were 18% false-negatives by these criteria. However, if the papillomas were dropped from this figure, the number of false-negatives fell to 7%. All of the missed carcinomas were either small and localized, or consisted of invasive carcinomas which were covered over with ulcerated mucosa containing fibrinous inflammatory exudate. These results support earlier data for bladder irrigation specimens by Tribukait and Esposti [6] and Collste et al. [30] that aneuploidy increased with the histological grade of the tumor, while Tribukait et al. [71], Jakobsen et al. [72] and Granberg-Öhman et al. [73] had reported similar data for biopsy specimens.

An attempt was made to correlate the results obtained by flow cytometry with those derived from routine cytologies and from cystoscopic observations. There were 4 groups recognized: First, were those where all three parameters correlated; this occurred in 220 of the 325 specimens – 64 positive in all cases and 156 negative in all cases. The second group consisted of those cases where only flow cytometric and cytologic analyses agreed; this occurred in only 39 specimens – 12 positives and 27 negatives. The third group contained those cases where only the flow cytometric data and cytoscopic examinations correlated; this occurred in 40 cases – 38 positives and 2 negatives. Group 4 was composed of those cases where flow cytometric data was not verified by either of the other procedures; this group consisted of 26 cases in which flow data were positive but could not be confirmed by the other two procedures. Twelve of the 21 patients from which these 26 samples in group 4 were taken subsequently developed positive cytologies or showed indentifiable tumor by cystoscopy within 1 year. Thus, flow cytometry, in combination with one or both of the other techniques, should prove valuable as an additional tool for detection of bladder cancer; it is possible that flow cytometric analysis of bladder irrigation specimens could be more sensitive than either of the other two procedures for early diagnosis of bladder cancer.

Klein et al. [32], in a related report, studied 123 patients with carcinoma *in situ*

(CIS) of the bladder. Eighty of these patients had flat CIS, while 43 had papillary tumors with foci of CIS or diffuse noninvasive papillary carcinomas. Analysis of bladder washings from these patients showed that flow cytometry correctly diagnosed flat CIS 98% of the time; the two false-negative cases had very small foci of tumor. Eighty-six percent of the positive cases had distinct non-tetraploid, aneuploid peaks while another 14% had tetraploid peaks which comprised greater than 15% of the total cells present. Eighty-eight percent of the cases which had papillary carcinomas *in situ* were positive by flow cytometry and 42% of these had non-tetraploid, aneuploid DNA profiles.

Gustafson et al. [74] also examined 20 patients with CIS and found that all 20 showed evidence of aneuploidy. This group also noted that tumor progression was apparent only in cases with multiple aneuploid DNA clones. Thus, flow cytometry appears to provide important clinical information about CIS which is not available from other sources. The results of these two laboratories clearly illustrate the utility of flow cytometry for recognition of carcinoma *in situ* within bladder irrigation specimens.

Melamed [70] and Melamed and Klein [36] recently summarized the flow cytometric results on bladder tumors obtained in their laboratory over the past several years. Using the criterian that the presence of an aneuploid population of cells by itself is a highly accurate indicator of an existing carcinoma, they were able to accurately predict 86% of the flat CIS cases and 42% of the cases of papillary CIS [32]. By this same criterian 67% of the invasive carcinomas were identified [31]. Modification of the requirements for identification of positive cases to include specimens which had a distinctive tetraploid population, or had greater than 15% hyperdiploid cells without an apparent aneuploid peak, resulted in recognition of nearly all the flat CIS, 80% of the papillary CIS, and 92% of the invasive carcinomas. False-positives have varied from 2 to 10% depending upon the number of cases which had severe cystitis. Approximately 12% of the benign papillomas contained aneuploid cells [34] and, by all of the criteria above, 46% of the patients with papillomas gave positive flow cytometric results. It is possible that there exists a division of the papillomas, signaled by these results from the flow cytometer, as to the potential for these tumors to progress. The necessary follow-up studies to ascertain this possibility have not been reported, however.

Jakobsen et al. [75] investigated 303 multiple biopsies on 45 patients with untreated bladder cancers. The biopsy specimens were minced with a scalpel and syringed to break up the tissue. The cells were stained with ethidium bromide in detergent [72] and trout erythrocytes (TRBCS) were used as an internal control. All but 2 specimens, classified as histological grade 0 by the Bergkvist criteria [76], were diploid. About half of the grade II specimens were diploid whereas 90% of the grade III and IV specimens were aneuploid. The frequency of aneuploidy, therefore, increased with the degree of atypia, an observation also noted for selected site samples taken from areas not adjacent to the primary tumor. The

DNA indices of the cells adjacent to the tumor were identical to that of the tumor in all cases examined. Samples from non-adjacent, selected sites, however, occasionally had different DNA stemlines at different locations.

Gustafson et al. [77] did a followup study on 229 patients with grade I and grade II tumors which had been surgically treated. Within this group 175 cases were initially diploid and 54 were aneuploid. They found no tumor progression in any of the 175 diploid cases as defined by 1) increase in the T-category (UICC), 2) development of flat CIS, or 3) local progression, such as papillomatosis, requiring further treatment. Their findings were similar to others in that the greatest number of aneuploids were found in the grade II tumors, with most of the grade I tumors being diploid. Examination of the degree of ploidy in patients with recurrent tumors indicated that there was a high level of consistency in that the recurrent tumors usually remained at the same degree of ploidy as the primary tumors during a lengthy period of observation. There were, however, 19 cases with primary diploid tumors which recurred as aneuploid tumors, and 8 cases which were initially aneuploid but reappeared as diploid tumors.

Many fewer flow cytometric studies have been performed on prostate carcinomas than on bladder tumors which is probably a reflection of the relatively greater difficulty in obtaining adequate material for examination in the flow cytometer. The clinical diagnosis of prostatic carcinoma is largely based upon histopathological analysis of biopsy material, often via fine-needle aspiration. This type of biopsy may not always be representative of the tumor which makes accurate classification of the disease difficult. There also appears to be a large variation in the clinical behavior of prostate tumors of the same histological type making prediction of the course of the disease very difficult [78]. Early investigations based upon absorption cytophotometry in the microscope had indicated that there was a correlation between the DNA content and prognosis of prostatic carcinomas [79–81]. Some of the initial flow cytometric studies on prostate carcinoma also indicated that there was a direct correlation between the DNA pattern and the state of differentiation [82–85].

Rönström et al. [86] reported the results of examination of 500 untreated patients with suspected prostatic cancer who submitted to transrectal fine-needle aspiration biopsies. Multiple biopsies were made of the same area for both flow cytometry and routine histological analysis. The samples for flow cytometric analysis were stained with ethidium bromide as described by Tribukait et al. [37]. Their results showed that benign prostatic tissues had a mean G2 + M content of 4.2%. They, therefore, cataloged any cell with a G2 + M fraction greater than 7% (mean + 2 standard deviations) as abnormal and highly suspicious of containing a tetraploid tumor stemline. Morphologically benign samples were generally diploid or tetraploid while 73% of the carcinomas were aneuploid; one third of the questionably malignant tumors had non-diploid DNA patterns. Only one case was found where a well-differentiated tumor showed evidence of having an aneuploid stemline. Half of the moderately-differentiated tumors were tetraploid while half were non-tetraploid, aneuploid; most of the poorly-differentiated tumors were non-tetraploid, aneuploid. Five percent of the moderately-differentiated tumors and 35% of the poorly-differentiated tumors had multiple aneuploid clones. The degree of aneuploidy also varied with the tumor progression: well- and moderately-differentiated tumors with aneuploid clones had an average peak position of 3.9c (3.9 times haploid chromosome DNA content) while the poorly-differentiated tumors had an average peak position of 3.6c (DNA Index roughly equal to 1.8). Thus, there was also a tendency toward triploidy with increasing degree of aneuploidy in the prostate tumors.

Tribukait et al. [87] examined the aneuploid tumors in greater detail placing special interest upon the distinction between tetraploid and non-tetraploid tumors. Examination of 300 patients showed exclusively diploid cell lines in 61% of the well-differentiated cases but only in 3% of the poorly-differentiated cases. They found that the percentage of the tetraploid tumors decreased with increasing cytologic grade (88% in well-differentiated tumors to 69% in moderately-differentiated and 33% in poorly-differentiated tumors). Likewise, multiple aneuploid clones were more common in poorly-differentiated tumors (0% in well-differentiated and 22% of the poorly-differentiated tumors). Thus, well-differentiated tumors could be separated into diploid and tetraploid tumors, poorly-differentiated tumors into tetraploid and aneuploid tumors, and moderately-differentiated tumors contained all three DNA classes. In addition, the percentage of non-diploid cells in relation to the total cells aspirated showed a direct correlation with the increasing tumor grade; the greatest effect was noted in the non-tetraploid, aneuploid tumors. Caution must be exercised in interpreting this data, however, since non-tetraploid, aneuploid tumors may be less cohesive than more highly differentiated tumors and thus be more apt to shed tumor cells by fine-needle aspiration. It is also possible that there were more diploid tumor cells in the tetraploid tumors than in non-tetraploid tumors. Support for this view comes from studies using absorption cytophotometry which suggests that tetraploid tumors may contain significant numbers of malignant diploid cells [79, 81].

Frankfurt et al. [88] recently reported a detailed analysis of 45 prostate carcinoma patients. They found a frequency of aneuploidy of 44.4% overall and that the frequency of aneuploidy increased with advancing stage of tumors. All of the tumors confined to the prostate gland (stage B) were diploid while most of the tumors with distant metastases were poorly-differentiated and usually had aneuploid DNA stemlines. Only 18.2% of the diploid tumors expressed distant metastases, whereas 2/3 of the aneuploid tumors had spread to the pelvic nodes and to distant sites; none of the aneuploid tumors were confined to the gland itself. Therefore, the presence of aneuploid cells appears to be a good indicator of tumor spread outside the prostate. There was also a direct correlation between the Gleason score [89, 90] and the degree of aneuploidy.

There have been relatively few additional flow cytometric studies of other urothelial tumors. Examination of kidney tumors has been hampered by the size and complexity, as well as by the relative rarity, of these tumors. Schwabe et al. [91] examined a small group of 36 patients with various renal tumors in an attempt to demonstrate a relationship between flow cytometric DNA analysis and histological grade using the grading system of Hermanek et al. [92]. Fourteen (39%) of the 36 tumors examined were aneuploid in patients who had undergone irradiation therapy on 4 consecutive preoperative days. Their study showed that grade I tumors were all diploid while grade II and grade III tumors were both diploid and aneuploid. There was no information about the uniformity of the kidney tumors in this study since cells from duplicate blocks of tissue were pooled for analysis. A microscope-based cytofluometry study by Bennington and Mayall [93] showed DNA profile differences between tumor and non-tumor regions of the kidney tumors and indicated that these differences increased with tumor grade. They could not, by flow cytometric DNA analysis alone, distinguish benign adenoma from grade I carcinoma, nor could they distinguish between clear cell and oncocytic tumors of the same grade. In general, however, they were able to predict the tumor grade from the cytometric data alone.

Baisch et al. [94] examined 46 renal carcinomas and found that 46% of these were aneuploid. All of the tumors of grade IIIb and grade IV were hyperdiploid (grading system of Syrjänen and Hjelt [95]). Almost half of the hyperdiploids and 89% of the diploids were from low grade tumors. In a 2 year follow-up 8 of 17 patients with hyperdiploid tumors and 1 of 14 with diploid tumors had either succumbed to the tumors or had relapsed with multiple metastases. Thus, as with several other tumor systems, there was an apparent direct relationship between ploidy and tumor progression.

Otto et al. [96] expanded upon this study of renal cell carcinomas by examining multiple site specimens from 68 patients with stages I to III tumors. Twenty of the 68 patients had received pre-operative irradiation. They did not distinguish between this group of patients and those who had not been irradiated since no flow cytometric DNA pattern differences were noted between the two groups. A total of thirty-five (51%) of the patients had aneuploid DNA contents and five of these had a nonhomogeneous DNA profile in different areas of the tumor. In general, they reported a tumor as being aneuploid if they found an aneuploid stemline in any portion of the kidney. Thirty-one (89%) of the 35 patients with aneuploid tumors had metastases during the observation period of 1 to 4 years, while only 7 (21%) of the patients with diploid tumors had metastases in the same period. Twenty-one of 22 grade III and grade IV tumors had metastases in this period while 5 of 15 grade I tumors and 12 of 29 grade II tumors metastasized. One interesting observation they reported was that 30% of the grade I tumors had aneuploid DNA contents indicating that the current schemes of grading renal tumors may have a high degree of inaccuracy; flow cytometry might, therefore, provide needed assistance in the grading process for renal tumors.

Chin et al. [97] recently reported flow cytometric data obtained on 54 renal cell carcinoma specimens from 50 patients. Aneuploid cells were detected in 31 of 43 primary and 9 of 11 metastatic lesions giving an overall incidence of aneuploidy of 74%. No significant difference in the appearance of aneuploidy was noted between clear cell and granular cell tumors, between primary and metastatic tumors, or between stage III and stage IV tumors (pathological staging procedure of Robson et al. [98]. There were relatively few stage I and stage II tumors examined, but two of the four stage I tumors and 1 of 2 stage II tumors were aneuploid. With one exception, they found complete agreement in the DNA indices of primary and metastatic lesions. The exceptional case, however, had diploid cells in the primary lesion and 2 different aneuploid stemlines in the metastatic lesion.

Ljungberg et al. [99] recently described a comprehensive examination of 25 renal cell carcinomas in which they examined up to 8 isolated sites per tumor. Their results showed that 52% of the tumors were aneuploid and that some of these had multiple aneuploid clones. Fourteen of the 25 tumors had homogeneous DNA patterns at all sites examined with 12 of these having diploid or near-diploid patterns. Eleven of the tumors (44%) had heterogeneous DNA patterns at different locations within the tumors; four of these 11 tumors had 2 to 3 different aneuploid clones growing in different locations. In general, the aneuploid samples exhibited significantly higher proliferative rates than did diploid cells. Low grade (I and II) tumors were largely diploid while grade IV tumors were usually aneuploid, as has been reported in several other tumor systems. No correlation between histological grade and DNA pattern was obtained for the grade III tumors. This study clearly illustrates the need to obtain multiple site samples from renal tumors in order to accurately describe the character of these tumors.

The bulk of the DNA analyses other than those involving the bladder, prostate and kidney have been concerned with examination of testicular tissue of patients with testicular cancer or with problems of male infertility. Evenson et al. [58] examined semen samples from 14 patients with stage I to stage III testicular tumors. The specimens were obtained at intervals of one day to 17 months following unilateral orchiectomy without further treatment. Control semen for comparison was collected from three normal subjects with proven fertility. The fresh semen from the normal volunteers gave a very homogeneous pattern in the flow cytometer after staining with acridine orange. This was in striking contrast to the results obtained with many of the semen specimens from the cancer patients where broad, non-symmetrical histograms were apparent. It was noted, by following these patients for several months, that the abnormal staining pattern persisted for periods up to one year after unilateral orchiectomy. A dramatic shift in the level of red fluorescence was noted in the sperm from the cancer patients when the sperm was heated prior to addition of the fluorescent dye. This increased red shift is apparently due to the accelerated unfolding of the helical DNA structure in the patient samples as compared to sperm from the normal subjects. Thus, flow cytometry can provide valuable information about the fragility of sperm DNA in these cancer patients following unilateral orchiectomy.

Rate of DNA proliferation in urological tumors

The proliferative rate of the cells in some tumors may have equal importance to the detection of aneuploid clones within the cell population since the rate of DNA synthesis is directly related to the rate of growth of a tumor. The value of DNA synthesis must be tempered, however, by consideration of the rate of cell death and of the rate that cells are shed from the tumor. In some tumor systems the evidence accumulated suggests that there is a direct relationship between the rate of DNA synthesis and the chances of early recurrence [100, 101]. The rate of DNA proliferation is usually determined from the thymidine labeling index (TLI), which is a measure of the incorporation of radioactively-labeled thymidine into the cellular DNA as gauged by autoradiography (reviewed by Meyer [102]). This procedure is very time consuming, taking several days for development of the autoradiograms and requiring cell-by-cell microscopic analysis by a trained investigator. Thus, attempts have been made to show a correlation between the results obtained by TLI with S-phase values from cell cycle analyses performed in the flow cytometer [19, 59]. A direct correlation of the S-phase values obtained for breast carcinoma tissues and the TLI results was obtained. It is now necessary to demonstrate that high values of S-phase accurately predict the recurrance of breast carcinomas, as is apparently the case for high TLI values [100]; this followup study is currently in progress (McDivitt and Stone, unpublished observations).

Several groups have reported S-phase determinations performed on urological tumor tissues. Tribukait et al. [64] examined 100 untreated, newly-diagnosed cancer cases for both the degree of ploidy and the percentage of cells in S-phase. Based on histological grade, the number of S-phase cells in aneuploid clones of grade 3 tumors was much greater than in aneuploid grade 2 tumors. Similar comparison of the percentage of S-phase cells in different grades of diploid tumors, however, showed no such variation. Tetraploid tumors, for reasons unknown, had the lowest proliferation rate. Based on the TNM system of clinical assessment of tumors [65], they found that the proportion of S-phase cells increased with the T-number. The results obtained by this group agreed well with mitotic index measurements made by Fulker et al. [103] for bladder tumors of different stages. It would thus appear that there is a generally higher rate of proliferation in bladder carcinomas with greater tumor involvement.

Frankfurt et al. [40] examined the percentage of cells in the S-phase of the cell cycle in biopsies of a number of different solid tumors, including several urological tumors. They reported that the median percentage S-phase cells was significantly higher in aneuploid tumors than in diploid tumors. However, they found no significant difference in the median S-phase percentages between primary and metastatic tumors. There was a tendency in bladder tumors for the S-phase percentage to increase with the degree of aneuploidy, whereas several other tumor systems failed to provide this type of correlation. Cell cycle analysis of diploid tumors presents some interesting problems, as indicated by these authors, since measurement of the cell cycle phases of these tumors includes the proliferative rates of both normal, uninvolved diploid cells as well as the diploid tumor cells. The combined result is therefore an average rate rather than an accurate measure of the tumor cell population. This is less problematic for aneuploid tumors since the histograms can often be dissected to separate the normal cell components from the tumor cell components. It is also possible that the percentage of cells which are normal in a diploid tumor can be quite variable. Therefore, without additional information such as that obtained from cytological or histological analysis, there is an uncertainty as to the valitidy of S-phase measurements on these tumors.

Farsund et al. [67, 68] studied multiple aspirates of tumors and surrounding bladder mucosa. Examination of the S-phase populations [67] showed that the percentage of cells replicating was significantly higher in grade 1 and grade 2 diploid tumors than in normal urothelium. There was an even greater increase in the percentage S-phase cells in aneuploid grade 2 and grade 3 tumors. The highest proliferative rate was in the grade 3 tumors where the percentage S-phase cells was more than 10 times that of normal bladder mucosa. They also noted that the S-phase percentage for the non-aneuploid mucosal cells of bladders containing aneuploid tumors was higher than for normal, uninvolved tissue, even though the cells appeared normal histologically. They found these diploid cells to have a higher S-phase value than either the grade 1 or grade 2 diploid tumor cells but still less than the values for the aneuploid cells themselves. It was previously noted by these authors that there was more extensive involvement of surrounding mucosa in cases where the aneuploid stemline was hypertriploid than hypotetraploid. The extensive involvement of surrounding mucosa in bladders having a tumor may be an important feature of this disease and the higher proliferative rate, of even the diploid mucosa in certain patients with aneuploid tumors, may reflect long range effects of the presence of the tumor. Whether this is merely a nonspecific effect on the total mucosa of the bladder or a early indication of further tumor development is not known at this time.

Gustafson et al. [74] examined 20 patients with CIS and found that all 20 had evidence of aneuploidy. When they followed these patients they found that cases which progressed to more extensive involvement generally had multiple aneuploid stemlines, a high percentage of aneuploid cells compared to diploid cells, and a high rate of proliferation. Gustafson et al. [77] also reported a follow-up study on 229 patients with grade 1–2 tumors which had been surgically treated. Within this group 175 cases were initially diploid and 54 were aneuploid. They found no tumor progression in any of the 175 diploid cases. The growth rate of tumors did not usually change upon recurrence, but the incidence of tumor progression increased in tumors with higher proliferation rates.

Roters et al. [104], while examining prostatic tumors, reported that all benign hyperplasias had G1 peaks comprising greater than 95% of the total cells; the G1 peaks of carcinomas, however, made up less than 95% of the cells. Since this is a reflection of the number of cells in other, possibly aneuploid, peaks and of cells in S-phase, this data indicated that malignant prostate tumors also have higher proliferative rates than the benign tumors.

Schwabe et al. [91] examined a small group of 36 patients with a variety of renal neoplasms and failed to show any correlation between either ploidy or the percentage of cells in S-phase with pathological tumor stage, lymph node involvement or metastatic spread. Chin et al. [97] also showed a wide variation in S-phase values for both diploid tumors and aneuploid tumors amongst a group of 50 patients with renal cell carcinomas. They found, however, that the median S-value was lower in diploid tumors than in aneuploid tumors and the values for metastatic aneuploid tumors was higher than for primary aneuploid tumors. Otto et al. [96] examined stage I to stage III renal cell carcinomas in the flow cytometer. Approximately 95% of the cells of diploid tumors were found in the G0/G1 region of the histogram and only 3% of the cells were in the S-phase. Aneuploid tumors showed a greater percentage of cells in S-phase having 88% of the cells in the G0/G1 peak and an average of 7% in the S-phase area of the histograms, although they reported a wide range of proliferative rates in the renal tumors. Ljungberg et al. [99] also reported that there was a significant difference in the percentage of renal carcinoma cells in S-phase between diploid and aneuploid tumors. It would thus appear that urological tumors other than bladder tumors might also show greater proliferative rates in a direct relationship to aneuploidy. It still not known how this tumor cell property relates to the progression of these tumors.

Analysis of low grade urological tumors

Low grade bladder tumors such as papillomas and some papillary carcinomas are recognized to be difficult to identify based on the results of DNA analysis from flow cytometry. Papillomas, by definition, are histologically benign and would not be expected to show gross nuclear alterations or to possess aneuploid stemlines, although there is some evidence that the rate of DNA synthesis, in at least some papillomas, is somewhat higher than found in normal urothelium (reviewed by Melicow [105]). Collste et al. [30] had reported a series of flow cytometric comparisons between bladder washings and bladder biopsies taken from 44 patients. Thirty-four of 39 positive tumors were detected in the bladder washings, but they reported four false-negatives by this technique. The 4 false-negative patients which were not detected by flow cytometric analysis of the irrigation fluids were all from well-differentiated papillomas. Likewise, the studies reported by Klein et al. [31] showed that the more a tumor progressed the more likely it was to be detected by flow cytometric analysis. Flow cytometric DNA analysis was positive for 31% of the papillomas, 86% of the noninvasive carcinomas, 97% of the flat carcinomas *in situ* (CIS) and 92% of the invasive carcinomas in this study.

Exfoliated cells from papillomas do, however, often differ from normal urothelium by proliferative activity, cell configuration, and amount of cytoplasm. Klein et al. [34] examined the combined RNA and DNA contents of cells obtained from bladder irrigations taken during endoscopic examination from 48 patients with papillomas. Urothelium from normal controls was found to have a uniform RNA content by flow cytometry; cellular RNA contents were considered to be abnormal if the histograms for RNA analysis were either asymmetrical or had numerous cells with higher than normal levels of RNA. The papillomas examined were divided into two groups dependent upon their histological appearance – 'orderly' or 'atypical'. By this criterian 20 of the cases were identified as orderly and 28 were atypical. DNA analysis alone identified 22 of the 48 (46%) cases using the criteria established by Klein et al. earlier for DNA analysis (see discussion above, Klein et al. [31–33]); six of the 22 cases had aneuploid stemlines, ten cases (21%]) were suspicious and 16 (33%) were normal. RNA analysis, however, was abnormal in 40 of the 48 cases (83%). Both the orderly and the atypical papillomas were equally identifiable by RNA analysis whereas DNA analysis alone could not reliably identify the orderly papillomas. All papillomas which were positive or suspicious by DNA analysis were also positive by RNA analysis. Since a greater number of atypical papillomas had an increased proportion of hyperdiploid and/or tetraploid cells Klein et al. [34] suggested that there is a greater proliferative activity within atypical than within orderly papillomas. The combined analysis of DNA and RNA, therefore, may have defined a division between the two groups of papillomas dependent upon the metabolic and proliferative activity of these cells.

Evaluation of therapeutic protocols

One important potential function of a flow cytometer is to follow the effects of a therapeutic protocol on a patient. This could be especially useful in the case of bladder tumors where periodic urinary cytologies or bladder washings can be made. There have been some preliminary studies which illustrate the potential usefulness of the flow cytometer for this type of study. Klein et al. [106] used the flow cytometer to follow 2 patients with aneuploid tumors who were on BCG therapy; the tumor of one of the patients responded to the therapy while the other did not. Bladder washings from the responder showed a loss of the aneuploid stemline and no recurrence of this group of cells. The second patient experienced an initial drop in the percentage of aneuploid cells but there was a subsequent recurrence of the clinical disease and re-appearance of aneuploid cells in the bladder washings. Therefore, the flow cytometric data correlated well with the clinical responses in these two patients. Staiano-Coico et al. [107] expanded upon this initial study by examining bladder irrigation specimens from 22 patients having low stage tumors which were treated with BCG therapy 3 to 5 weeks following local tumor resection. BCG was instilled in the bladder at weekly intervals over a period of 6 weeks with a follow-up examination performed 6 weeks after the last BCG treatment (12 week sample). Before each treatment, voided urines were collected for cytology and bladder irrigations were performed to obtain samples for flow cytometry. Twelve of the 22 patients were still free of tumor 15 months after the initiation of therapy and, in most cases, flow cytometry had correctly predicated the patient response to therapy by the 12 week checkup. Adolphs et al. [108], however, noted that normal cytological profiles do not reappear in the bladder for several months following BCG therapy. The overall results of these studies indicated that flow cytometry could be used to follow the effectiveness of this type of therapy.

Farsund et al. [109] followed the effects of chemotherapy on bladder tumors by flow cytometry. Two patients with bladder tumors having aneuploid stemlines were treated by repeated intravesical instillation of either doxorubicin or mitomycin C in the bladder for 1–2 hours. The patients were then followed by selective site sampling of bladder mucosa taken during routine cystoscopic examination. Successful treatment was indicated in both cases by reduction in the ratio of aneuploid to diploid peaks in the histograms. There was still some question following the apparently successful treatment of these tumors since the diploid cells present after loss of the aneuploid stemlines did not display blood group isoantigens A, B and H as expected for normal mucosal cells.

Klein et al. [110] also used the flow cytometer to follow the effects of irradiation on bladder tumors in 28 patients with invasive carcinomas. Bladder irrigation specimens were taken prior to integrated irradiation and then again at the time of cystectomy 1 to 14 days later (average was 2 days). All patients were positive for tumor by flow cytometry with evidence of aneuploid stemlines prior to irradiation. Five of the patients showed improved tumor grading following irradiation and 4 of these 5 showed complete disappearance of the aneuploid stemlines by flow cytometry. Twenty of the 28 patients showed no difference in staging of the tumor following irradiation, but 8 of these patients showed complete loss of the aneuploid stemline by flow cytometry. Three of the patient tumors were staged higher after treatment, and none of these showed loss of the aneuploid stemline. Their results indicated that flow cytometry detected an overall downstaging response of 43%, suggesting that flow cytometry might be useful for following the effects of irradiation therapy on bladder tumors. The use of bladder washings for this purpose was questioned by these authors, however, since only the superficial cells can be analyzed by this means so that the technique provides no information about the state of a tumor deeply invading the bladder wall.

Wijkström et al. [111] examined bladder washes and biopsies from 61 patients with carcinoma who underwent preoperative irradiation followed by cystectomy. They used two courses of irradiation. In one treatment protocol they gave 36 Gy of irradiation over a 4 week period followed by a 4 week interval before surgery, while in the second procedure they gave 20 Gy of irradiation over a 5 day period followed by immediate surgery. The first protocol resulted in clinical downstaging of all patients while, in the latter procedure, they had downstaging in only 11 of 52 cases. The downstaging of the patients receiving 20 Gy was thought to be either the results of errors in the initial staging or the result of complete tumor resection during the initial examination. DNA analyses on the patients receiving 20 Gy of irradiation showed that, in some cases, there was an apparent loss of aneuploid stemlines even though there was still tumor present in the bladder. They suggested that, in these cases, there had been both aneuploid and diploid tumor cells present in the original tumor and that the aneuploid cells were more radiosensitive than the diploid tumor cells; the diploid tumor cells having therefore survived the treatment protocol. The overall results from this study, however, indicated that neither proliferation rate, presence or absence of aneuploid cells, nor degree of aneuploidy were of value to identify tumors destined to become progressive. Only the presence of multiple aneuploid stemlines in a tumor seemed to correlate with tumor progression. There was a suggestion, however, that the loss of an aneuploid stemline could have positive prognostic significance.

Investigations based upon absorption cytophotometry in the microscope indicated that there was a correlation between the DNA content and prognosis of prostatic carcinomas [79–81]. In addition, these studies suggested a direct correlation between the effectiveness of hormone therapy and the presence of a diploid-tetraploid tumor. Aneuploid tumors had a very poor response to the hormonal therapy. Kjaer et al. [112] reported an early flow cytometric study on prostate carcinomas where fine-needle biopsies were taken from 8 patients with untreated prostatic carcinoma and again at frequent intervals during hormone therapy with estradiol and estramustine phosphate. Four of six tumors which had an initial hyperdiploid population changed to a diploid pattern within 3 and 6 months after initiation of the treatment protocol. There was also a concomitant cytological change from malignant cells to a mixture of degenerating and benign cells in the later samples. Diploid tumors showed no change in DNA pattern during treatment, but there was an obvious cytological change during this time. Two of the six hyperdiploid tumors showed no change in DNA pattern and one can infer from their data that there was likewise no regressive change noted clinically or cytologically.

Schwabe et al. [113] reported a study of urinary sediments taken during chemotherapy for malignancies of the gonads. These examinations showed that there was an increased abnormality in the histograms obtained from patients under treatment. There was a generalized, time-dependent cell cycle arrest in the S- and G2/M-phases of the cell cycle of exfoliated urothelial cells obtained from these patients being treated with multidrug therapy. The drugs used in various combinations were vinblastine, bleomycin, cis-platinum, ifosfamide and eposide (VP_{16}). The authors believe that this cell cycle arrest might prove to be a good indicator of the effectiveness of the chemotherapeutic regimen.

The preliminary results obtained from several laboratories indicate, therefore, that flow cytometry might provide an additional means to assess the effectiveness of a therapeutic regimen used to treat a patient. At present, the most likely feature to follow would be changes in the ploidy of the tumor DNA. Re-appearance of an aneuploid stemline after surgery or chemotherapy could be used to predict the recurrence of active tumor growth. This procedure, however, is not sufficient in itself since recurrence of tumors can occur with DNA profiles which do not appear abnormal by flow cytometry. Therefore, it is necessary to utilize flow cytometry along with some independent procedure to properly identify these tumors.

Further applications of flow cytometry

The overwhelming majority of applications of flow cytometry to problems in urologic cancer has involved cell cycle analysis. These studies have adequately demonstrated the sensitivity of the flow cytometer for detection of abnormal cells within bladder irrigation specimens, and in the detection of prostate cancer using fine-needle aspirates. Somewhat less success has been achieved examining renal tumors due to the relative rarity and complexity of the tumors; however, preliminary data accumulated by several laboratories indicate that flow cytometry might also play an important role in characterizing these tumors as well, once sufficient numbers of renal tumors have been systematically examined. It would appear that knowledge of tumor ploidy and/or proliferative rate might yield important prognostic information about the tumors and lead to more effective treatment protocols. This same type of analysis might also be utilized to follow the effects of therapeutic regimens in many of the urological tumor systems since a change in ploidy to a diploid stemline from an aneuploid stemline could signal the result of an effective treatment protocol. There are, of course, obvious pitfalls in this approach since diploid or near-diploid tumors can not always be recognized by DNA analysis alone. Combined use of flow cytometry with alternative techniques which follow other tumor specific markers could, however, increase the effective accuracy of each procedure.

Frankfurt et al. [88] discussed an interesting observation which has been made by several laboratories studying DNA ploidy in human tumors. There is an apparent stability in the DNA profile found in these various tumors as expressed in the limited number of stemlines observed in most tumors. Multiple stemlines are usually found in only a small percentage of the tumors examined. This is somewhat surprising since karyotypic analysis indicates that the number of chromosomes in metaphases varies substantially from cell to cell [114]. Frankfurt suggests that many of the cells with variant DNA must be lost during mitosis in order to produce the result seen by flow cytometry. Support for this type of interpretation comes from the relative stability of DNA contents observed in tumors which have been followed over an extended period and the frequency of finding the same ploidy in primary and metastatic tumors. It is possible that aneuploidy is a consequence of an earlier, more basic tumorigenic event and that by the time a measurable tumor exists, the aneuploid stemline is a stable characteristic of these cells.

There are several other issues which also have not been resolved concerning these studies. For instance, there is a great deal of uncertainty in the identification of low grade and benign tumors by DNA analysis alone. This is an area where future emphasis should be placed since accurate, early diagnosis of these tumors is vital to the future health of the patient. The preliminary studies of Klein et al. [34] indicated that there was a difference in the level of RNA synthesis of papillary tumor cells as compared to normal urothelium. This type of analysis should serve as an indicator for further studies of cellular differences between the low grade tumors and the normal precursor cells which might be applicable to examination in the flow cytometer. The recent widespread production of monoclonal antibodies to a variety of cellular antigens may yield probes suitable for this analysis in the near future.

Another area that deserves greater research effort is that of proper identification of the cells being examined in the flow cytometer. Melamed and coworkers have utilized the differential staining of acridine orange and light scatter characteristics of bladder tumor cells in order to gate contaminating cells such as lymphocytes, dead cells and squamous epithelial cells out of their histograms [29]. Farsund et al. [109], on the other hand, prepared a stained slide of each specimen so that the cellular composition could be ascertained from these slides and the data normalized to reflect this composition. An alternative approach is now available using an immunological reaction to cellular intermediate filaments in conjunction with the DNA probes in order to identify the carcinoma cells in the presence of other, contaminating, cell types [115–118]. Most human tissues contain specific intermediate filaments characteristic to those tissues or class of tissues. There are now commercially-available antisera specific to several of these intermediate filaments so that the tissue origin of different types of cells can be ascertained. For instance, vimentin is generally found in cells of mesenchymal origin, cytokeratins in different types in epithelial cells, desmin in muscle cells, and neurofilaments in neural tissues [117, 119–123]. In the majority of cases, the type of intermediate filaments characteristic to a given tissue class is a feature that is preserved even after the cells become neoplastic. Therefore, it is possible to use information about the profile of intermediate filaments to identify the tissue of origin of many of the metastatic tumors. There are, however, exceptions to this generalization where uncharacteristic intermediate filaments appear in tumor cells [124] and in some tissue cultured cells [125–128]. In these cases, however, it is generally the appearance of vimentin, in addition to the anticipated presence of tissue specific intermediate filaments, that occurs so that the characteristic intermediate filaments are not lost. Therefore, identification of the tumor cells should still be possible in many of these exceptional cases also. The immunological labeling of intermediate filaments has been used in the flow cytometer to separate a mixed population of epithelial cells from other contaminating cells [129, 130]. This technique should be useful in many tumor systems to effectively gate contaminating cells from the resulting histograms and thereby increase the accuracy of measurements performed on the tumor cell population.

There has been an increased level of interest in the immunological characteristics of urological tumors since the advent of hybridoma techniques for monoclonal antibody production [131]. A number of reports have been published detailing the isolation and identification of several new antibodies to urological tissues and tumors [132–140]. Several of these antibodies should be useful in flow cytometric analyses of cells washed or scraped from tumor cell surfaces. One might expect that future development of monoclonal banks could better define the low grade urological tumors and lead to better detecton and treatment of these tumors.

One of the most powerful techniques available on most flow cytometers is the capability to analyze multiple parameters simultaneously on single cells. The integrated analysis of multiple parameters such as combination of DNA analysis with an immunological analysis of tumor specific markers [141], or of pairs of tumor-specific antigenic markers, should yield important data concerning the origin and biology of individual tumors. Multiparametric analysis in the flow cytometer can be used to isolate specific tumor cells from mixed cell populations and should receive increased attention in the future. There are important questions that could be addressed concerning antigenic modulation of tumor cells which might be related to the proliferative capacity of the cells, to the cell lineage, or to the ploidy of the individual cells.

Multiparameter analyses are not limited to examination of immunological phenomena since any unique property of a tumor cell might yield useful information such as rate of an enzymatic reaction [142–144], amount of total protein or RNA [34, 145–147], binding of specific lectins [148, 149], or the presence or absence of receptor molecules [150–154].

It is also now possible to do retrospective flow cytometric analyses on tissues which have been embedded in paraffin blocks [155] using a procedure developed by Hedley et al. [156, 157] for sectioning and rehydrating the tissue samples with the eventual release of stained nuclei from the fixed tissues. The procedure allows limited analysis of the ploidy level of the tumors but may not be sufficiently sensitive to yield other cell cycle information as it is presently used.

Flow cytometry, as a laboratory procedure, is currently undergoing a rapid period of evolution as many new advancements in instrumentation are introduced with relative frequency. There is, at the same time, an ever increasing volume of literature detailing new applications of this instrument to important problems in biology and medicine. Clearly, flow cytometry should become a very important routine laboratory procedure in many hospitals as the cost of the instrumentation falls and the confidence in the resulting data produced by the flow cytometer increases.

264

References

1. Melamed MR, Mullaney PF: An historical review of the development of flow cytometers and sorters. In: Flow Cytometry and Sorting, Melamed MR, Mullaney PF, Mendelsohn ML (eds). John Wiley and Sons, New York, 3–9, 1979
2. Koss LG: Analytical and quantitative cytology. A historical perspective. Anal Quant Cytol 4: 251–256, 1982
3. Gray JW, Coffino P: Cell cycle analysis by flow cytometry. Methods Enzymol 58: 233–248, 1979
4. Melamed MR, Mullaney PF, Mendelsohn ML: Flow Cytometry and Sorting, John Wiley and Sons, New York, 1979
5. Kachel V, Menke E: Hydrodynamic properties of flow cytometric instruments. In: Flow Cytometry and Sorting, Melamed MR, Mullaney PF, Mendelsohn ML (eds). John Wiley and Sons, New York, 41–59, 1979
6. Horan PK: Hematology. Single-cell analysis enters the space age. Diagnostic Medicine 4(Oct): 63–85, 1981
7. Lovett EJ III, Schnitzer B, Keren DF, Flint A, Hudson JL, McClatchey KD: Application of flow cytometry to diagnostic pathology. Lab Invest 50: 115–140, 1984
8. Loken MR, Lanier LL: Three-color immunofluorescence analysis of leu antigens on human peripheral blood using two lasers on a fluorescence-activated cell sorter. Cytometry 5: 151–158, 1984
9. Böhmer R-M, King NJC: Flow cytometric analysis of immunogold cell surface label. Cytometry 5: 543–546, 1984
10. Segal DM, Stephany DA: The measurement of specific cell: cell interactions by dual-parameter flow cytometry. Cytometry 5: 169–181, 1984
11. Arndt-Jovin DJ, Grimwade BG, Jovin TM: A dual laser flow sorter utilizing a cw pumped dye laser. Cytometry 1: 127–131, 1980
12. Parks DR, Hardy RR, Herzenberg LA: Three-color immunofluorescence analysis of mouse B-lymphocyte subpopulations. Cytometry 5: 159–168, 1984
13. Weichel W, Liesegang B, Gehrke K, Göttlinger C, Holtkamp B, Radbruch A, Stackhouse TK, Rajewsky K: Inexpensive upgrading of a FACS I and isolation of rare somatic varients by double-fluorescence sorting. Cytometry 6: 116–123, 1985
14. Shapiro HM: Multistation multiparameter flow cytometry: A critical review and rationale. Cytometry 3: 227–243, 1983
15. Baisch H, Beck H–P, Christensen IJ, Hartmann NR, Fried J, Dean PN, Gray JW, Jett JH, Johnston DA, White RA, Nicolini C, Zeitz S, Watson JV: A comparison of mathematical methods for the analysis of DNA histograms obtained by flow cytometry. Cell Tissue Kinet 15: 235–249, 1982
16. Dean PN, Gray JW, Dolbeare FA: The analysis and interpretation of DNA distributions measured by flow cytometry. Cytometry 3: 188–195, 1982
17. Ritch PS, Shackney SE, Schuette WH, Talbot TL, Smith CA: A practical graphical method for estimating the fraction of cells in S in DNA histograms from clinical tumor samples containing aneuploid cell populations. Cytometry 4: 66–74, 1983
18. Mann RC, Hand Jr RE, Braslawsky GR: Parametric analysis of histograms measured in flow cytometry. Cytometry 4: 75–82, 1983
19. McDivitt RW, Stone KR, Craig RB, Meyer JS: A comparison of human breast cancer cell kinetics measured by flow cytometry and thymidine labeling. Lab Invest 52: 287–291, 1985
20. Del Bino G, Bruni C, Koch G, Mazzini G, Costa A, Silvestrini R: Validation of a mathematical procedure for computer analysis of flow cytometric DNA data in human tumors. Cytometry 6: 31–36, 1985
21. Culpin D, Morris VB: Pattern of DNA synthesis and its effect on the classification of cells by flow cytometry. Cell Tissue Kinet 18: 1–12, 1985

22. Jakobsen A: The use of trout erythrocytes and human lymphocytes for standardization in flow cytometry. Cytometry 4: 161–165, 1983

23. Vindeløv LL, Christensen IJ, Nissen NI: Standardization of high-resolution flow cytometric DNA analysis by the simultaneous use of chicken and trout red blood cells as internal reference standards. Cytometry 3: 328–331, 1983

24. Schroff RW, Bucana CD, Klein RA, Farrell MM, Morgan Jr AC: Detection of intracytoplasmic antigens by flow cytometry. J Immunol Methods 70: 167–177, 1984

25. Goerttler K, Stöhr M: Automated cytology. The state of the art. Arch Path Lab Med 106: 657–661, 1982

26. Darzynkiewicz Z, Traganos F, Sharpless TK, Melamed MR: Conformation of RNA *in situ* as studied by acridine orange staining in automated cytofluorometry. Exp Cell Res 95: 143–153, 1975

27. Coulson PB, Bishop AO, Lenarduzzi R: Quantitation of cellular deoxyribonucleic acid by flow microfluorometry. J Histochem Cytochem 25: 1147–1153, 1977

28. Bauer KD, Dethlefsen LA: Total cellular RNA content: Correlation between flow cytometry and ultraviolet spectroscopy. J Histochem Cytochem 28: 493–498, 1980

29. Collste LG, Darzynkiewicz Z, Traganos F, Sharpless TK, Devonec M, Claps MLK, Whitmore Jr WF, Melamed MR: Cell-cycle distribution of urothelial tumour cells as measured by flow cytometry. Br J Cancer 40: 872–877, 1979

30. Collste LG, Devonec M, Darzynkiewicz Z, Traganos F, Sharpless TK, Whitmore Jr WF, Melamed MR: Bladder cancer diagnosis by flow cytometry. Correlation between cell samples from biopsy and bladder irrigation fluid. Cancer 45: 2389–2394, 1980

31. Klein FA, Herr HW, Sogani PC, Whitmore Jr WF, Melamed MR: Detection and follow-up of carcinoma of the urinary bladder by flow cytometry. Cancer 50: 389–395, 1982

32. Klein FA, Herr HW, Whitmore Jr WF, Sogani PC, Melamed MR: An evaluation of automated flow cytometry (FCM) in detection of carcinoma *in situ* of the urinary bladder. Cancer 50: 1003–1008, 1982

33. Klein FA, Herr HW, Sogani PC, Whitmore Jr WF, Melamed MR: Flow cytometry of normal and nonneoplastic diseases of the bladder: An estimate of the false positive rate. J Urol 127: 946–948, 1982

34. Klein FA, Melamed MR, Whitmore Jr WF, Herr HW, Sogani PC, Darzynkiewicz Z: Characterization of bladder papilloma by two-parameter DNA-RNA flow cytometry. Cancer Res 42: 1094–1097, 1982

35. Devonec M, Darzynkiewicz Z, Kostyrka-Claps ML, Collste L, Whitmore Jr WF, Melamed MR: Flow cytometry of low stage bladder tumors: correlation with cytologic and cytoscopic diagnosis. Cancer 49: 109–118, 1982

36. Melamed MR, Klein FA: Flow cytometry of urinary bladder irrigation specimens. Human Path 15: 302–305, 1984

37. Tribukait B, Moberger G, Zetterberg A: Methodological aspects of rapid-flow cytofluorometry for DNA analysis of human urinary bladder cells. In: First International Symposium on Pulse-cytophotometry, Haanen CAM, Hilen HFP, Wessels JMC (eds). European Press Medikon, Ghent, Belgium, 50–60, 1975

38. Farsund T: Selective sampling of cells for morphological and quantitative cytology of bladder epithelium. J Urol 128: 267–271, 1982

39. Krishan A: Flow cytometry: long-term storage of propidium iodide/citrate-stained material. Stain Tech 52: 339–343, 1977

40. Frankfurt OS, Slocum HK, Rustum YM, Arbruck SG, Pavelic ZP, Petrelli N, Huben RP, Pontes EJ, Greco WR: Flow cytometric analysis of DNA aneuploidy in primary and metastatic human solid tumors. Cytometry 5: 71–80, 1984

41. Arndt-Jovin DJ, Jovin TM: Analysis and sorting of living cells according to deoxyribonucleic acid content. J Histochem Cytochem 25: 585–589, 1977

266

42. Hamori E, Arndt-Jovin DJ, Grimwade BG, Jovin TM: Selection of viable cells with known DNA content. Cytometry 1: 132–135, 1980

43. Latt SA: Fluorescent probes of DNA microstructure and synthesis. In: Flow Cytometry and Sorting, Melamed MR, Mullaney PF, Mendelsohn ML (eds). John Wiley and Sons, New York, 263–284, 1979

44. Darzynkiewicz Z: Acridine orange as a molecular probe in studies of nucleic acids *in situ*. In: Flow Cytometry and Sorting, Melamed MR, Mullaney PF, Mendelsohn ML (eds). John Wiley and Sons, New York, 285–316, 1979

45. Cooper EH, Levi PE, Anderson CK, Williams RE: The evolution of tumor cell populations in human bladder cancer. Br J Urol 41: 714–717, 1969

46. Falor WH: Chromosomes in noninvasive papillary carcinoma of the bladder. J Am Med Assoc 216: 791–794, 1971

47. Spooner ME, Cooper EH: Chromosome constitution of transitional cell carcinoma of the urinary bladder. Cancer 29: 1401–1412, 1972

48. Sandberg AA: Chromosome markers and progression in bladder cancer. Cancer Res 37: 2950–2956, 1977

49. Falor WH, Ward RM: Prognosis in early carcinoma of the bladder based on chromosomal analysis. J. Urol 119: 44–48, 1978

50. Levi PE, Cooper EH, Anderson CK, Williams RE: Analyses of DNA content, nuclear size and cell proliferation of transitional cell carcinoma in man. Cancer 23: 1074–1085, 1969

51. Fosså SD: DNA-variations in neighbouring epithelium in patients with bladder carcinoma. Acta Pathol Microbiol Scand [A] 85: 603–610, 1977

52. Fosså SD, Kaalhus O, Scott-Knudsen O: The clinical and histopathological significance of Feulgen DNA-values in transitional cell carcinoma of the human urinary bladder. Eur J Cancer 13: 1155–1162, 1977

53. Wijkström H, Granberg-Öhman I, Tribukait B: Chromosomal and DNA patterns in transitional cell bladder carcinoma. A comparative cytogenetic and flow-cytofluorometric DNA study. Cancer 53: 1718–1723, 1984

54. Granberg-Öhman I, Tribukait B, Wijkström H, Alim A, Berlin T: Chromosome and DNA cytometric study of a papillary carcinoma of the bladder with a high stemline and numerous double minutes. Cancer Genet Cytogenet 5: 227–235, 1982

55. Barlogie B, Raber MN, Schumann J, Johnson TS, Drewinko B, Swartzendruber DE, Göhde W, Andreeff M, Freireich EJ: Flow cytometry in clinical cancer research. Cancer Res 43: 3982–3997, 1983

56. Darzynkiewicz Z, Traganos F, Kapuscinski J, Staiano-Coico L, Melamed MR: Accessibility of DNA *in situ* to various fluorochromes: Relationship to chromatin changes during erythroid differentiation of Friend leukemia cells. Cytometry 5: 355–363, 1984

57. Evenson DP, Melamed MR: Rapid analysis of normal and abnormal cell types in human semen and testis biopsies by flow cytometry. J Histochem Cytochem 31 (suppl 1A): 248–253, 1983

58. Evenson DP, Klein FA, Whitmore WF, Melamed MR: Flow cytometric evaluation of sperm from patients with testicular carcinoma. J Urol 132: 1220–1225, 1984

59. McDivitt RW, Stone KR, Meyer JS: A method for dissociation of viable human breast cancer cells that produces flow cytometric kinetic information similar to that obtained by thymidine labeling. Cancer Res 44: 2628–2633, 1984

60. Frankfurt OS, Greco WR, Slocum HK, Arbuck SG, Gamarra M, Pavelic ZP, Rustum YM: Proliferative characteristics of primary and metastatic human solid tumors by DNA flow cytometry. Cytometry 5: 629–635, 1984

61. Tribukait B, Esposti PL: Quantitative flow-microfluorometric analysis of the DNA in cells from neoplasms of the urinary bladder: Correlation of aneuploidy with histological grading and the cytological findings. Urol Res 6: 201–205, 1978

62. Pedersen T, Larsen JK, Krarup T: Characterization of bladder tumours by flow cytometry on bladder washings. Eur Urol 4: 351–355, 1978

63. Vindeløv LL: Flow microfluorometric analysis of nuclear DNA in cells from solid tumors and cell suspensions. A new method for rapid isolation and staining of nuclei. Virchows Arch B Cell Pathol 24: 227–242, 1977

64. Tribukait B, Gustafson H, Esposti P-L: The significance of ploidy and proliferation in the clinical and biological evaluation of bladder tumours. A study of 100 untreated cases. Br J Urol 54: 130–135, 1982

65. UICC (Union International Contre le Cancer): TNM classification of malignant tumours. Geneva: International Union Against Cancer, 1974

66. WHO (World Health Organization): International histological classification of tumours, No. 10. In: Histological Typing of Urinary Bladder Tumors. Mostofi FK, Sobin LH, Torloni H (eds). World Health Organization, Geneva, 1973

67. Farsund T, Laerum OD, Høstmark J: Ploidy disturbance of normal-appearing bladder mucosa in patients with urothelial cancer: relationship to morphology. J Urol 130: 1076–1082, 1983

68. Farsund T, Hoestmark JG, Laerum OD: Relation between flow cytometric DNA distribution and pathology in human bladder cancer. A report on 69 cases. Cancer 54: 1771–1777, 1984

69. Farsund T, Høstmark J: Mapping of cell sycle distribution in normal human urinary bladder epithelium. Scand J Urol Nephrol 17: 51–56, 1983

70. Melamed MR: Flow cytometry of the urinary bladder. Urol Clinics of North America 11: 599–608, 1984

71. Tribukait B, Gustafson H, Esposti P: Ploidy and proliferation in human bladder tumors as measured by flowcytofluorometric DNA-analysis and its relation to histopathology and cytology. Cancer 43: 1742–1751, 1979

72. Jakobsen A, Bichel P, Sell A: Flow cytometric investigations of human bladder carcinoma compared to histological classification. Urol Res 7: 109–112, 1979

73. Granberg–Öhman I, Tribukait B, Wijkström H, Berlin T, Collste LG: Papillary carcinoma of the urinary bladder. A study of chromosomal and cytofluorometric DNA analysis. Urol Res 8: 87–93, 1980

74. Gustafson H, Tribukait B, Esposti PL: The prognostic value of DNA analysis in primary carcinoma *in situ* of the urinary bladder. Scand J Urol Nephrol 16: 141–146, 1982

75. Jakobsen A, Mommsen S, Olsen S: Characterization of ploidy level in bladder tumors and selected site specimens by flow cytometry. Cytometry 4: 170–173, 1983

76. Bergkvist A, Ljungqvist A, Moberger G: Classification of bladder tumours based on the cellular pattern. Acta Chir Scand 130: 371–378, 1965

77. Gustafson H, Tribukait B, Esposti PL: DNA profile and tumour progression in patients with superficial bladder tumours. Urol Res 10: 13–18, 1982

78. Whitmore Jr WF: The natural history of prostatic cancer. Cancer 32: 1104–1112, 1973

79. Tavares AS, Costa J, Costa Maia J: Correlation between ploidy and prognosis in prostatic carcinoma. J Urol 109: 676–679, 1973

80. Zetterberg A, Esposti P-L: Cytophotometric DNA-analysis of aspirated cells from prostatic carcinoma. Acta Cytol 20: 46–57, 1976

81. Zetterberg A, Esposti PL: Prognostic significance of nuclear DNA levels in prostatic carcinoma. Scand J Urol Nephrol 55 (suppl): 53–58, 1980

82. Sprenger E, Michaelis WE, Vogt-Schaden M, Otto C: The significance of DNA flow-through fluorescence cytophotometry for the diagnosis of prostate carcinoma. Beitr Path 159: 292–298, 1976

83. Bichel P, Frederiksen P, Kjoer T, Thommesen P, Vindeløv LL: Flow microfluorometry and transrectal fine-needle biopsy in the classification of human prostatic carcinoma. Cancer 40: 1206–1211, 1977

84. Frederiksen P, Thommesen P, Kjoer TB, Bichel P: Flow cytometric DNA analysis in fine needle

aspiration biopsies from patients with prostatic lesions. Diagnostic value and relation to clinical stages. Acta Pathol Microbiol Scand (A) 86: 461–464, 1978

85. Zimmermann A, Truss F: Comparative cytologic and flow-through cytophotometric studies in prostate cells. Urologe A 17: 391–394, 1978

86. Rönström L, Tribukait B, Esposti P-L: DNA pattern and cytological findings in fine-needle aspirates of untreated prostatic tumors. A flow-cytofluorometric study. Prostate 2: 79–88, 1981

87. Tribukait B, Rönström L, Esposti P-L: Quantitative and qualitative aspects of flow DNA measurements related to the cytologic grade in prostatic carcinoma. Anal Quant Cytol 5: 107–111, 1983

88. Frankfurt OS, Chin JL, Englander LS, Greco WR, Pontes JE, Rustum YM: Relationship between DNA ploidy, glandular differentiation, and tumor spread in human prostate cancer. Cancer Res 45: 1418–1423, 1985

89. Gleason DF: Classification of prostatic carcinomas. Cancer Chemotherapy Reports 50: 125–128, 1966

90. Gleason DF, Mellinger GT and V.A. Research Group: Prediction of prognosis for prostatic adenocarcinoma by combined histological grading and clinical staging. J Urol 111: 58–64, 1974

91. Schwabe HW, Adolphs H-D, Vogel J: Flow-cytophotometric studies in renal carcinoma. Urol Res 11: 121–125, 1983

92. Hermanek P, Sigel A, Chlepas S: Histological grading of renal cell carcinoma. Eur Urol 2: 189–191, 1976

93. Bennington JL, Mayall BH: DNA cytometry on four-micrometer sections of paraffin-embedded human renal adenocarcinomas and adenomas. Cytometry 4: 31–39, 1983

94. Baisch H, Otto U, König K, Klöppel G, Köllermann M, Linden WA: DNA content of human kidney carcinoma cells in relation to histological grading. Br J Cancer 45: 878–886, 1982

95. Syrjänen K, Hjelt L: Grading of human renal adenocarcinoma. Scand J Urol Nephrol 12: 49–55, 1978

96. Otto U, Baisch H, Huland H, Klöppel G: Tumor cell deoxyribonucleic acid content and prognosis in human renal cell carcinoma. J Urol 132: 237–239, 1984

97. Chin JL, Pontes JE, Frankfurt OS: Flow cytometric deoxyribonucleic acid analysis of primary and metastatic human renal cell carcinoma. J Urol 133: 582–585, 1985

98. Robson CJ, Churchill BM, Anderson W: The results of radical nephrectomy for renal cell carcinoma. J Urol 101: 297–301, 1969

99. Ljungberg B, Stenling R, Roos O: DNA content in renal cell carcinoma with reference to tumor heterogeneity. Cancer 56: 503–508, 1985

100. Meyer JS, Hixon B: Advanced stage and early relapse of breast carcinomas associated with high thymidine labeling indices. Cancer Res 39: 4042–4047, 1979

101. Hansson L, Tribukait B, Lewensohn R, Ringborg U: Flow cytofluorometric DNA analyses of metastases of human malignant melanomas. Anal Quant Cytol 4: 99–104, 1982

102. Meyer JS: Growth and cell kinetic measurements in human tumors. Pathol Annual 16 (pt 2): 54–81, 1981

103. Fulker MJ, Cooper EH, Tanaka T: Proliferation and ultrastructure of papillary transitional cell carcinoma of the human bladder. Cancer 27: 71–82, 1971

104. Roters M, Laemmel A, Kastendieck H, Becker H: DNA distribution pattern of prostatic lesions measured by flow cytometry. Acta Pathol Microbiol Scand (suppl 274): 431–435, 1981

105. Melicow MM: Tumors of the bladder: A multifaceted problem. J Urol 112: 467–478, 1974

106. Klein FA, Herr HW, Whitmore Jr WF, Pinsky CH, Oettgen HT, Melamed MR: Automated flow cytometry to monitor intravesical BCG therapy of superficial bladder cancer. Urol 17: 310–314, 1981

107. Staiano-Coico L, Huffman J, Wolf R, Pinsky CM, Herr HW, Whitmore Jr WF, Oettgen HF, Darzynkiewicz Z, Melamed MR: Monitoring intravesical Bacillus Calmette-Guer in treatment of bladder carcinoma with flow cytometry. J Urol 133: 786–788, 1985

108. Adolphs HD, Schwabe HW, Helpap B, Volz C: Cytomorphological and histological studies on the urothelium during and after chemoimmune prophylaxis. Urol Res 12: 129–133, 1984

109. Farsund T, Laerum OD, Høstmark J, Jordfald G: Local chemotherapeutic effects in bladder cancer demonstrated by selective sampling and flow cytometry. J Urol 131: 22–32, 1984

110. Klein FA, Whitmore Jr WF, Wolf RM, Herr HW, Sogani PC, Staiano-Coico L, Melamed MR: Presumptive downstaging from preoperative irradiation for bladder cancer as determined by flow cytometry: Prelimanry report. Int J Radiat Oncol Biol Phys 9: 487–491, 1983

111. Wijkström H, Gustafson H, Tribukait B: Deoxyribonucleic acid analysis in the evaluation of transitional cell carcinoma before cystectomy. J Urol 132: 894–898, 1984

112. Kjaer TB, Thommesen P, Frederiksen P, Bichel P: DNA content in cells aspirated from carcinoma of the prostate treated with oestrogenic compounds. Urol Res 7: 249–251, 1979

113. Schwabe HW, Adolphs H-D, Hartlapp J: Flow-cytophotometric studies on urine sediments of patients treated with anti-cancer-drugs. Urol Res 11: 159–162, 1983

114. Kraemer PM, Petersen DF, Van Dilla MA: DNA constancy in heteroploidy and the stem line theory of tumors. Science 174: 714–717, 1971

115. Gown AM, Vogel AM: Monoclonal antibodies to intermediate filament proteins of human cells: Unique and cross-reacting antibodies. J Cell Biol 95: 414–424, 1982

116. Gown AM, Vogel AM: Monoclonal antibodies to human intermediate filament proteins: II. Distribution of filament proteins in normal human tissues. Am J Path 114: 309–321, 1984

117. Ramaekers F, Huysmans A, Moesker O, Kant A, Jap P, Herman C, Vooijs P: Monoclonal antibody to keratin filaments, specific for glandular epithelia and their tumors. Use in surgical pathology. Lab Invest 49: 353–361, 1983

118. Achtstätter T, Moll R, Moore B, Franke WW: Cytokeratin polypeptide patterns of different epithelia of the human male urogenital tract: Immunofluorescence and gel electrophoretic studies. J Histochem Cytochem 33: 415–426, 1985

119. Osborn M, Weber K: Intermediate filaments: Cell-type-specific markers in differentiation and pathology. Cell 31: 303–306, 1982

120. Ramaekers FCS, Haag D, Kant A, Moesker O, Jap PHK, Vooijs GP: Coexpression of keratin- and vimentin-type intermediate filaments in human metastatic carcinoma cells. Proc Nat Acad Sci, USA 80: 2618–2622, 1983

121. Miettinen M, Lehto V-P, Virtanen I: Antibodies to intermediate filament proteins in the diagnosis and classification of human tumors. Ultrastruct Pathol 7: 83–107, 1984

122. Nelson WG, Battifora H, Santana H, Sun T-T: Specific keratins as molecular markers for neoplasms with a stratified epithelial origin. Cancer Res 44: 1600–1603, 1984

123. Settle SA, Hellström I, Hellström KE: A monoclonal antibody recognizing cytoskeletal keratins of stratified epithelia and bladder carcinomas. Exp Cell Res 157: 293–306, 1985

124. Ramaekers F, Puts J, Moesker O, Kant A, Jap P, Vooijs P: Demonstration of keratin in human adenocarcinomas. Am J Pathol 111: 213–223, 1983

125. Franke WW, Schmid E, Winter S, Osborn M, Weber K: Widespread occurrence of intermediate-sized filaments of the vimentin-type in cultured cells from diverse vertebrates. Exp Cell Res 123: 25–46, 1979

126. Virtanen I, Lehto V-P, Lehtonen E, Vartio T, Stenman S, Kurki P, Wager C, Small JV, Dahl D, Badley RA: Expression of intermediate filaments in cultured cells. J Cell Sci 50: 45–63, 1981

127. Connell ND, Rheinwald JG: Regulation of the cytoskeleton in mesothelial cells: reversible loss of keratin and increase in vimentin during rapid growth in culture. Cell 34: 245–253, 1983

128. Ben-Ze'ev A: Cell density and cell shape-related regulation of vimentin and cytokeratin synthesis. Inhibition of vimentin synthesis and appearance of a new 45 kD cytokeratin in dense epithelial cell cultures. Exp Cell Res 157: 520–532, 1985

129. Ramaekers FCS, Beck H, Vooijs GP, Herman CJ: Flow-cytometric analysis of mixed cell populations using intermediate filament antibodies. Exp Cell Res 153: 249–253, 1984

130. Oud PS, Henderik JBJ, Beck HLM, Veldhuizen JAM, Vooijs GP, Herman CJ, Ramaekers FCS:

Flow cytometric analysis and sorting of human endometrial cells after immunocytochemical labeling for cytokeratin using a monoclonal antibody. Cytometry 6: 159–164, 1985

131. Köhler G, Milstein C: Continuous cultures of fused cells secreting antibody of predefined specificity. Nature 256: 495–497, 1975

132. Frankel AE, Rouse RV, Herzenberg LA: Human prostate specific and shared differentiation antigens defined by monoclonal antibodies. Proc Nat Acad Sci, USA 79: 903–907, 1982

133. Cordon-Cardo C, Bander NH, Fradet Y, Finstad CL, Whitmore WF, Lloyd KO, Oettgen HF, Melamed MR, Old LJ: Immunoanatomic dissection of the human urinary tract by monoclonal antibodies. J Histochem Cytochem 32: 1035–1040, 1984

134. Lowe DH, Handley HH, Schmidt J, Royston I, Glassy MC: A human monoclonal antibody reactive with human prostate. J Urol 132: 780–785, 1984

135. Raynor RH, Hazra TA, Moncure CW, Mohanakumar T: Characterization of a monoclonal antibody, KR-P8, that detects a new prostate-specific marker. J Nat Cancer Inst 73: 617–625, 1984

136. Bander NH, Cordon-Cardo C, Finstad CL, Whitmore Jr WF, Vaughan Jr ED, Oettgen HF, Melamed M, Old LJ: Immunohistologic dissection of the human kidney using monoclonal antibodies. J Urol 133: 502–505, 1985

137. Finstad CL, Cordon-Cardo C, Bander NH, Whitmore WF, Melamed MR, Old LJ: Specificity analysis of mouse monoclonal antibodies defining cell surface antigens of human renal cancer. Proc Nat Acad Sci, USA 82: 2955–2959, 1959

138. Hamburger AW, Reid YA, Pelle B, Milo GE, Noyes I, Krakauer H, Fuhrer JP: Isolation and characterization of a monoclonal antibody specific for epithelial cells. Cancer Res 45: 783–790, 1985

139. Brawer MK, Peehl DM, Stamey TA, Bostwick DG: Keratin immunoreactivity in the benign and neoplastic human prostate. Cancer Res 45: 3663–3667, 1985

140. Chopin DK, deKernion JB, Rosenthal DL, Fahey JL: Monoclonal antibodies against transitional cell carcinoma for detection of malignant urothelial cells in bladder washing. J Urol 134: 260–265, 1985

141. Czerniak B, Darzynkiewicz Z, Staiano-Coico L, Herz F, Koss LG: Expression of Ca antigen in relation to cell cycle in cultured human tumor cells. Cancer Res 44: 4342–4346, 1984

142. Dolbeare F: Dynamic assay of enzyme activities in single cells by flow cytometry. J Histochem Cytochem 27: 1644–1646, 1979

143. Martin JC, Swartzendruber DE: Time: A new parameter for kinetic measurements in flow cytometry. Science 207: 199–201, 1980

144. Haskill S, Kivinen S, Nelson K, Fowler Jr WC: Detection of intratumor heterogeneity by simultaneous multiparameter flow cytometric analysis with enzyme and DNA markers. Cancer Res 43: 1003–1009, 1983

145. Schwabe HW, Adolphs H-D: Improved application of impulse cytophotometry for the diagnosis of urinary bladder carcinoma. Urol Res 10: 61–66, 1982

146. Pollack A, Moulis H, Block NL, Irvin GL III: Quantitation of cell kinetic responses using simultaneous flow cytometric measurements of DNA and nuclear protein. Cytometry 5: 473–481, 1984

147. Clevenger CV, Bauer KD, Epstein AL: A method for simultaneous nuclear immunofluorescence and DNA content quantitation using monoclonal antibodies and flow cytometry. Cytometry 6: 208–214, 1985

148. Paulie S, Hansson Y, Lundblad M-L, Perlmann P: Lectins as probes for identification of tumor-associated antigens on urothelial and colonic carcinoma cell lines. Int J Cancer 31: 297–303, 1983

149. Ghazizadeh M, Kagawa S, Izumi K, Kurokawa K: Immunohistochemical localization of T antigen-like substance in benign hyperplasia and adenocarcinoma of the prostate. J Urol 132: 1127–1130, 1984

150. Van NT, Raber M, Barrows GH, Barlogie B: Estrogen receptor analysis by flow cytometry. Science 224: 876–879, 1984

151. Maron R, Jackson RA, Jacobs S, Eisenbarth G, Kahn CR: Analysis of the insulin receptor by anti-receptor antibodies and flow cytometry. Proc Nat Acad Sci, USA 81: 7446–7450, 1984

152. Donnelly BJ, Lakey WH, McBlain WA: Estrogen receptor in human benign prostatic hyperplasia. J Urol 130: 183–187, 1983

153. Donnelly BJ, Lakey WH, McBlain WA: Androgen binding sites on nuclear matrix of normal and hyperplastic human prostate. J Urol 131: 806–811, 1984

154. Benson Jr RC, Utz DC, Holicky E, Veneziale CM: Androgen receptor binding activity in human prostate cancer. Cancer 55: 382–388, 1985

155. Schutte B, Reynders MMJ, Bosman FT, Blijham GH: Flow cytometric determination of DNA ploidy level in nuclei isolated from paraffin-embedded tissue. Cytometry 6: 26–30, 1985

156. Hedley DW, Friedlander ML, Taylor IW, Rugg CA, Musgrove EA: Method for analysis of cellular DNA content of paraffin-embedded pathological material using flow cytometry. J Histochem Cytochem 31: 1333–1335, 1983

157. Hedley DW, Friedlander ML, Taylor IW, Rugg CA, Musgrove EA: DNA flow cytometry of paraffin-embedded tissue. Cytometry 5: 660, 1984

Editorial Comment

JEFFRY L. HUFFMAN

Automated flow cytometry (FMC) has made a substantial impact on the approach to urologic carcinoma, specifically regarding the diagnosis and follow-up of bladder, prostatic, renal and adrenal tumors. The most common application has been in bladder carcinoma with its advantage of availability of obtaining bladder specimens by a relatively non-invasive urethral catheterization. Dr. Kenneth R. Stone has clearly reviewed the history and multiple applications of flow cytometry. The purpose of this commentary is to review some of the limitations of the technology and present recent applications.

One advantage of FCM has been its ability to analyze multiple parameters simultaneously on single cells. Not only can the relative DNA content and distribution be evaluated, but cellular RNA, presence or absence of cellular antigens along with other intra-cellular components, and enzymatic reactions can be evaluated.

FCM also is an objective method allowing sequential specimens to be compared in a quantitative fashion. This is of value during treatment of disease allowing the effects of therapy to be monitored along with evaluating progression or regression of disease.

Limitations of flow cytometry

Many medical centers have accumulated a tremendous amount of laboratory and clinical data within their flow cytometry facilities and have developed standardized methods of cell collection, preparation, staining, and computer-generated analysis. However, there are relatively few controls employed at each step of the analysis. Experienced centers may argue correctly that exhaustive controls are not necessary based on their record of clinical correlations; but when results between centers are compared, standardization and built-in controls at every stem become necessary.

The methods of sample collection are poorly controlled. Bladder barbotage is the usual method to obtain bladder washings, however, the exfoliation of cells is not constant. Since the flow cytometry reading is based on percentages of cells in different populations, the effect of the barbotage on cell exfoliation is highly relevant. For example, if cancerous cells exfoliate more readily than normal cells, the relative populations within the sample will be skewed towards the carcinima cells. Again, this may not be a problem within one center if the same methods of collection are employed; however, as stated above, comparison between centers becomes difficult. Samples obtained from patients in an outpatient clinic by barbotage through a 16F catheter are relatively less cellular than those obtained endoscopically under anesthesia using a resectoscope sheath and Ellik evacuator. This same argument can be used to question the results of a study employing flow cytometry to judge the effect of radiation therapy. Does radiation therapy influence exfoliation of one type of cell over another? Will enough 'normal cells' be exfoliated to hide an aneuploid population, thus leading to a false-negative result? Satisfactory answers to these questions will require much more clinical investigation.

A serious limitation of FCM is the large numbers of cells required for each sample. An improvement in the application to bladder cancer would be the ability to perform analyses on voided specimens. However, a larger number of cells is required for analysis than that available with voided samples. Most centers perform their computer analysis using 5,000 counted cells, far more than present in voided samples. Thus, bladder barbotage is used and more than 5,000 cells are obtained.

Antigen analysis by FCM quantitative immunofluorescence requires approximately 25,000 cells per specimen form the sample collection resulting in 5,000 cells for analysis after multiple transfers, incubations and filtrations of the cell suspension. Do these 5,000 measured cells represent a satisfactory cross-section of the original population? Theoretically, some of the unanalyzed 20,000 cells may contain information not identified in the 5,000 counted cells.

Another limitation of FCM in bladder cancer is the influence of non-urothelial cells, e.g., inflammatory or stromal cells, on the flow cytometric measurement. Although some methods, e.g., treatment with Triton-X, are used to limit the numbers of inflammatory cells in the sample, nucleated, non-urothelial cells remain in specimens. This is especially true in those patients who have had intravesical therapy with agents such as BCG, mitomycin or doxorubicin, which often generate an intense inflammatory response reflected in the urine. The potential influence of lymphocytes on the flow cytometry analysis is readily apparent. The cytometer views a lymphocyte the same as a normal urothelial cell, both having identical DNA content. In fact, many centers use human peripheral bood lymphocytes as diploid control. Therefore, if there is an abundance of lymphocytes in the washing, the percentage of normal diploid cells would be falsely elevated. This may obscure an aneuploid stemline with relatively few cells or significantly alter the percent of hyperdiploid cells.

As Dr. Stone points out, attempts have been made to isolate only the cells of interest, i.e., urothelial cells, within mixed cell populations using FCM [1–3]. A mouse monoclonal antibody identifying intermediate filament proteins or cytokeratin has been used with early success. Cytokeratin is found only in epithelial cells and not in connective tissue, smooth muscle, endothelium, blood cells, or other non-epithelial elements. With the help of computer-generated histograms, the population of cells staining positive for cytokeratin can be separated and reanalyzed specifically for DNA (Fig. 1A-D). The simplest and most reliable parameter for analysis by FCM is DNA content. At some centers, this is as accurate as conventional exfoliative cytology for the diagnosis of bladder cancer [4]. The diagnosis of carcinoma by FCM is based on the presence of cells with an abnormal DNA content (aneuploidy). This may be identified by a discrete multimodal distribution of DNA which is extremely accurate for the diagnosis of carcinoma. However, in a fairly substantial number of samples, there may not be a distinguishable peak but rather an increased number of cells with a hyperdiploid DNA content. There may also be a peak at the 4C level which cannot be separated from a normal tetraploid peak of G2, mitotic, or binucleated cells. Thus in these instances, the diagnosis of carcinoma is difficult. In fact, some centers have empirically established an abnormal value as one having greater than 15% of cells hyperdiploid. This value is based on experience with many cases of carcinoma. Within centers with a large experience, these results have been very reliable; however, direct comparison with results from centers not employing identical methods of sample collection, cell staining, and computer analysis may be misleading.

Future applications of flow cytometry

The current expense of automated flow cytometry instrumentation and the need for engineering and computer assistance makes this technique not routinely applicable to the practicing urologist. Thus, for flow cytometry to be an applicable clinical technique to a urology practice, it is necessary to transport specimens to a core FCM facility capable of performing the measurements. At the present time, basic studies have not been completed regarding the stability of cells and reproducibility of results

274

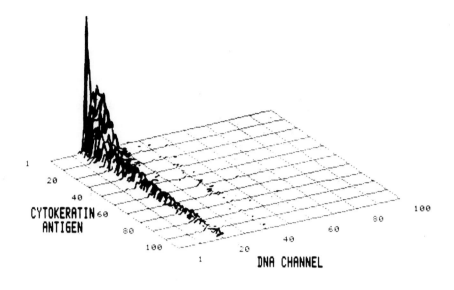

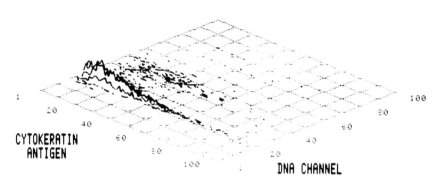

Figure 1. These pseudo-three dimensional histograms demonstrate cytokeratin antigen detection by FCM in bladder washings of patients with bladder papilloma (A), invasive carcinoma (B), and chronic cystitis (c). Histogram D (human lymphocytes) shows no detection as expected. Note the high percentage of cytokeratin-negative or non-urothelial cells in the diploid population of the histogram of the patient with chronic cystitis (C).

at one center compared to another. Therefore, if cells are to be transported from one hospital to another or from one city to another, controls and methods of transport will be very important.

The ease of transport is the appealing aspect of the applications of flow cytometry to paraffin-fixed specimens; early experimental results using prostate cancer models have been encouraging [5]. Once a biopsy or bladder washing is collected and fixed, it can be transported for subsequent analysis. However, adequate clinical controls at multiple centers have not yet been completed to allow satisfactory comparison of results.

The applications of flow cytometry as a research tool in urologic oncology are multiple. Many constituents of the cell can be examined using a variety of specific probes including mouse monoclonal antibodies. This technique employs a DNA stain, e.g., propidium iodide, and fluorescein isothiocyan-

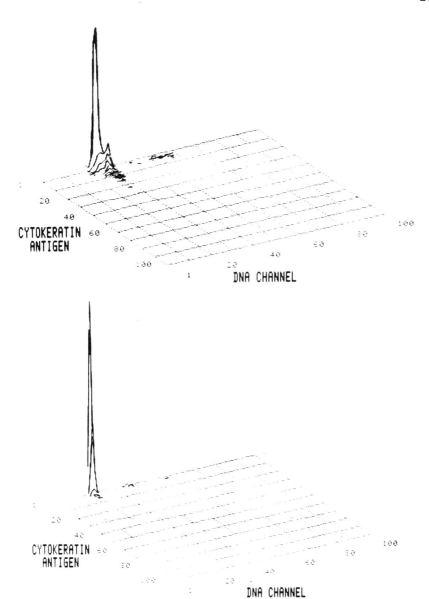

ate (FITC)-conjugated goat anti-mouse IgG which labels the monoclonal antibodies. In addition to the FCM immunofluorescence work with cytokeratin, preliminary work identifying cellular antigens related to human bladder carcinoma has also been completed.

This FCM process allows simultaneous measurement of DNA and cellular antigens and has been used to characterize histologically similar bladder cancers and to assess response in patients undergoing intravesical BCG therapy for carcinoma in situ [6]. The BCG study employed a mouse monoclonal antibody defining a highly restricted differentiation antigen of the urothelium (Om5). Bladder washings from 15 patients undergoing BCG therapy were analyzed for the presence or absence of the Om5 antigen. Thirteen of 15 patients had Om5 detected in exfoliated cells prior to initiation of BCG therapy. Nine of the 13 patients had persistently detectable Om5 after therapy and of these, 8 had

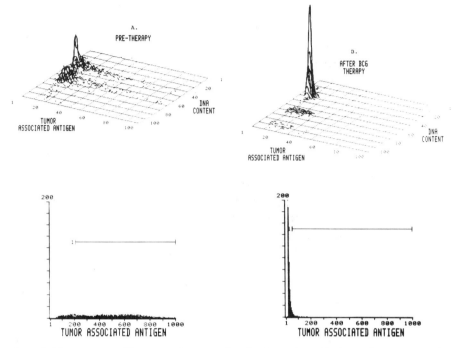

Figure 2. Flow cytometry histograms demonstrating the change in antibody binding to Om5 and in DNA content of exfoliated bladder epithelial cells from a patient with multifocal carcinoma in-situ treated with BCG. Note the loss of antibody binding cells in the histogram following BCG therapy (B), a (normal) tetraploid DNA population and the absence of aneuploid cells.

recurrent cancer by biopsy, positive urinary cytology, or both. Four patients lost OM5-labeled cells after therapy, and all of these patients were without evidence of recurrent disease by biopsy and cytology (Fig. 2A-D).

Microscopic immunofluorescence techniques to judge antibody binding are relatively subjective. Thus, the specific advantage of FCM quantitative immunofluorescence is the resultant percentage of cells exhibiting the antigen. This quantitative method allows direct comparison of sequential samples from the same patient and may help predict response to therapy or progression of disease.

The heterogeneity of human bladder carcinoma is well known; thus combinations of two or more antibodies may be necessary to stain all tumor cells and to discriminate subsets or tumor populations with differing characteristics. Whatever combination of antibodies that eventually proves must useful, it is now clear (1) that human bladder tumors can be characterized by monoclonal antibodies on the basis of cellular antigen expression, (2) that this characterization may be used to assess biological properties of the tumor and perhaps clinical status and response to therapy, and (3) that multiparameter measurements such as these are possible with flow cytometry. In fact, using a dual laser system with fluorescence emission at differing wavelengths [1], it is conceivable that more than one antigen can be evaluated simultaneously within a cell.

In summary, automated flow cytometry has thus far been a useful adjunct in the diagnosis and follow-up of many patients with urologic cancers. Its practicality for the practicing urologist has yet to be determined, mostly due to the expense of the instrumentation and the unavailability of satisfactory transport mechanisms to core facilities. Once transport mechanisms are refined and satisfactory controls determined, clinical utility may be seen. Certainly as a research tool, this technology has been exciting, and I expect such applications only to increase.

References

1. Sun T, Eichner R, Nelson WG, Tseng SCG, Weiss RA, Jarinen M, Woodcock-Mitchell J: Keratin Classes: Molecular markers for different types of epithelial differentiation. J Investing Dermatol 81: 109–115, 1983
2. Ramaekers FCS, Beck H, Vooijs GP, Herman CJ: Flow cytometric analysis of mixed cell population using intermediate filament antibodies. Exp Cell Res 153: 249–253, 1984
3. Huffman JL, Gerin-Chesa P, Gay H, Whitmore Jr WF, Melamed MR: Flow cytometric characterization of human bladder cells using a cytokeratin monoclonal antibody. Bull N Y Acad Med (in press)
4. Melamed MR: Flow cytometry of the urinary bladder. Urol Clin North Amer 11: 599–608, 1984
5. deVere White R, Naus GJ, Olsson CA, Deitch AD: Flow cytometry in fresh and formalin-fixed prostate tissue. Surg Forum 35: 659–661, 1984
6. Huffman JL, Fradet Y, Cordon-Cardo C, Herr HW, Pinskey CM, Oetlgen HF, Old LJ, Whitmore Jr WF, Melamed MR: Effect of intravesical BCG on detection of a urothelial differentiation antigen in exfoliated cells of carcinoma in situ of the human urinary bladder. Can Res 45: 5201–5204, 1985
7. Shapire HM, Schildkraut ER, Curbelo R, Turner RB, Webb RH, Brown DC, Block MJ: Cytomat-R: A computer-controlled multiple laser source multiparameter flow cytophotometer system. J Histochem Cytochem 25: 836–844, 1977

12. Approaches to the treatment of renal cell carcinoma

HOWARD N. WINFIELD and TIMOTHY L. RATLIFF

The over-riding fact today in the treatment of renal cell carcinoma (RCC) is that surgical excision is the only modality which can offer the patient a real change for cure. Evidence of metastatic spread beyond Gerota's fascia markedly limits the therapeutic role of surgery. Alternative methods of therapy such as radiotherapy, chemotherapy, and immunotherapy have demonstrated less than optimal results. Unfortunately, one-third of patients with RCC will present with metastases at diagnosis and approximately 50% of those patients operated on for cure will subsequently develop metastases. Despite this gloomy picture, medical centers throughout the world are making great efforts to develop new techniques of early diagnosis of RCC and modes of therapy to control or cure the more advanced tumor.

An attempt has been made to summarize current approaches in the management of RCC and to delineate some of the forefronts of treatment for this unpredictable malignancy.

Surgical options

Radical nephrectomy

This cancer operation is indicated for clinical Stage I, II, and IIIA. If there is pre-operative clinical evidence of local lymph node involvement (Stage IIIB or IIIC) or advanced disease (Stage IV), the role of radical nephrectomy for cure is not indicated and will be discussed later (see Table 1).

Radical nephrectomy involves an intraperitoneal laparotomy to rule out metastases, early ligation of the renal artery and vein, and then removal of the kidney and adrenal within an intact surrounding Gerota's fascia. The ureter and ipsilateral gonadal vein should be taken down to the level of the common iliac artery.

The rationale for performing a radical rather than a simple nephrectomy is based on the series by Robson and associates [1]. In this study of 88 patients

Ratliff, T.L. and Catalona, W.J. (eds), Genitourinary Cancer. ISBN 0–89838–830–9
© *1987, Martinus Nijhoff Publishers, Boston. Printed in the Netherlands.*

operated on between 1949 and 1964, it was demonstrated that tumor had spread into the peri-renal fat in 46% of case and to the ipsilateral adrenal in 6%. Thus, a simple nephrectomy would have compromised the chance of cure in over 50% of cases.

The surgical approaches to the kidney are diverse. The main objective is clear exposure of the tumor-containing kidney and ipsilateral adrenal so as to prevent tumor spillage and to obtain complete control of the renal pedicle and great vessels. There are advocates of the anterior transperitoneal, thoracoabdominal intrapleural and extrapleural approaches. The subcostal incision has been used for low lying tumors. The role of the posterior lumbotomy approach for cancer surgery is minimal. The advantages and disadvantages of each approach is summarized (see Table 2).

The technical aspects of these surgical procedures are beyond the scope of this review [2]. The operative mortality of a radical nephrectomy has been reported between 2–5% and up to 25% for major vascular tumor involvement [3, 4].

The five year survival rate after surgical intervention is closely related to the stage of the disease [1, 5–7] (see Table 3).

Role of lymph node dissection

Considerable controversy surrounds the role of retroperitoneal lymph node dissection (RPLND) in the management of renal cell carcinoma (RCC). Questions are: 1) does the lymph node dissection have a therapeutic or diagnostic purpose and; 2) is an extensive dissection more beneficial than a limited one?

The lymphatic drainage of the kidneys was exquisitely described by Parker [8] and later reviewed by Marshall [9]. A complete regional lymph node dissection for a right-sided kidney tumor should start at the diaphragm superiorly and extend inferiorly to the bifurcation of the inferior vena cava (IVC). It should include lateral caval, pre-caval, post-caval, and inter-aortocaval nodes. For a left sided tumor, the dissection should extend from the left crus of the diaphragm and

Table 1[a]. Staging of Renal Cell Carcinoma

Stage I	tumor confined to renal capsule.
Stage II	tumor extension beyond the renal capsule but still confined to Gerota's fascia.
Stage IIIA	tumor within Gerota's fasica but involving the renal vein and/or inferior vena cava.
Stage IIIB	tumor extension involving local lymph nodes.
Stage IIIC	tumor involvement of local lymph nodes and renal vein and/or IVC.
Stage IVA	tumor involvement of adjacent organs other than adrenal.
Stage IVB	distant metastases.

[a] Staging of Renal Cell Carcinoma — as per Robson, Churchill and Anderson, 1969

extend inferiorly to the bifurcation of the aorta, anterior and posterior to the aorta [9].

With increasing size of the RCC, especially if there is renal vein or IVC tumor thrombus, there will be parasitic vessels which feed the kidney in a completely disorganized fashion. The lymphatics which accompany this neovascularity provide unpredictable drainage for tumor dissemination [10].

Robson proposed performing complete RPLND. In this series of 88 cases, tumor involvement of lymph nodes was found in 22.7% [1]. Other series where extensive RPLND have been performed have shown an incidence of positive regional nodes varying from 6–32% [3, 6, 11, 12]. Other advocates of the extensive dissection claim a 5-year survival with positive nodes as high as 45% compared to 26% without node dissection [13]. However, most studies concerned with the role of RPLND are retrospective, not randomized, consisting of small

Table 2. Surgical approaches to radical nephrectomy

	Advantages	Disadvantages
Anterior transperitoneal Midline vertical Chevron Subcostal	– good control of renal pedicle – patients with thoracic spinal deformity – minimal circulatory compromise – bilateral tumors – ex-vivo bench surgery – thrombus in IVC	– difficult to visualize and mobilize large upper pole tumors from under diaphragm
Thoracoabdominal Extrapleural	– early control of renal pedicle – good exposure of upper pole kidney – minimal pulmonary compromise - no chest tube	– post-op pain – circulatory compromise in this position
Intrapleural	– for IVC control: infrahepatic suprahepatic – for solitary pulmonary metastases – choice of rib interspace required for best exposure to upper pole	– post-op pain – pulmonary complication – chest tube – positional circulatory compromise
Posterior lumbotomy	– decreased post-op pain	– poor pedicle control – poor access to peritoneal cavity

case series with variation in staging and unclear surgical limits. The diagnostic imaging for metastatic disease is considerably improved since the early study of Flocks [14].

Lymph node invasion usually indicates systemic spread [15]. Many patients with negative lymph nodes will die of disseminated tumor indicating blood borne metastases [10]. There may be an occasional patient with one or two positive nodes who may be cures by RPLND. Whether these rare patients justify extensive RPLND, with its associated morbidity, being performed in all patients is questionable. The alternative modes of non-surgical therapy are, unfortunately, limited.

The overall impression is that until a prospective randomized study clearly demonstrates improved survival with extensive RPLND, a limited regional dissection as described by deKernion should be performed [10]. This should provide information in staging the patient without increasing the morbidity. For the occasional patient with limited early nodal disease, this dissection may be curative.

Surgical management of tumor in the inferior vena cava

Tumor extending into the renal vein and inferior vena cava (IVC) occurs in 25% and 5–10% of cases of RCC respectively [16, 17]. Initially, reports of IVC tumor involvement were very pessimistic. Later reports by Marshall and Skinner encouraged more aggressive surgical approaches with reported 5 year survivals of 45–55% [18, 19]. The non-surgical approach had a dismal survival of less than 1 year. However, after interpreting the result further, it appears that the proximal extent of the tumor in the IVC has important prognostic significance. Assuming no evidence of metastatic disease at presentation, Sosa and associates reviewed the records of 24 patients with IVC involvement [20]. He found that with surgical therapy, mean survival was 61 months for infrahepatic vena caval involvment as opposed to 23 months for tumor thrombus extending to the level of the hepatic veins or beyond the diaphragm. In this latter group, there was a likelihood of discovering tumor in the regional lymph nodes and/or perinephric fat, thus obviating cure in most cases. The occurence of metastatic disease in addition to intracaval tumor thrombus portends a dismal prognosis [21]. There are studies which claim 5 year survival of up to 35% after surgical resection in which IVC

Table 3. 5-Year survival rates after radical nephrectomy

Stage I	56- 82%
Stage II	43-100%
Stage III	8- 51%
Stage IV	0- 13%

tumor involvement is accompanied by a solitary metastasis [15, 21, 22]. Needless to say, the solitary metastasis is frequently followed by further foci of metastases.

Therefore, due to the lack of alternative successful forms of therapy, aggressive surgical intervention is suggested in Stage IIIA renal cell carcinoma. One may subdivide the degree of caval involvement according to Table 4, to determine surgical approach and prognosis.

For infradiaphragmatic tumor thrombus, a midline or thoracoabdominal incision allows good control of the IVC above and below the tumor thrombus as well as the contralateral renal vein. Mobilization of the liver is sometimes requires [23]. Should tumor be found invading into the wall of the IVC, resection of the involved wall is required along with the nephrectomy specimen [24]. Prior to this, however, the collateral venous circularion of the remaining kidney must be assessed. In most cases, this circulation is adequate for the left kidney after acute interruption of venous return, but insufficient for right kidney drainage [16]. Renal venous pressures greater than 40mm pressure following soft clamping will require some form of venous diversion to avoid destruction of the remaining kidney. Surgical options consist of utilization of a saphenous vein graft to the portal vein or other major venous channel [25], autotransplantation of the remaining kidney, or the new technique of pericardial patch graft [26].

For supradiaphragmatic involvement of the IVC with tumor thrombus, a chest approach is required. Preliminary abdominal laparotomy should reveal no evidence of local or distant metastatic disease. Then a midline sternotomy will allow access to the mediastinum and heart as needed. If the tumor thrombus has not entered the right atrium, the IVC may be clamped where it traverses the pericardium. The Pringle manoeuver reduces blood loss (soft clamping the entire porta hepatis). Should the venous return be insufficient by the superior vena cava alone, then cardiopulmonary bypass is required. For tumor extending into the heart, bypass surgery is required. A free floating tumor thrombus can often be gently milked from the IVC with a minimal amount of difficulty. The major complications of massive hemorrhaging and tumor emboli have been reduced in recent years by numerous new surgical technical improvements and approach [18–20, 27–29].

For tumor thrombus infiltrating the wall of IVC above the diaphragm, the tumor is considered unresectable in certain centers. However, the use of the pericardial patch as a tube like graft has been proposed [26], but the risk seem

Table 4. Renal Cell Carcinoma tumor thrombus in Inferior Vena Cava (IVC)

A	Infradiaphragmatic (subhepatic)	non-infiltrating wall infiltrating wall
B	Supradiaphragmatic (and hepatic veins)	non-infiltrating wall infiltrating wall

awesome. In some cases, the tumor may be adherent in only a few areas of the cava and can be dissected free after suitable vascular control.

The operative mortality for IVC involvement below the hepatic veins and the diaphragm is approximately 6.5% as opposed to hepatic vein or supradiaphragmatic caval involvement where the intraoperative mortality is at least 25% [20, 21, 24].

Role of surgery in bilateral renal cell carcinoma

Bilateral RCC may occur either simultaneously or sequentially in both kidneys. It is unclear whether bilateral RCC reflects two separate primary lesions or is a metastatic process from one kidney to the other. In pathological studies, the latter phenomenon is reported to occur in 30% of cases [30]. However, in clinical practice, bilateral RCC (synchronous and asynchronous) occurs in 1.8–4% cases [7, 31]. The incidence is higher in patients with Von Hippel-Lindau disease [32].

Aggressive surgical treatment allows reasonably good success provided there is no other evidence of metastatic disease. The surgical options are delinated in Table 5. The advancement in techniques for partial nephrectomy with use of intra-operative mannitol, renal cooling and minimal renal vascular pedicle occlusion have improved the success in the management of bilateral RCC. Whether one should perform radical nephrectomy first and then the partial nephrectomy at a later date or vice versa is controversial [33, 34]. There are advocates of performing surgery on both kidneys at the same time. They claim that serum creatinine will initially rise but dialysis usually is not required [31]. Overall, however, the survival does not seem to be dependent on whether a single or combined operative approach is used [35].

The use of 'bench surgery' utilizing intracellular perfusate (Collin's solution) is applicable for large complex central lesions. Total bilateral nephrectomy and dialysis is sometimes required when both kidneys are extensively involved with tumor. This extirpative surgery may seem overly heroic, however, one should consider that the 5 year survival rate of patients with end stage disease on chronic hemodialysis is 40–50%, which is well above that of untreated renal carcinoma.

Table 5. Surgical options for bilateral Renal Cell Carcinoma or Carcinoma in solitary kidney

1	Partial nephrectomy in situ
2	Partial nephrectomy ex vivo — bench surgery with autotransplantation
3	Total bilateral radical nephrectomy and dialysis. Possible renal transplantation (Allograft)
4	Tumor enucleation
5	Adjuvant laser therapy to tumor bed (for partial nephrectomy or tumor enucleation)

Should there be no evidence of metastatic disease after one year, subsequent renal transplantation is an alternative [36]. Although there are reported cases of this practice, the risk of immunosuppression and resultant exacerbation of preexisting clones of malignant cells is a real threat. Enucleation of the renal tumor runs the risk of leaving behind tumor cells which have penetrated beyond the tumor capsule. In the future, laser beam treatment to the tumor bed reduce the chance of residual viable tumor cells.

It has been suggested that patients with synchronous bilateral RCC have a favorable survival (69–78%–5 year survival) when treated by aggressive surgical approaches [37–39]. This is compared to less favorable results (38%–5 year survival) for asynchonous lesions.

Other authors do not agree that the prognosis depends on synchronous versus asynchronous RCC or the fate of the contralateral kidney [35, 40, 41]. Survival rates seem to depend on the adequacy of tumor resection. More specifically, survival depends on the stage of the lesion in each kidney or the solitary kidney at presentation. The problem with most studies analyzing survival results for bilateral RCC is that the series are small, the staging may vary, and the grading of the tumor is not usually reported. There are no prospective randomized studies and the natural course of renal carcinoma is extremely variable.

The reported 5 year survival rates for bilateral RCC of up to 78% appears as good as Stage I disease. No doubt, the improved diagnostic tools and aggressive surgical techniques have contributed to this success.

Role of surgery in metastatic renal cell carcinoma

Of patients first presenting with RCC, approximately 25–33% are found to have evidence of metastases before any form of therapy. Subsequently, up to 50% of patients operated on for cure for apparent low stage RCC will later manifest metastases.

One must differentiate between nephrectomy done for palliation versus adjunctive nephrectomy for possible cure in metastatic disease.

Palliative nephrectomy is performed to improve the quality of remaining life by relieving the symptoms of the primary tumor. It does not significantly increase the quantity of life in the vast majority of cases. The indications for palliative nephrectomy are listed in Table 6. It is rare today to be required to perform palliative nephrectomy; most of the complications of metastatic RCC can be managed medically with relative ease.

It has been shown by numerous investigators that nephrectomy alone for metastatic RCC provides little or no prolongation of life survival compared to no surgical treatment if one clearly eliminates the patient selection factor [42]. Bottiger showed that of patients with stage IV RCC, 50% were dead within 1 year and the 5 year survival was only 5% [5]. Johnson studied 93 patients and found the median survival to be 11.3 months with nephrectomy and 7.9 months if no surgery was performed [41]. The presence of limited osseous metastases had an improved survival of slightly greater than 6 months [43, 44].

Adjunctive nephrectomy for metastatic RCC implies performing a radical nephrectomy in the presence of limited or solitary metastases. Control of the limited metastases is by either further aggressive surgical ablation, immunological or chemotherapeutic modes of therapy. It has been reported that in patients with minimal metastatic disease to the lungs which could be completely resected, the 5 year survival was as high as 58% [42, 45]. However, the end result is usually the same; death is from metastatic disease [4, 45–47].

The concept of spontaneous remission or regression which has been bantered around for years as a possible indication for nephrectomy in metastatic RCC is mentioned only to be condemned [48]. There are perhaps 80 to 100 cases of spontaneous regression of metastatic disease reported in the literature, occuring with a frequency of 0.8% after nephrectomy. However, biopsy confirmation of the metastases was often not obtained in these studies. When one considers the fact that the operative mortality for radical nephrectomy ranges from 2.3–15%, it is difficult to support this form of treatment for the purpose of inducing regression of metastatic foci.

In summary, radical nephrectomy is justified for stage IV RCC only if a solitary or limited easily resectable metastatic foci are present (preferably lung). Palliative nephrectomy is solely for control of symptoms, biochemical or hormonal manifestations.

Role of pre-operative renal artery embolization

The concept of renal artery embolization in the treatment of human RCC came into vogue after the initial studies of Lalli and Almgard [49, 50]. Since then numerous devices have been advocated for pre-operative renal artery embolization (Table 7). Following renal artery embolization, if nephrectomy is not performed immediately, the patient experiences symptoms of the post infarction

Table 6. Metastatic Renal Cell Cancer indications for palliative nephrectomy

---

Uncontrollable hemorrhage
Persistent pain
Fever
Endocrinological causes — PTH, ACTH, Polycythemia
GI dysfunction
Hepatic dysfunction
Cardiac dysfunction
Psychological factors

---

syndrome — loin pain, nausea, vomiting, fever, hematuria, and ileus. There may be a mild increase in blood pressure and a leukocytosis. The syndrome usually abates over 3 days. The major risk of pre-operative embolization is displacement of the material into a vessel other than the renal artery [51–53]. The use of absolute alcohol has been advocated as being the most effective but it also has been associated with colonic infarction if an occlusion balloon catheter was not used [54, 55].

Pre-operative renal artery embolization in RCC has been proposed for 2 major purposes: 1) to facilitate surgery in patients with large RCC and; 2) to augment the host immunological response to the tumor.

There are surgeons who strongly believe that the ease of tumor resection is augmented by pre-operative embolization [55, 56]. Others have shown no great advantage as far as blood loss, decreased operative time, or ease of nephrectomy is concerned [55]. The survival rate does not appear to be affected [57]. Finally, there is the theoretical risk of pre-operative embolization in which there is tumor thrombus in the renal vein or IVC. With interruption of the parasitic vascular supply to the thrombus, it may become dislodged and embolize to the lungs. Overall, the use of pre-operative embolization to facilitate nephrectomy appears to be a personal preference of the individual surgeon with no strong objective evidence to support its clear cut benefit.

The use of pre-operative arterial embolization and infarction followed 3 to 7 days later by radical nephrectomy for metastatic RCC was advocated in the mid 1970's [58–60]. It was proposed that the massive release of tumor antigens following the infaction would stimulate the immunological response and in fact initial studies did appear to demonstrate this. In animal studies, it has been suggested that following dearterialization, there is stimulation of natural killer (NK) cell activity [61, 62].

Swanson and associates from M.D. Anderson initially reported a 36% response rate in 50 patients with metastatic RCC who underwent angioinfarction of the primary tumor followed 1 week later by radical nephrectomy and administration

Table 7. Angiographic occlusive devices of the renal artery

Autologous muscle [49]
Absorbable gelatin sponge [52]
Steel coils [45]
Blood clot
Inflatable balloon
Mitomycin C capsules
BCG
^{125}I seeds [65]
Gold particles
Absolute alcohol [53]

---

of progestational agents [63]. Followup of these patients and enlarging their series (100 patients), they showed a decline to a response rate of 28% [64]. Patients with only pulmonary metastases had the best survival of 64% at one year. The 5 year survival, however, was only 13%, not much improved compared to no surgery at all.

In summary, pre-operative renal artery embolization for metastatic RCC has not demonstrated any clear cut advantage in treatment compared to nephrectomy alone.

Radiation therapy

Radiotherapy has not shown significant activity against RCC and thus plays a limited role in treatment. Studies by van der Werf-Messing and other authors have demonstrated that pre-operative radiotherapy (3000 rads over 3 weeks) has not improved survival or influenced local recurrence in any stage of RCC [66, 67]. In fact, the group receiving nephrectomy alone appeared to have longer survival.

Similarily post-operative radiation therapy did not improve survival of local and distant recurrence in randomized studies [68, 69]. The risk of radiation hepatitis following radiotherapy became apparent for right-sided lesions. Injury to spinal cord, bowel, and contralateral kidney are real concerns.

Radiation therapy has a role in palliation of metastatic lesions, primarily to bony lesions. Doses of up to 4000 rads over 2 to 4 weeks are generally administered.

Hormonal therapy

Growth of renal tumors in syrian hamsters was shown to be induced by diethylstilbestrol. This phenomenon could be inhibited by the use of progestational agents [70]. Based on these findings, Bloom used progestational agents in the treatment of metastatic RCC. In reviewing the literature, he claimed an objective response rate of 16% and subjective improvement in 55% of cases [71]. However, this study was not randomized and response criteria varied. The high objective response rate has not been replicated by other authors [45, 72]. It has been suggested that renal tumors containing significant numbers of progesterone receptors may be more sensitive to the use of progestational agents [73]. However, it has been reported that kidneys harbouring adenocarcinoma may in fact contain a lower content of progesterone receptors compared to autologous or control kidneys [74, 75]. This finding may explain the poor response to progesterone therapy.

Due to the lack of effective alternative therapeutic modalities in the management of metastatic RCC, progestational agents are still prescribed. The side effects are minimal and the sense of helplessness of both the patient and physician may be partly allayed.

Other hormonal agents such as testosterone, tamoxifen, nafoxidine, and estramustine phosphate have been tried with little success [76, 77]. At the present time, the administration of hormonal therapy appears to have minimal activity in the treatment of RCC.

Role of chemotherapy

Due to the unpredictable growth pattern of RCC, chemotherapeutic drugs have demonstrated little success in the treatment of metastatic disease. Single agents such as vinblastine have demonstrated a 25% response rate [78]. Other single cytotoxic agents such as methyl-GAG, adriamycin, and chloroethyl-cyclohexy-nitrosurea (CCNU) have a response rate of 20% or less [7]. Cis platinum has not been shown to be effective in RCC [79].

Multiple agent chemotherapeutic protocols have not been shown to be superior to single agents. Recent reports have suggested that high dose methotrexate with leucovorin rescue alone or in combination with vinblastine may account for up to 30% overall response rate. The median survival appeared prolonged up to 110 weeks [80, 81]. The toxicity from these agents is considerable.

The lack of impact of chemotherapeutic agents on advanced RCC has prompted extensive research into the development of in vitro tests which could identify suitable cytotoxic agents. The clonogenic assay for human RCC stimulated considerable excitement, but with time, has not produced the success expected due to difficulties in culturing tumor cells and the present lack of effective chemotherapeutic agents [82–84]. In addition, the clonogenic assay is an expensive tool and presently is being used only in centers with sufficient financial support towards research [72]. However, only with continued efforts to determine effective chemotherapeutic agents, single or combination, will any impact in the treatment of metastatic RCC be realized.

Role of immunotherapy

Immunotherapy has been tested extensively in the management of metastatic RCC. However, despite the initial enthusiasm for this mode of therapy, immunotherapy has not been demonstrated to date, to be clearly superior to any other mode of therapy in the treatment of this unpredictable malignancy.

As listed in Table 8, immunotherapy has been tried in various forms:

1) Active Specific Immunotherapy
This is the use of tumor vaccines where by an immune response is stimulated

within the host. The use of a vaccine prepared from polymerized insoluble autologous tumor extracts has been tried with reported regression of pulmonary metastases [85]. Schapira and associates used irradiated autologous cells mixed with corynebacterium parvum injected intradermally in 3 patients [86]. This protocol is now being used in a phase III trial [72].

2) Active Nonspecific Immunotherapy

This form of immunotherapy attempts to activate the intrinsic host defense mechanism using various agents. This approach has been the most popular.

Bacillus Calmette-Guerin (BCG) first proposed by Morales and collegues was administered intradermally along with cytoreductive surgery in 10 patients [87, 88]. There were no complete responses and 40% objective responses. Metastatic deposits in bone appeared to be less responsive to BCG therapy than those in soft tissues. Limitations of these studies, of course, were the small number of patients in a non-randomized selection.

Montie attempted to combine a few nonspecific immunotherapy agents for metastatic RCC and found an objective response rate of 14–22% in 60 patients, which was not much better than hormonal therapy alone [89].

3) Passive Immunotherapy

The use of immune ribonucleic acid (I-RNA), extensively studies by deKernion and associates, is the technique of administering intradermal injections of purified RNA to patients with metastatic RCC. The purified RNA is extracted from the lymphoid organs of sheep which have previously been immunized with human RCC [72]. Thus, one is attempting to transfer cell-mediated immunity. The initial results of this treatment modality were reported as stabilizing metastases with some partial regression [90, 91]. It seemed to have its best applicability in patients who had minimal metastatic disease limited to the lungs [92].

However, later studies have suggested that the immune RNA is actually inactivated by host circulating enzymes. Thus, it is unlikely that it could have any effect on host lymphocytes and tumor progression. The initial apparent success with this technique appears to be solely a reflection of the usual variation in the natural history of metastatic RCC [93].

Attempts to stimulate autologous lymphocytes by immune RNA in an ex-vivo setting with delayed transfer back into the host has not demonstrated improved results [94, 95].

Table 8. Forms of immunotherapy in Renal Cell Carcinoma (RCC)

1	Active Specific
2	Active Non-specific
3	Passive
4	Interferon

The use of transfer factor, a polypeptide substance capable of transferring delayed hypersensitivity responses, has been tried in metastatic RCC with little or no substantial effect [96].

Hybridoma technology has developed rapidly in the last few years. Attempts are being made to produce monoclonal antibodies specific for RCC expressed antigens. The variation in tumor associated anigens may hamper this technique, but great efforts are being made in this area of research.

4) Interferon

Interferon is a form of active non-specific immunotherapy which has, up to the present, held the greatest hope for success in the treatment of metastatic RCC. Interferons are glycoproteins which are produced by human cells in response to viral infection or other inducers [99]. They have been shown to have antiviral and antineoplastic activity. The latter activity may be mediated by direct tumor toxicity and/or indirect cytotoxicity through natural killer cell stimulation.

It has been suggested that interferon may decrease growth rate of tumor cells by loss of activities of polyamine biosynthetic enzymes such as ornithine decarboxylase and s-adenosylmethionine decarboxylase [99, 100].

deKernion and associates have used human leukocyte -interferon in 43 patients with metastatic RCC [97]. They found one complete responder, 14% partial response, and 23% minimal response or stabilization of disease for greater than 3 months. These results seemed to be superior to hormonal or chemotherapy. As in other modes of immunotherapy, the responders had limited tumor burden with metastases primarily to the lung. Previous nephrectomy and good performance status was noted. The major side-effects of interferon therapy were anorexia, fatigue, fever, depression and occassional hematologic depression. Quesada reported similar results in a series of 19 patients where 5 patients (26%) showed partial responses with the use of human leukocyte interferon [98].

To date, interferons seem to offer improved treatment of metastatic RCC if the tumor burden is limited, especially involving the lungs. It appears to be superior to any other form of adjunctive therapy and hopefully, suitable protocols will be developed using it in combination with other agents.

The immunological system is very complex and certainly much more must be discovered. Compounding this complexity is the fact that renal cell carcinoma varies in its aggressiveness and its expression of antigenicity in different patients [93]. It is, therefore, not surprising that series employing immunotherapy have shown generally equivocal results. Only by utilizing well randomized studies with large numbers of patients can the physician feel justified in utilizing a form of immunotherapy.

Frontiers in management of renal cell carcinoma

One easily recognizes the major limitations of the treatment options for renal cell carcinoma. Surgical therapy is potentially curative provided that the tumor has not spread beyond the confines of Gerota's fascia. Radiotherapy and chemotherapy have had minimal impact in the treatment of advanced RCC. Immunotherapy has generated great expectations, but has not yet had the impact hoped for.

Research into the use of interferon in combination with other agents has shown early good results. In the murine model, interferon has been combined with difluoromethyl ornithine (DFMO) [101, 102]. DFMO is a specific enzyme-activated irreversible inhibitor of ornithine decarboxylase, which reduces polyamine biosynthesis and promotes accumulation of methylglyoxal bisguanyl hydrozone (MGBG) in experimental tumor models [103].

Results are still preliminary, but there is a suggestion that this combination significantly inhibits growth of various human RCC cell lines in the in vitro setting [104]. Whether this will apply in vivo will have to be determined. Finally, combination of DFMO and MGBG significantly inhibited renal cell tumor growth in treated mice compared to control animals [105].

With persistent efforts in the laboratory setting, hopefully, a major break through in the management of advanced RCC will be developed. This, along with improved diagnostic tools will provide early and effective treatment for renal cell carcinoma.

References

1. Robson CJ, Churchill BM, Anderson W: The results of radical nephrectomy for renal cell carcinoma. J Urol 101: 297, 1969
2. Crawford ED, Borden TA: Genitourinary Cancer Surgery. Lee and Febiger, Philadelphia Chs 4–6, 1982
3. Waters WB, Richie JP: Agressive surgical approach to renal cell carcinoma: review of 130 cases. J Urol 122: 306, 1979
4. Skinner DG, Colvin RB, Vermillion CD, Pfister RC, Leadbetter WF: Diagnosis and management of renal cell carcinoma. A clinical and pathological study of 309 cases. Cancer 28: 1165, 1971
5. Bottiger LE: Prognosis in renal carcinoma. Cancer 26: 780, 1970
6. Skinner DG, Vermillion CD, Colvin RB: The surgical management of renal cell carcinoma. J Urol 107: 705, 1972
7. McDonald MW: Current therapy for renal cell carcinoma. J Urol 127: 211, 1982
8. Parker AE: Studies on the main posterior lymph channels of the abdomen and their connections with the lymphatics of the genitourinary system. Amer J Anat 56: 409, 1935
9. Marshall FF, Powell K: Lymphadenectomy for renal cell carcinoma: anatomical and therapeutic considerations. J Urol 128: 677, 1982
10. deKernion JB: Lymphadenectomy for renal cell carcinoma. Therapeutic implications. Urol Clin N Amer 7: 697, 1980

11. Petkovic SD: An anatomical classification of renal tumors in the adult as a basis for prognosis. J Urol 81: 618, 1959

12. Hulten L, Rosencrantz M, Seeman T, Wahlqvist L, Ahrne Ch: Occurence and localization of lymph node metastases in renal carcinoma. A lymphographic and histopathological investigation in connection with nephrectomy. Scand J Urol Nephrol 3: 129, 1969

13. Peters PC, Brown GL: The role of lymphadenectomy in the management of renal cell carcinoma. Urol Clin N Amer 7: 705, 1980

14. Flocks RH, Kadesjy MC: Malignant neoplasms of the kidneys: an analysis of 353 patients followed five years or more. J Urol 79: 196, 1958

15. deKernion JB, Berry D: The diagnosis and treatment of renal cell carcinoma. Cancer suppl 45: 1947, 1980

16. Clayman RV, Gonzalez R, Fraley EE: Renal cell cancer invading the inferior vena cava: clinical review and anatomical approach. J Urol 123: 157, 1980

17. Marshall VF, Middleton RG, Holswade GR, Goldsmith EI: Surgery for renal cell carcinoma in the vena cava. J Urol 103: 414, 1970

18. Skinner DG, Pfister RF, Colvin R: Extension of renal cell carcinoma into the vena cava: the rationale for aggressive surgical management. J Urol 107: 711, 1972

19. Marschal FF, Reitz BA, Diamond DA: A new technique for management of renal cell carcinoma involving the right atrium: hypothermia and ardiac arrest. J Urol 131: 103, 1984

20. Sosa RE, Muecke EC, Vaughan Jr ED, McCarron Jr JP: Renal cell carcinoma extending into the inferior vena cava: the prognostic significance of the level of vena caval involvement. J Urol 132: 1097, 1984

21. Sogani PC, Herr HW, Bains MS, Whitmore Jr WF: Renal cell carcinoma extending into inferior vena cava. J Urol 130: 660, 1983

22. Tolia BM, Whitmore Jr WF: Solitary metastasis from renal cell carcinoma. J Urol 114: 836, 1975

23. McCullough DL, Gittes RF: Vena cava resection for renal cell carcinoma. J Urol 112: 162, 1974

24. Kearney GP, Waters WB, Klein LA, Richie JP, Gittes RF: Results of inferior vena cava resection for renal cell carcinoma. J Urol 125: 769, 1981

25. Lome LG, Bush IM: Resection of the vena cava for renal cell carcinoma: an experimental study. J Urol 107: 717, 1972

26. Marshall FF, Reitz BA: Supradiaphragmatic renal cell carcinomatumor thrombus: indications for vena caval reconstruction with pericardium. J Urol 133: 266, 1985

27. Freed SZ, Gliedman ML: The removal of renal carcinoma thrombus extending into the right atrium. J Urol 113: 163, 1975

28. Klein FA, Vernon Smith MJ, Greenfield LJ: Extracorporeal circulation for renal cell carcinomawith supradiaphragmatic vena caval thrombi. J Urol 131: 880, 1984

29. Krane RJ, deVere White R, Davis Z, Sterling R, Dobnik DB, McCormick JR: Removal of renal cell carcinoma extending into the right atrium using cardiopulmonary bypass, profound hypothermia and circulatory arrest. J Urol 131: 945, 1984

30. Bastable JRG: Bilateral carcinoma of the kidneys. Brit J Urol 32: 60, 1960

31. Viets DH, Vaughan Jr ED, Howards SS: Experience gained from the management of 9 cases of bilateral renal cell carcinoma. J Urol 118: 937, 1977

32. Malek RS, Utz DC, Culp OS: Hypernephroma in the solitary kidney: experience with 20 cases and review of the literature. J Urol 116: 553, 1976

33. Vermooten V: Indications for conservative surgery in certain renal tumors: a study based on the growth pattern of clear cell carcinoma. J Urol 64: 200, 1950

34. Klein TW, Lamm D, Gittes RF: Renal autotransplantation: influence of contralateral nephrectomy on the damaging of warm ischemia during transplantation. Invest Urol 15: 256, 1977

35. Smith RB, deKernion JB, Ehrlich RM, Skinner DG, Kaufman JJ: Bilateral renal cell carcinoma and renal cell carcinoma in the solitary kidney. J Urol 132: 450, 1984

36. Stroup RF, Shearer JK, Traurif AR, Lytton B: Bilateral adenocarcinoma of the kidney treated nephrectomy: a case report and review of the literature. J Urol 111: 272, 1974

37. Wickham JEA: Conservative renal surgery for adenocarcinoma. The place of bench surgery. Brit J Urol 47: 25, 1975

38. Zincke H, Swanson SK: Bilateral renal cell carcinoma: influence of synchronous and asynchronous occurence on patient survival. J Urol 128: 913, 1982

39. Jacobs SC, Berg SI, Lawson RK: Synchronous bilateral renal cell carcinoma: total surgical excision. Cancer 46: 2341, 1980

40. Schiff Jr M, Bagley DH, Lytton B: Treatment of solitary and bilateral renal carcinomas. J Urol 121: 581, 1979

41. Johnson DE, VonEschenbach A, Sternberg J: Bilateral renal cell carcinoma. J Urol 119: 23, 1978

42. Appelqvist P: The role and value of surgery in metastatic renal adenocarcinoma: a retrospective clinical study of 106 nephrectomized cases. J Surg Oncol 26: 138, 1984

43. Johnson DE, Kaesler KE, Samuels ML: Is nephrectomy justified in patients with metastatic renal carcinoma? J Urol 114: 27, 1975

44. Montie JE, Stewart BH, Straffon RA, Banowsky LHW, Hemitt CB, Montague DK: The role of adjunctive nephrectomy in patients with metastatic renal cell carcinoma. J Urol 117: 272, 1977

45. deKernion JB, Ramming KP, Smith RB: The natural history of metastatic renal cell carcinoma: a computer analysis. J Urol 120: 148, 1978

46. Middleton RG: Surgery for metastatic renal cell carcinoma. J Urol 97: 973, 1967

47. Tolia BM, Whitmore Jr WF: Solitary metastases from renal cell carcinoma. J Urol 114: 836, 1975

48. Katz SE, Schapira HE: Spontaneous regression of genitourinay cancer — an update. J Urol 128: 1, 1982

49. Almgard LE, Fernstrom I, Haverling M, Ljungqvist A: Treatment of renal adenocarcinoma by embolic occlusion of the renal circulation. Brit J Urol 45: 474, 1973

50. Lalli AF, Peterson N, Bookstein JJ: Roentgen-guided infarctions of kidneys and lungs. A potential therapeutic technic Radiol 93: 434, 1969

51. Gianturco C, Anderson JH, Wallace S: Mechanical devices for arterial occlusion. Amer J Roentgen 124: 428, 1975

52. Barth KH, Strandberg JD, White Jr RI: Long term follow-up of transcatheter embolization with autologous clot, oxycel and gelfoan in domestic swine. Invest Rad 12: 273, 1977

53. Ellman BA, Parkhill BJ, Curry III TS, Marcus PB, Peters PC: Ablation of renal tumors with absolute ethanol: a new technique. Radiol 141: 619, 1981

54. Mebust WK, Weigel JW, Lee KR, Cox GG, Jewell WR, Krishnan EC: Renal cell carcinoma — angioinfarction. J Urol 131: 231, 1984

55. Klimberg I, Hunter P, Hawkins IF, Drylie DM, Wajsman I: Preoperative angioinfarction of localized renal cell carcinoma using absolute ethanol. J Urol 133: 21, 1985

56. Kaisary AV, Williams G, Riddle PR: The role of preoperative embolization in renal cell carcinoma. J Urol 131: 641, 1984

57. Christensen K, Fyreborg U, Anderson JF, Nissen HM: The value of transvascular embolization in the treatment of renal carcinoma. J Urol 133: 191, 1985

58. Bracken RB, Johson DE, Goldstein HM, Wallace S, Ayala AG: Percutaneous transfemoral renal artery occlusion in patients with renal carcinoma. Preliminary report. Urology 6: 6, 1975

59. Freed SZ, Halperin JP, Gordon M: Idiopathic regression of metastases from renal cell carcinoma. J Urol 118: 538, 1977

60. Mohr SJ, Whitesel JA: Spontaneous regression of renal cell carcinoma metastases after preoperative embolization of primary tumor and subsequent nephrectomy. Urology 14: 5, 1979

61. Johnson G, Kalland T: Enhancement of mouse natural killer cell activity after dearterialization of experimental renal tumors. J Urol 132: 1250, 1984

62. Johnson G, Kalland T: Characterization of effector cells mediating the augmentation of spontaneous cell-mediated cytotoxicity induced by therapeutic infarction of human renal carcinomas. Urol Int 39: 236, 1984

63. Swanson DA, Wallace S, Johson DE: The role of embolization and nephrectomy in the treatment of metastatic renal carcinoma. Urol Clin N Amer 7:719, 1980

64. Swanson DA, Johnson DE, von Eschenbach AC, Chuang VP, Wallace S: Angioninfarction plus nephrectomy for metastatic renal cell carcinoma — an update. J Urol 130: 449, 1983

65. Lang EK, deKernion JB: Transcatheter embolization of advanced renal cell carcinoma with radioactive seeds. J Urol 126: 581, 1981

66. van der Werf-Messing B: Carcinoma of the kidney. Cancer 32: 1056, 1973

67. Juusela H, Malmio K, Alfthan O, Oravisto KJ: Preoperative irradiation in the treatment of renal adenocarcinoma. Scand J Urol Nephrol 11: 277, 1977

68. Peeling WB, Mantell RS, Shepheard BGF: Postoperative irradiation in the treatment of renal cell carcinoma. Brit J Urol 41: 23, 1969

69. Finney R: The value of radiotherapy in the treatment of hypernephroma — a clinical trial. Brit J Urol 45: 258, 1973

70. Bloom HJG: Medroxyprogesterone acetate (Provera) in the treatment of metastatic renal cancer. Brit J Cancer 25: 250, 1971

71. Bloom HJG: Hormone-induced and spontaneous regression of metastatic renal cancer. Cancer 32: 1006, 1973

72. deKernion JB: Treatment of advanced renal cell carcinoma — traditional methods and innovative approaches. J Urol 130: 2, 1983

73. Concolino G, Marocchi A, Conti C, Tenaglia R, Di Silverio F, Bracci U: Human renal cell carcinoma as a hormone-dependent tumor. Cancer Res 38: 4340, 1978

74. McDonald MW, Diokno AC, Seski JC, Menon KMJ: Measurement of progesterone receptor in human renal cell carcinoma and normal renal tissue. J Surg Oncol, 22: 164, 1983

75. Mukamel E, Bruhis S, Nissenkorn I, Servadio C: Steroid receptors in renal cell carcinoma: relevance to hormonal therapy. J Urol 131: 227, 1984

76. Glick JH, Wein A, Torri S, Alavi J, Harris D, Brodovsky H: Phase II study of tamoxifen in patients with advanced renal cell carcinoma. Cancer Treat Rep 64: 343, 1980

77. Swanson DA, Johnson DE: Estramustine phosphate (Emcyt) as treatment for metastatic renal carcinoma. Urology 17: 344, 1981

78. Hrushesky WJ, Murphy GP: Current status of the therapy of advanced renal carcinoma. J Surg Oncol 9: 277, 1977

79. Rodriquez LH, Johnson DE: Clinical trial of cisplatinum (NSC 119875) in metastatic renal cell carcinoma. Urology 11: 344, 1978

80. Bell DR, Aroney RS, Fisher RJ, Levi JA: High-dose methotrexate with leucovorin rescue, vinblastine, and bleomycin with or without tamoxifen in metastatic renal cell carcinoma. Cancer Treat Rep 68: 587, 1984

81. Baumgartner G, Heinz R, Arbes H, Lenzhofer R, Pridun N, Schuller J: Methotrexate-citrovorum factor used alone and in combination chemotherapy for advanced hypernephromas. Cancer Treat Rep 64: 41, 1980

82. Salmon SE, Hamburger AW, Soehnlen B, Durie BGM, Alberts DS, Moon TE: Quantitation of differential sensitivity of human-tumor stem cells to anticancer drugs. New Engl J Med 298: 1321, 1978

83. Lieber MM, Kovach JS: Soft agar clonogenic assay for primary human renal carcinoma: in vitro chemotherapeutic drug sensitivity testing. Reas at annual meeting of American Urologic Association, abstract 531, Boston, Massachusetts, May 10–14, 1981

84. Lieber MM: Update on in vitro chemosensitivity testing. Read at annual meeting of South Central Section, American Urological Association, New Orleans, Louisianna, September 12–16, 1982

85. Tallberg T, Tykka H, Halttunen P, Mahlberg K, Uusitalo R, Uusitalo H, Carlson O, Sandstedt B, Oravisto KJ, Lehtonen T, Sarna S, Strandstrom H: Cancer immunity. The effect in cancer-immunotherapy of polymerised autologus tumour tissue and supportive measures. Scand J Clin Lab Invest 39 (151): 1–35, 1979

86. Schapira DV, McCune CS, Henshaw EC: Treatment of advanced renal cell carcinoma with specific immunotherapy consisting of autologous tumor cells and c. parvum. Proc Amer Assoc Cancer Res Amer Soc Clin Oncol, abstract C-234, 20: 348, 1979

87. Morales A, Wilson JL, Pater JL, Loeb M: Cytoreductive surgery and systemic bacillus Calmette-Guerin therapy in metastatic renal cancer: a phase II trial. J Urol 127:230, 1982

88. Morales A, Eidinger D: Bacillius Calmette-Guerin in the treatment of adenocarcinoma of the kidney. J Urol 115: 377, 1976

89. Montie JE, Bukowski RM, James RE, Straffon RA, Stewart BH: A critical review of immunotherapy of disseminated renal adenocarcinoma. J Surg Oncol 21: 5, 1982

90. Ramming KP, deKernion JB: Immune RNA therapy for renal cell carcinoma: survival and immunologic monitoring. Ann Surg 186: 459, 1977

91. Brower PA, deKernion JB, Ramming KP: Immune cytolysis of human renal carcinoma mediated by xenogeneic immune ribonucleic acid. J Urol 115: 243, 1976

92. deKernion JB, Ramming KP: The therapy of renal adenocarcinoma with immune RNA. Invest Urol 17: 378, 1980

93. Droller MJ: Immunotherapy in genitourinary neoplasia. J Urol 133: 1, 1985

94. Richie JP, Wang BS, Steele Jr GD, Wilson RE, Mannick JA: In vivo and in vitro effects of xenographic immune ribonucleic acid in patients with advanced renal cell carcinoma: a phase I study. J Urol 126: 24, 1981

95. Richie JP, Steele Jr GD, Wilson RE, Ervin T, Wang BS, Mannick JA: Current treatment of metastatic renal cell carcinoma with xenogenic immune ribonucleic acid. J Urol 131: 236, 1984

96. Montie JE, Bukomwski RM, Deodhar SD, Hewlett JS, Stewart BH, Straffon RA: Immunotherapy of disseminated renal cell carcinoma with tranfer factor. J Urol 117: 553, 1977

97. deKernion JB, Sarna G, Figlin R, Lindner A, Smith RB: The treatment of renal cell carcinoma with human leukocyte alpha-interferon. J Urol 130: 1063, 1983

98. Quesada JR, Swanson DA, Trindade A, Gutterman JU: Renal cell carcinoma: antitumor effects of leukocyte interferon. Cancer Res 43: 940, 1983

99. Lee E, Sreevalsan T: Interferon as an inhibitor of polyamine enzymes. Advances in Polyamine Res 3: 175, 1981

100. Sekar V, Atmar VJ, Joshi AR, Krim M, Kuehn GD: Inhibition of ornithine decarboxylase in human fibroblast cells by type I and type II interferons. Biochem Bioph Res Comm 114: 950, 1983

101. Sunkara PS, Prakash NJ, Mayer GD, Sjoerdma A: Tumor suppression with a combination of -difluoromethylornithine and interferon. Science 219: 851, 1983

102. Heby O: Role of polyamines in the control of cell proliferation and differentiation. Differentiation 19: 1, 1981

103. Kingsnorth AN, McCann PP, Diekema KA, Ross JS, Malt RA: Effects of -difluoromethylornithine on the growth of experimental Wilms' tumor and renal adenocarcinoma. Cancer Res 43: 4031, 1983

104. Ratliff TL: personal communication

105. Herr HW, Kleinert EL, Conti PS, Burchenal JH, Whitmore Jr WF: Effects of -difluoromethylornithine and methylglyoxal Bis (guanylhydrazone) on the growth of experimental renal adenocarcinoma in mice. Cancer Res 44: 4381, 1984

Editorial Comment

JEAN B. deKERNION

The staging system of renal cell carcinoma has traditionally been after the method of Robson et al as indicated in the text and illustrated in Table 1. However, our new understanding of the prognostic factors of renal cell carcinoma demand a more detailed staging scheme. Stage III includes renal vein and vena caval involvement as well as lymph node involvement and these represent very different risks for local recurrence and metastatic disease. The TNM system avoids these pitfalls and stratifies the extent of vena caval involvement as well as extent of lymph node involvement.

In spite of years of research and many clinical trials, surgery remains the only treatment for this tumor. The surgical approach is clearly stated by the author. It is our preference to perform a supracostal eleventh rib incision for small tumors and tumors in the lower pole. Involvement or suspected involvement of the renal vein with limited extension into the vena cava in a patient with a small primary tumor can often be very nicely managed through a subcostal incision which extends across the midline into the other rectus muscle, and offers an added advantage of simplicity, rapidity and easy access to the vena cava and aorta. Large upper pole tumors are best managed through a thoracoabdominal approach. Extensive vena caval involvement is best approached, in our opinion, through a median sternotomy incision joined to a midline abdominal incision.

The extent of the surgical field, for the first time in several decades, is being reassessed. The authors rightly state that the current treatment appears to be a standard radical nephrectomy with Gerota's fascia and its contents. However, a realistic reappraisal of this principle seems appropriate on the basis of the experience with partial nephrectomy for tumors in solitary kidneys, and conservative excision of multiple tumors. In the opinion of this writer, the current information is insufficient to warrant the risk of abandoning radical nephrectomy as treatment of a tumor for which there is no alternative to surgery. Nonetheless, in selected patients with small polar tumors, partial nephrectomy may become a viable option. With respect to lymph node excision, patients with extensive involvement will seldom be benefited. However, early extension to nodes in or near the renal hilum may not preclude surgical cure and we agree with the authors' recommendation for limited unilateral lymph node dissection.

Aggressive treatment of patients with vena caval extension is appropriate in the modern era. Extension into the right atrium can be managed surgically but few patients achieve a long-term survival and the indication for surgery in these patients should be primarily relief of symptoms. We have recently, after the suggestion of our transplant surgeons, learned to dissect along the vena cava from below to a point close to the hepatic veins. This requires great caution and some experience, but allows a direct approach which can be managed through an abdominal incision and does not require mobilization of the liver. Large vena caval thrombi are often associated with extensive bland non-tumor thrombus into the opposite renal vein and distally into the iliac vein. Removal of the renal vein bland thrombus is essential. We occasionally have attempted to remove the distal bland thrombus, with limited success. The vena cava in such patients should either be ligated (if total occlusion has existed for some time) of clipped below the level of the renal veins.

Management of bilateral tumors or tumor in the solitary kidney has been fairly well standardized and every attempt should be made for surgical excision with preservation of renal tissue sufficient to obviate the need for renal dialysis. The use of workbench surgery has markedly decreased and almost all tumors can be well managed in situ. At our institution, ex vivo surgery has not been required for approximately the last twenty patients with tumors in solitary kidneys. Current debate involves the role of enucleation versus partial nephrectomy. In my opinion, enucleation is indicated only when partiel nephrectomy with a margin of normal tissue is not feasible, as in the patient with multiple small tumors in a solitary kidney.

The futility of nephrectomy for patients with diffuse mletastatic disease has been clearly demonstrated and is amply reiterated by the author. Patients with severe sumptoms may be candidates for nephrectomy when the tumor appears to be resectable. In the absence of symptoms, nephrectomy still seems appropriate when the patient has a treatable (either by excision or radiation) solitary metastatic site. We have recently been willing to perform adjunctive nephrectomy in patients who fulfill specific criteria: small, completely resectable primary lesion; absence of regional metastases; normal performance status; and limited pulmonary metastases. Most such patients will have a life expectancy of more than one year and might be well served by the removal of the primary lesion. All such patients are then placed on experimental treatment protocols since this group of patients is the group most likely to respond to systemic therapies. In the absence of an approved experimental systemic therapy, one must seriously question the wisdom of adjunctive nephrectomy. Regardless of therapy, most such patients will eventually succumb from metastatic disease. The addition of preoperative angio-infarction has not proven to be of any benefit in these patients and is practiced at very institutions. The added side effects and cost do not warrant its use except under strict experimental conditions.

The treatment of metastatic disease remains a difficult and frustrating problem for the urologist. No good chemotherapeutic agent has been identified, through we continue to use intravenous vinblastine in selected patients. Hormones have no objective effect although a subjective response can sometimes be achieved with minimal toxicity. Immunotherapy is still experimental as are the interferons. In a total of approximately 140 patients with measureable metastatic renal carcinoma treated in the past five years at our institution with either immunotherapy or various interferons, only three complete responses have been recorded and the total objective response rate (partial response plus complete response) is static at approximately sixteen percent. Almost all responders were patients in the favorable prognostic category, with normal performance status and minimal tumor burden confined to the lungs. The influence of the tumor's natural history in this group of patients must be questioned and the true efficacy of these agents will only be determined after randomized trials. No clear survival benefit from any of these treatments has been recorded. Further careful clinical studies with the interferons and with other immunostimulants still seem appropriate since the level of response to these agents is higher than what has been recorded in careful clinical studies with other agents.

In summary, reassessment of the extent of the surgical treatment should be a concern of urologic oncologists for at least the next several years. Continued careful controlled trials with existing and new systemic treatments offers the only hope for improving survival of patients with metastatic disease.

Index

Ᵹ

Ϝ